COMBINATORIAL CHEMISTRY

COMBINATORIAL CHEMISTRY

Synthesis and Application

Edited by

STEPHEN R. WILSON
New York University

ANTHONY W. CZARNIK
IRORI Quantum Microchemistry

A Wiley-Interscience Publication
JOHN WILEY & SONS, INC.
New York • Chichester • Weinheim • Brisbane • Singapore • Toronto

This text is printed on acid-free paper.

Copyright © 1997 by John Wiley & Sons, Inc.

All rights reserved. Published simultaneously in Canada.

Reproduction or translation of any part of this work beyond
that permitted by Section 107 or 108 of the 1976 United
States Copyright Act without the permission of the copyright
owner is unlawful. Requests for permission or further
information should be addressed to the Permissions Department,
John Wiley & Sons, Inc., 605 Third Avenue, New York, NY
10158-0012.

Library of Congress Cataloging in Publication Data

Combinatorial chemistry : synthesis and application / edited by
    Stephen R. Wilson and Anthony W. Czarnik.
        p.   cm.
    Includes index.
    ISBN 0-471-12687-X (cloth : alk. paper)
    1. Combinatorial chemistry.   I. Wilson, Stephen R. (Stephen
Ross), 1946–   .   II. Czarnik, Anthony W., 1957–   .
RS419.C666   1997
615'.19—dc20   96-44718

Printed in the United States of America

10 9 8 7 6 5 4 3 2

CONTENTS

LIST OF CONTRIBUTORS

Robert W. Armstrong, Department of Chemistry and Biochemistry, University of California, Los Angeles, California 90095

Stephen Benkovic, Pennsylvania State University, University Park, Pennsylvania 16802

Sylvie E. Blondelle, Torrey Pines Institute for Molecular Studies, 3550 General Atomics Court, San Diego, California 92121

S. David Brown, Department of Chemistry and Biochemistry, University of California, Los Angeles, California 90095

Joseph H.-L. Chau, Department of Chemistry, P. M. Gross Chemical Laboratory, Duke University, Durham, North Carolina 27708-0346

Jrlung Chen, Department of Chemistry, P. M. Gross Chemical Laboratory, Duke University, Durham, North Carolina 27708-0346

Anthony W. Czarnik, IRORI Quantum Microchemistry, 11205 N. Torrey Pines Road, Suite 100, La Jolla, California 92037

Shelia Hobbs DeWitt, BioOrganic Chemistry Section, Department of Chemistry, Parke-Davis Pharmaceutical Research Division of Warner-Lambert Company, Ann Arbor, Michigan 48105

Barbara Dörner, Torrey Pines Institute for Molecular Studies, 3550 General Atomics Court, San Diego, California 92121

Richard A. Houghten, Torrey Pines Institute for Molecular Studies, 3550 General Atomics Court, San Diego, California 92121

Thomas A. Keating, Department of Chemistry and Biochemistry, University of California, Los Angeles, California 90095

Mark J. Kurth, Department of Chemistry, University of California, Davis, California 95616

Grove P. Miller, Pennsylvania State University, University Park, Pennsylvania 16802

Michael P. Nova, IRORI Quantum Microchemistry, 11025 N. Torrey Pines Road, Suite 100, La Jolla, California 92037

John M. Ostresh, Torrey Pines Institute for Molecular Studies, 3550 General Atomics Court, San Diego, California 92121

Michael C. Pirrung, Department of Chemistry, P. M. Gross Chemical Laboratory, Duke University, Durham, North Carolina 27708-0346

Wolfgang E. Rapp, Rapp Polymere, Ernst Simon Str. 9, D 72072 Tübingen, Germany

Julius Rebek, Jr., Skaggs Institute for Chemical Biology, The Scripps Research Institute, La Jolla, California 92037

Jeff Smiley, Pennsylvania State University, University Park, Pennsylvania 16802

Irving Sucholeiki, Sphinx Pharmaceuticals, A Division of Eli Lilly & Company, 840 Memorial Drive, Cambridge, Massachusetts 02139

Carol M. Taylor, Department of Chemistry, University of Auckland, Private Bag 92019, Auckland, New Zealand

Paul A. Tempest, Department of Chemistry and Biochemistry, University of California, Los Angeles, California 90095

Stephen R. Wilson, Department of Chemistry, New York University, New York, New York 10003

Edward A. Wintner, Skaggs Institute for Chemical Biology, The Scripps Research Institute, La Jolla, California 92037

Xiao-yi Xiao, IRORI Quantum Microchemistry, 11025 N. Torrey Pines Road, Suite 100, La Jolla, California 92037

Wenyan Zong, Pennsylvania State University, University Park, Pennsylvania 16802

PREFACE

This book will explore the subject of combinatorial chemistry with particular emphasis on organic applications. Combinatorial chemistry has emerged over the last few years as an exciting new paradigm for drug discovery. A flurry of papers, meetings, and conferences have appeared in the last few years. In a very short time, the topic has become the focus of considerable scientific interest and research effort. What is combinatorial chemistry? This book was conceived with two purposes in mind. First, it is our hope that the book will be a way for newcomers to enter the field with some confidence and perspective. Second, the book serves as a forum for leaders in the field to define and describe some of their specialized positions. Any area of science that is very "hot" quite naturally suffers somewhat from inflated claims and overenthusiastic statements. With the selection of authors, we have tried to present a cross section of many of the organic chemistry technologies available at the time of this writing. Although combinatorial chemistry had its origins in peptide chemistry, we have intentionally focused this book on nonpeptide organic applications, with only a few exceptions.

One of us (A. W. C.) has said that "the only limitation to the kinds of chemistry we can accomplish combinatorially is our willingness to view the development of high-volume synthesis as an activity worthy of study." This book—which reports the state-of-the-art developments in 1996—should be considered just the beginning.

S. R. WILSON

New York, New York

A. W. CZARNIK

La Jolla, California

ix

COMBINATORIAL CHEMISTRY

1

INTRODUCTION TO COMBINATORIAL LIBRARIES: CONCEPTS AND TERMS

STEPHEN R. WILSON

Department of Chemistry, New York University, New York, New York 10003

In the past few years, combinatorial chemistry has become the popular and often misunderstood "new wave" in drug discovery. In some cases, combinatorial chemistry is presented as being in direct competition with rational, or computer-aided, drug design. Nothing could be further from the truth. Combinatorial chemistry encompasses many strategies and processes for the rapid synthesis of large, organized collections of compounds called libraries. When planned intelligently, combinatorial methods produce collections of molecularly diverse compounds that can be used for rapidly screening for biological activity. Without planning, the GIGO (garbage in–garbage out) principle applies. Whether or not a library has in some way been designed or made more or less at random depends on the reasons for preparing the compounds. Combinatorial chemistry as a laboratory practice cannot replace computer modeling as an exercise in refining our basic understanding of molecular interactions. It is likely that both rational drug design and combinatorial chemistry will be used, in concert when appropriate, or directly applied to the problems best suited to each method.

Combinatorial chemistry includes many research areas—new analytical methods, new computer modeling and database-related challenges, new synthetic approaches, new types of reagents, and new types of assays. Although this chapter will provide current leads into all these fields, the basic groundwork for combinatorial chemistry is still being laid. Many new research areas have yet to be explored.

Combinatorial chemistry has its conceptual roots in the immune system. In the body, when a new antigen comes in contact with the preexisting large collection of antibodies, the antibody that binds best is selected and reproduced in large numbers

1

to effect the immune response. In a similar way, combinatorial chemistry involves the synthesis of a large number of compounds. (This collection can be a chemical mixture, a physical mixture, or individual pure components.) The collection is then tested for biological activity. Finally the active compound is identified and made in quantity as a single compound. This type of overall approach is not unlike a bioassay guided search for useful natural products.

Thus, combinatorial chemistry approach has two phases: (1) making a library and (2) finding the active compound. Screening mixtures for biological activity has been compared to finding a needle in a haystack. This approach may seem unlikely to improve the likelihood of finding new drug leads. The fact that it appears to work has generated all the excitement.

This introductory chapter will review several methods for haystack construction and needle searching. For example, the best way to prepare a mixture is in some type of array or coded form. Then, it is easy to locate and decode the structure of the active compound. Combinatorial chemistry has also prompted a resurgence of interest in rapid synthesis methods, particularly in the area of solid-phase synthesis. Many related topics such as automated synthesis, methods for identifying the structure of the active compound on a small scale, and handling the massive amounts of data sometimes obtained (i.e., computer databases) are also discussed. The main portion of the book continues with specific topics written by experts in the field.

1.1   HISTORY

The first report describing combinatorial chemistry appeared in 1984 in a study by Mario Geyson (1) titled, "Use of Peptide Synthesis to Probe Viral Antigens for Epitopes to a Resolution of a Single Amino Acid." Another early pioneer was Furka (2) who introduced the commonly used pool-and-split methods. The 1980s was a period of rapid development in solid-phase peptide synthesis—Bruce Merrifield won the Nobel prize in chemistry in 1984 for his work on solid-phase synthesis (3). During this time, automated peptide synthesizer technology was in its infancy, and the preparation of individual peptides was a challenge. In 1985 Richard Houghten introduced the "tea bag" method for rapid multiple peptide synthesis (4). These and other advances in manual multiple-peptide synthesis (5) fed the beginnings of a wave of rapid bioassays based on the developing area of molecular biology. Mass screening of peptide ligands as a tool for drug discovery allowed the development of high-throughput bioassays (6,7).

Because, historically, biological assays from natural products screening were often carried out on mixtures, early pioneers in combinatorial chemistry developed the concept of intentionally making mixtures for the purpose of testing. This approach had the benefit of more rapid screening. For example, if a mixture showed no activity, then all compounds in the mixture could be assumed to be inactive. (This assumes that compound A in the mixture does not effect the assay of compound B or even react with compound B.) Instead of the usual method of individual peptide synthesis, it is possible to couple a mixture of all 20 amino acids to another mixture of 20 amino acids to produce 400 dipeptides. If these newly formed 400 dipeptides are reacted with a mixture of 20 additional amino acids, 8,000 tripeptides are obtained. This process describes the original formulation of combinatorial chemistry. The mixture of 8,000 tripeptides would be called a combinatorial library. The combinatorial possibilities for the number of compounds is seen to increase exponentially as shown in Figure 1.1, that is, N reactions can produce $N \times N$ compounds.

Although it is easy to see how the rapid production of many compounds in a mixture works, it is not so easy to see how to make this process work in drug discovery. There are several problems. For example, in the process shown in Figure 1.1, what would happen if one or more of the amino acids does not react or reacts sluggishly to give a low yield? The mixture would then not contain 8,000 tripeptides but a lower number. The peptides would not be present in the idealized statistical distribution (i.e., equimolar ratios). Additionally, how does one find a single active peptide in a mixture with 7,999 inactive ones?

The first problem is always a sticky one and will be discussed in more detail later. The second problem has the following solution, called deconvolution. Imagine constructing the library not with all 20 amino acids but starting with only 19 amino acids, leaving out one specific (known) residue. After subsequent coupling with 20 times 20 amino acids, this leads to a library of only 7,600 tripeptide compounds. If this library is now inactive, we have learned that position 1 of the

Number of different peptides increases exponentially with length of molecule

Number of amino acid residues	Peptide	Number of distinct peptides
2	$NH_2\text{-}X_1X_2\text{-}COOH$	400
3	$NH_2\text{-}X_1X_2X_3\text{-}COOH$	8,000
4	$NH_2\text{-}X_1X_2X_3X_4\text{-}COOH$	160,000
5	$NH_2\text{-}X_1X_2X_3X_4X_5\text{-}COOH$	3,200,000
6	$NH_2\text{-}X_1X_2X_3X_4X_5X_6\text{-}COOH$	64,000,000
7	$NH_2\text{-}X_1X_2X_3X_4X_5X_6X_7\text{-}COOH$	1,280,000,000
8	$NH_2\text{-}X_1X_2X_3X_4X_5X_6X_7X_8\text{-}COOH$	25,600,000,000

X_n represents individual amino acids residues.
Numbers of distinct peptides are based on
20 residues at each position

Figure 1.1 Combinatorial peptide chemistry. The number of different peptides increases exponentially with length.

tripeptide has the residue that was omitted from the synthesis. If you continue this process, methodically omitting one amino acid after another, a single combination still has the active compound. Thus a maximum of 20 experiments are needed to define position 1. Now, with the active first residue fixed, 20 more experiments are carried out to define the best residue in position 2. There are $20 + 20 + 20 = 60$ omission experiments required to define the complete tripeptide sequence of the active component in 8,000 compounds. This mathematical principle is the parallelism advantage: $20 + 20 + 20 = 60$ (linear) versus $20 \times 20 \times 20 = 8000$ (exponential) that underlies the principle of combinatorial chemistry (8,9). This iterative synthesis and screening strategy has been discussed in detail by Dooley and Houghten (8). A careful analysis of methods for deconvolution of libraries and their intrinsic problems is described by Freier and co-workers (10).

As you can see from this example, this strategy for combinatorial chemistry relies on two important points. First, the synthesis of the mixture must be fast and efficient because you need to prepare many variations of the libraries. Second, the testing must also be fast and easy, because you need to rapidly test many compound mixtures to find the active sequences. Because it is not always the case that both synthesis and testing are fast and efficient, these two key points return again and again. In addition, complications involving multiple active components (more than one needle in each haystack) often confuse the issue. On the other hand, the classic combinatorial situation in Figure 1.1 is a basic method with which one can contrast other approaches.

Fast and easy synthesis and testing suggests automation and robotics. Over the past few years, combinatorial chemistry has grown so quickly, in part because good automation exists in both areas. Section 1.7 on robotic instrumentation will review some advances in robotics that have enabled fast and easy preparation of compounds. A discussion of the automation of bioassays, that is, high-throughput screening, is beyond the scope of this book, and readers are referred to other reviews of advances in assay processes (6).

1.2   REVIEW OF THE LITERATURE

Combinatorial chemistry is an approach to synthetically produce *molecular diversity*. Traditionally, molecular diversity was primarily obtained from natural products. Two early reviews contrast natural products diversity (11) with molecular diversity obtained from peptide combinatorial chemistry (12). Two other early reviews in 1993 on applications of combinatorial chemistry barely mention organic chemistry (13,14). It was not until 1994 that new comprehensive literature reviews of combinatorial chemistry were published covering both peptide combinatorial methods (15) and organic chemical applications (16). Since that time many other reviews have appeared directly addressing organic combinatorial chemistry (17–26). A comprehensive bibliography of combinatorial chemistry references is available on the World Wide Web (http://vesta.pd.com) (27).

1.3 SOLID-PHASE ORGANIC SYNTHESIS

Until the revolution in high-speed bioassays, the testing of new compounds was the rate-limiting step in the drug discovery process. While it might take a chemist one or two weeks to synthesize a single compound, it required a much longer time to carry out the biological assays. Now modern high-speed assays using robotic samplers can screen more than 10,000 compounds per week. The biological assay has evolved from the rate-limiting step to the driving force in the need for large numbers of compounds, and thus the driving force of combinatorial chemistry. In some cases, where compounds are prepared attached to polymer supports, bioassays are still not very well adapted.

In the area of high-speed automated synthesis, peptide chemistry has already arrived. In 1963, Merrifield reported the first examples of solid-phase synthesis of peptides using chloromethylated-polystyrene containing immobilized N-protected amino acid building blocks (3). This chemistry developed over the ensuing decade and became the basis for much of the progress in peptide chemistry.

Figure 1.2 shows the Merrifield approach. An insoluble polymer bead containing—CH_2Cl groups is prepared by chloromethylation of the copolymer of styrene and *p*-divinylbenzene. These chloromethyl groups can be esterified with N-protected amino acid building blocks. The amino group is iteratively deprotected and coupled with new N-protected amino acids to build the growing chain. Merrifield used the *tert*-butyloxycarbonyl protecting group (BOC group) to protect the free amino terminus during the coupling step. This allows deprotection with acid (CF_3COOH) before coupling with the next N-protected residue. The cycle can be continued until the desired sequence is obtained. By-products and excess reagents are not bound by the resin and can be removed from the resin beads during washing cycles.

An entire industry has developed to serve the peptide synthesis field. There are many instrument companies that provide automated peptide synthesizers, as well as other companies that provide peptide building blocks, reagents, and supplies (17). Solid-phase synthesis techniques do not, per se, mean fast synthesis. On the other hand, there are many years of experience in automating bead-based synthetic approaches because it is easy to extend the principles to organic applications.

Although peptide chemistry advanced using solid-phase techniques, applications of polystyrene bead-supported approaches to traditional organic molecules did not go far in the earlier days. Some work appeared in the 1970s, but an early review by Rapoport had a negative tone (28). Although later successes by Leznoff (29), Neckers (30), Frechet (31), and others clearly showed that polystyrene bead-supported organic chemistry worked quite well, interest in the field largely disappeared (32). This might have been due to several factors. First, solid-phase chemistry often produced only small quantities of compound. Pre-1980 nuclear magnetic resonance (NMR) instrumentation required much larger amounts of compound for characterization than is needed with today's high-field Fourier transform (FT) machines. Second, the high-speed testing of small amounts of compound that launched

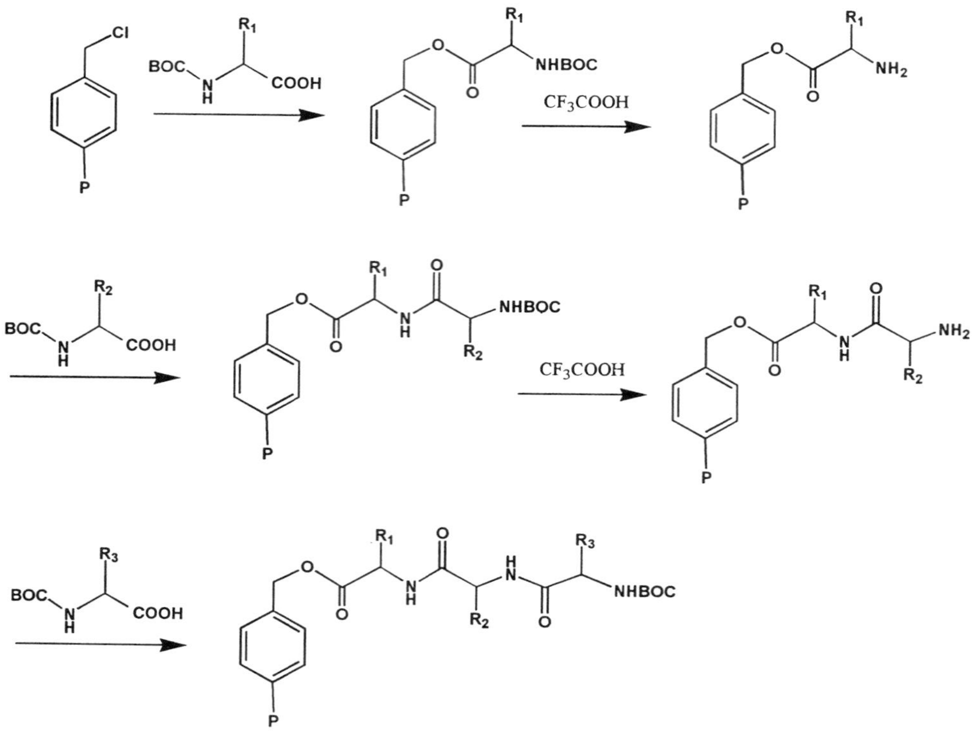

Figure 1.2   Merrifield solid-phase peptide synthesis (3).

the field of combinatorial chemistry had not emerged. The late 1970s and 1980s was a period of tremendous growth in the development of selective reagents and methods for solution-phase organic synthesis. There were plenty of new targets and new synthesis methodology to occupy the attention of organic chemists. Thus, while solid-phase peptide methods rapidly matured and led to instrumentation for automation of chemistry, solid-phase methods for organic synthesis all but faded away. Until 1992, the combinatorial library field was exclusively the domain of peptide and oligonucleotide-based chemistry.

The situation changed in 1992 with the report by Bunin and Ellman of the preparation of combinatorial libraries of organic molecules (33). The report of solid-phase synthesis of Diversomers by the Parke-Davis group (34) shortly thereafter stimulated considerable interest in reexamination of solid-phase organic synthesis. Within the past few years, a number of reports have appeared that point to great potential for solid-phase organic synthesis. An excellent recent review of the literature of solid-phase organic synthesis has recently been published (35).

Bunin and Ellman's (33) solid-phase synthesis of 1,4-benzodiazopines is an excellent illustration of the process of combinatorial library production using organic templates (Fig. 1.3). The chemistry is very similar to the Parke-Davis Diversomer

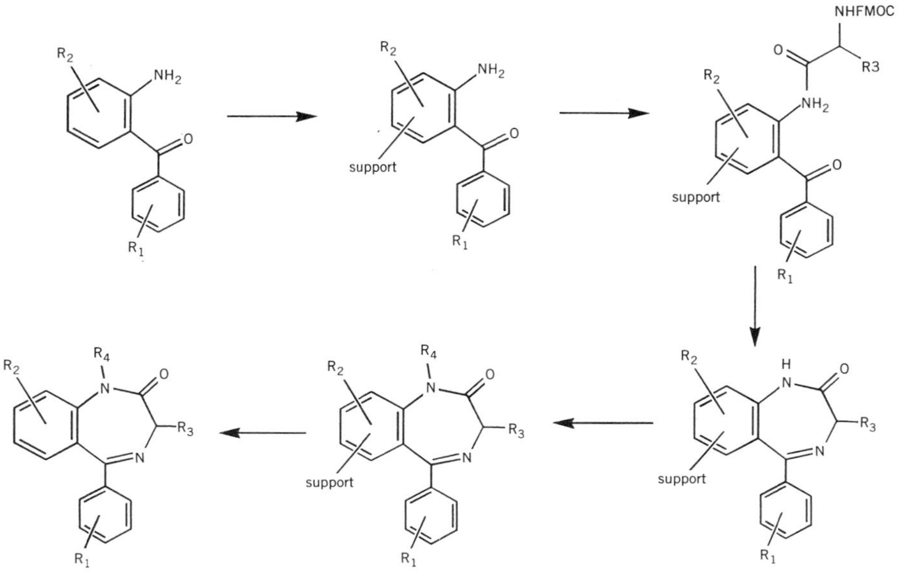

Figure 1.3 Ellman solid-phase 1,4-benzodiazepine synthesis.

approach (34) detailed in Chapter 2, except that Bunin and Ellman's compounds were not cleaved from the solid support. 1,4-Benzodiazepines are constructed from three components: 2-aminobenzophenones, N-protected amino acids, and alkylating agents. As one can see in Figure 1.3, the preparation of a combinatorial library on solid-phase synthesis beads requires several things. First, a selection of building blocks are needed with R_1, R_2, R_3, and R_4 that can be permuted. Second, a reaction scheme that is suitable for interative conversion, in a similar manner to peptide synthesis, is required. Third, a method for linking one of the building blocks to a solid support and conditions for cleaving the compound(s) off the support at the end of the cycle must be found.

The variation of groups R_1–R_4 give a matrix of different structures (Fig. 1.4). These compounds are the combinatorial library and the chemistry is sometimes called matrix chemistry. Besides chemistry issues, keeping track of a large collection of structures is often difficult. Section 1.8 discusses some of these points as well as software solutions that attempt to deal with multidimensional collections of pharmacophores.

From only a few studies in 1992, the number of publications reporting applications of the use of solid-phase organic chemistry has increased dramatically. So many new applications of organic reactions on a solid support have been reported that only a partial list of the types of reactions carried out on a solid support can be provided here (Table 1.1).

Besides the reaction itself, solid-phase synthesis methods also require consideration of several new technical issues. Table 1.2 reports some characteristics of the

Template	R_1	R_2	R_3	R_4
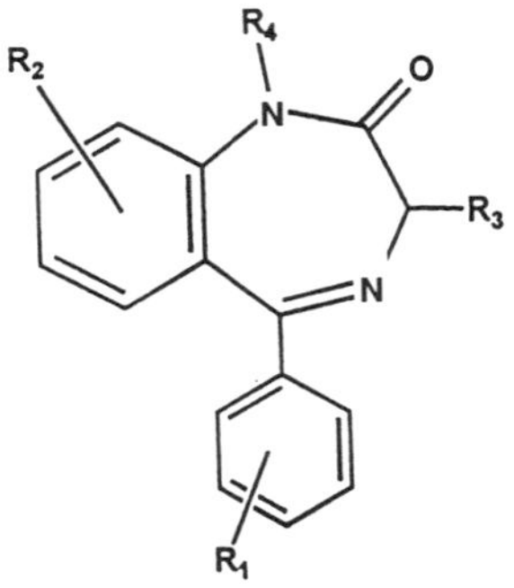	OH	Cl	CH_3	H
	OH	Cl	CH_3	$CH_3 CH_2$
	OH	Cl	CH_3	$CH_3 CH_2 CH_2$
	OH	Cl	$CH_3 CH_2$	H
	OH	Cl	$CH_3 CH_2$	$CH_3 CH_2$
	OH	Cl	$CH_3 CH_2$	$CH_3 CH_2 CH_2$

Figure 1.4 Typical molecular spread sheet of benzodiazepine derivatives.

most common form of resin bead: crosslinked polystyrene. In planning a synthesis, one must consider loading, the level of substitution on the beads and swelling characteristics of the resin. As can be seen in Table 1.2, crosslinked polystyrene beads swell quite a bit in volume with different solvents. The physical size of the beads used in a solid-phase synthesis, of course, also effects the weight of each bead

TABLE 1.1 Organic Reactions on Polystyrene Solid Supports (35)

Reaction	Reference
Dieckman cyclization	28
Diels-Alder reaction	36
Micheal reaction	37
Aldol condensation	38
Mitsunobu reaction	39
Pausen-Khand cycloaddition	40
Organometallic additions	41
Stille reaction	42
Suzuki reaction	43
Heck reaction	44 and 45
Suzuki coupling	46
Urea synthesis	47
Thiazoline synthesis	48
Solid-phase Steroid synthesis	49
Wittig reaction	37

TABLE 1.2 **Data for Polystyrene-Bead Solid Support (50, 51)**

Styrene–divinylbenzene copolymer: 1–2% crosslinked; 1 g of 200–400 mesh resin has ~4–10 × 10⁶ beads

Thermal stability: 105–130°C

Bead sizes: 100 mesh (212 μm), 140 mesh (150 μm), 200 mesh (106 μm), 325 mesh (75 μm), 400 mesh (45 μm)

Swelling: DMF (3.5 mL/g), THF (5.1 mL/g), CH₃OH (1.5 mL/g), H₂O (1.5 mL/g), CH₂Cl₂ (5.3 mL/g), CHCl₃ (5.9 mL/g)

Loading: 0.1–0.4 mmol/g resin, ~100–400 pmol per bead

and therefore the amount of product on each bead. Although crosslinked polystyrene resin beads (Merrifield-type resin) are the most common for historical reasons, a popular new material called TentaGel is now coming into wide use (52). This new material contains a polystyrene core with polyethylene glycol spacer arms (PS–PEG). TentaGel (although physiomechanically less robust than polystyrene) has very desirable characteristics for synthesis because the attached reacting groups project out in solution rather than being anchored close to the polymer backbone. This provides for better reactivity and for reactivity more closely paralleling

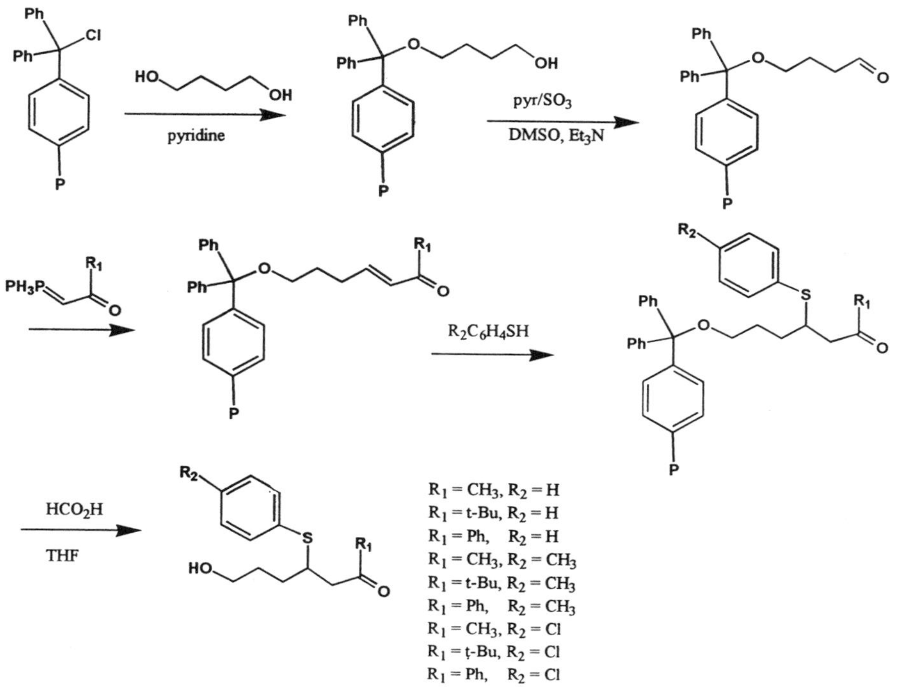

Figure 1.5 Solid-phase synthesis of small molecule combinatorial libraries (37).

solution-phase chemistry. Applications of TentaGel in combinatorial chemistry is the subject of Chapter 4.

A good example to illustrate the use of well-known organic reactions is Chen and co-workers' report of the preparation of a small collection of compounds from a trityl resin-linked alcohol (Fig. 1.5) (37). The diol was linked to trityl polystyrene and then oxidized with SO_3/pyridine to the aldehyde. The resulting polystyrene-linked aldehyde could be reacted with three different Horner-Emmons reagents (R_1 = Me, t-Bu, and Ph). Using the split-mix method, these enones were combined in equal amounts, split into three separate reaction vessels, and reacted in a Michael addition reaction with three different R_2-SH compounds. Nine different compounds were formed, a very small but prototypical combinatorial library. After product cleavage, each of the nine compounds could be isolated and completely characterized. In addition, the use of Fourier transform–infrared (FT-IR) and gas chromatography–mass spectroscopy (GC–MS) for analysis of products attached to beads was demonstrated. This work and its extensions are more fully described in Chapter 3.

1.4 ANALYTICAL TECHNIQUES FOR SOLID-PHASE SYNTHESIS

The principle of solid-phase synthesis requires that the product remain attached to the resin bead. A disadvantage of the technique is that it is more difficult to characterize the product at intermediate stages of the synthesis. Methods used to identify reaction products from solid-phase synthesis typically involve elemental analysis, titration of reactive groups, or simply weight gain (35). Sometimes, a small amount of the intermediate resin beads are removed, and the attached product cleaved and analyzed in the usual manner. For product identification, organic chemists usually use spectroscopic methods such as IR, NMR, or MS. Scheme 3.15 in Chapter 3 shows the FT-IR of starting material and product in a typical solid-phase reaction; the conversion to product can be clearly observed by changes in the spectrum.

The mainstay of organic structural analysis, however, is NMR. Unfortunately, the heterogeneous environment of resin-attached compounds leads to very broad ^{1}H-NMR lines. Recent work suggests that the use of magic-angle spinning ^{1}H-NMR (53,54) and ^{13}C-NMR (34) with polystyrene resin-bound compounds may be useful. The use of ^{13}C-NMR with synthetic compounds bound to TentaGel resin beads (PS–PEG) was shown to give excellent line widths for compounds where no signal could be observed for the same compounds directly attached to polystyrene (55). The use of ^{13}C-enriched building blocks also provided high-quality spectra with less interference from the polymer and solvent.

Finally, the use of mass spectroscopy for evaluating solid-phase synthesis has been explored. Methods usually require cleavage of the product from the resin and analysis of the resulting microsample in the usual manner. Several examples have been reported involving direct GC–MS of the product from a single bead. A single 100–200 mesh polystyrene "Merrifield" bead weighs approximately 0.1–0.2 μg. At a usual loading, each bead contains ~400 pmol of compound, more than enough for a mass spectrum. Figure 3.20 in Chapter 3 shows a typical single-bead result.

Several reports have also appeared using direct matrix-assisted laser desorption (MALDI) of combinatorial library beads (56–58). The most elegant approach to mass spectral analysis of synthesis beads was the report of the molecular weight imaging of individual beads using time-of-flight secondary ion mass spectrometry. The structure of small peptides could be seen directly from individual 30–60 μm polystyrene beads after cleaving the resin–peptide link with trifluoroacetic acid (TFA) (59).

The combination of affinity selection for active receptor ligands with electrospray mass spectroscopy shows promise for the rapid identification of active compounds in a combinatorial library (Fig. 1.6) (60). A small molecule combinatorial library containing 600 compounds was incubated with purified receptor and then separated by size-exclusion chromatography. The receptor containing bound ligand was collected, and the ligand was released and analyzed by electrospray mass spectroscopy. Figure 1.6 shows the low-molecular-weight (MW) region of the spectrum reveals a tight-binding ligand from the library at MW = 708. Specific binding of this compound can be determined by evaluating its competition with a known receptor ligand. It is likely that further developments of this "affinity selection" technique could speed up isolation and identification of leads from combinatorial libraries.

1.5   ENCODING OF BEADS

The combinatorial method for producing mixtures of thousands or millions of compounds has always presented an awkward deconvolution process. In principle, a better strategy would be to prepare the compounds in pure form, in separate, labeled bottles. What if each compound was attached to a separate bead—one compound per bead (61)? The mixture of beads then represents a physically separable collection of compounds. This approach has been widely used and only requires a means to determine what is attached to a single bead. Instead of direct structure determination of the compound attached to a single bead, the synthesis history of the bead is recorded on the bead—*encoding*. Each bead can be derivatized with a "tag" that contains information on the structure attached to the bead. Therefore, instead of identifying the compound, one identifies the code. This concept was first described for beads encoded with a genetic DNA tag (62). This elegant approach allows amplification of the encoded "signal" by polymerase chain reaction (PCR) for analysis.

A more practical approach for organic chemistry is the tagging strategy developed by Ohlmeyer and co-workers (63). The use of the split-synthesis method provides a final library wherein each bead has a single compound attached. This method (Fig. 1.7) involves attachment (at the level of a few percent of the real compound) of a binary code of chlorophenyl groups at each synthesis step. Using electron-capture GC analysis, 0.1 pmol of code attached to a single 50–80 μm bead is more than enough for detection (64). The presence or absence of one of the four GC separable chlorophenyl derivatives (Fig. 1.7, $n = 1$–4) gives a binary code of 0 or 1. Thus the binary codes such as 0000, 0001, 0010, 0100, and so forth can be

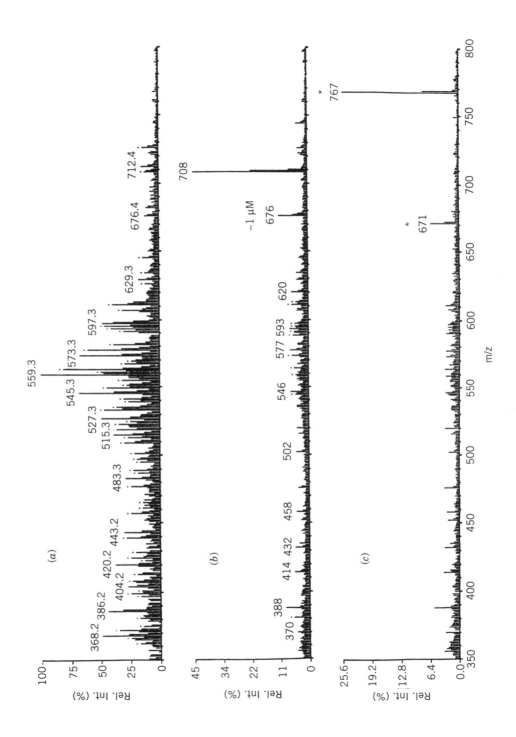

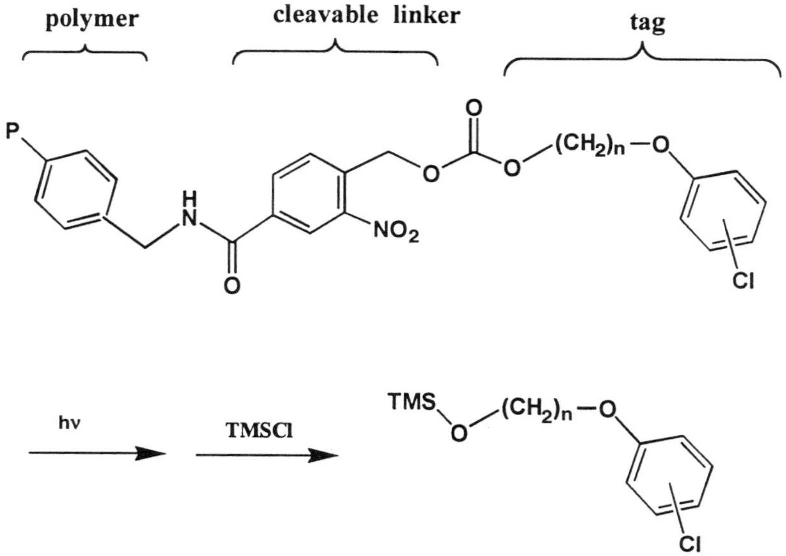

Figure 1.7 Still bead encoding method from combinatorial libraries (41). The synthesis polymer is derivitized with a photocleavable linker and a tag containing a choloroaryl group. The tags can be removed from the beads, the resulting alcohols silylated and then detected by GC.

used to define the synthetic steps applied to the bead. The compound synthesis proceeds on the beads as usual. After each step a coding reaction is carried out on the bead at a trace level ($\sim 1\%$). Usually the code is linked using a photocleavable linker so that the code can be removed without damaging the valuable (perhaps active) compound attached to that bead. Details of the use of an encoded library to locate ligands for a synthetic (unnatural) receptor molecule has been reported (65). Further development and commercialization of this coding method is now in the hands of Pharmacopoeia (66) and a review of the Still coding method has just appeared (67).

Another coding method uses peptide sequences for a reaction code (68). Two orthogonally protected points of extension allow the primary peptide (or organic) molecule to be formed at one point and a coding sequence built at the second. The code can be "read" by selective cleavage of the coding peptide, followed by sequencing. The coding sequence was claimed not to effect binding of the primary structure.

Figure 1.6 (*a*) Electrospray MS of a 600-compound small molecule library. (*b*) Library from (*a*) after affinity selection with an excess of receptor. Note the strong enrichment and selection of the compound at MW = 708 (MH+). (*c*) Mixture after affinity selection in the presence of a strong competitive ligand. This figure shows that the compound at 708 MH+/Z can be competed off the receptor by this peptide ligand.

Finally, an intriguing new coding method has just appeared. TentaGel polymer beads containing a memory storage device are used in synthesis. The synthesis code can be written into the memory chip with radiofrequency pulses (69). The memory chips are similar to EPROM chips (erasable, programmable, read-only memory.) A more comprehensive discussion of this technology is covered in Chapters 7 and 8.

1.6   POSITIONALLY ADDRESSABLE SPATIAL ARRAYS

Another approach to separation/identification of combinatorial library collections is based on preparing each compound immobilized on a separate spot on a surface. This method then allows the x/y coordinates of the spot to be related to the structure. This process was pioneered by the Affymax group and described in detail in a classic *Science* article: "Light-Directed, Spatially Addressable Parallel Chemical Synthesis" (70). In this technology, solid-phase synthesis is carried out on surface-derivatized glass substrates using photolabile protecting groups and photo-lithographic techniques. Light-directed peptide or oligonucleotide synthesis could be carried out using a 50-μm checkerboard mask for selected photo-deprotection of spots. About 40,000 compounds can be prepared in a 1-cm^2 area using these techniques.

Recently, details of an application of the Affymax method to organic synthesis appeared. The light-directed synthesis of a collection of biotin analogs were prepared and immobilized in checkerboard fashion to a glass plate. This array was then screened using imaging of the binding of fluorescent avidin to the surface of the plate (71). A review of the Affymax method has recently appeared (72).

A more accessible version of this general concept uses simultaneous parallel synthesis on cellulose disks (73). Peptide synthesis on a 50-nmol scale can be achieved in an array of 100 spots on a 1-cm^2 area. Reagents and protected amino acids can be delivered to the spots either manually or using a commercially x/y-programmable thin-layer chromatography (TLC) spotter. The spot synthesis of peptides was used for rapid antibody binding studies and thus far has not been extended to organic compounds.

1.7   ROBOTIC INSTRUMENTATION: THE INDUSTRIAL REVOLUTION OVERTAKES ORGANIC SYNTHESIS

Organic synthesis is labor intensive and its operations have not substantially changed since the turn of the century. Although there were some developments in automated synthesis in the early 1980s (74,75), major interest never materialized. The Zymark Corporation introduced its sample handling robot in 1981, and despite the slow applications to synthetic chemistry, automation of sample handling for high-speed bioassay caught on (7).

The extensive use of peptide synthesis for drug discovery, monoclonal antibodies, vaccines, and diagnostics contributed to the continued development of automation in the peptide field. Many companies developed commercial synthe-

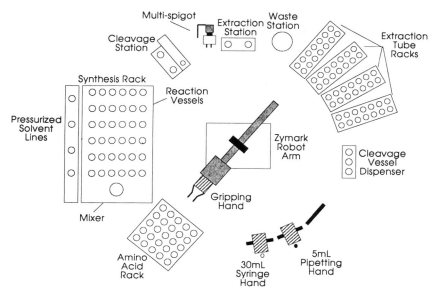

Figure 1.8 Equimolar peptide mixture synthesizer. A Zymark robot arm is surrounded by a synthesis station and cleavage/protection station.

sizers including ABI, Waters/Millipore, Advanced ChemTech, and Biosearch. At the same time, instrumentation for DNA synthesis, which is very similar in its technical approach, also flourished.

It was not until recently that interest in solid-phase organic synthesis returned, driven largely by combinatorial chemistry. The design and construction of a robotic combinatorial library synthesizer (Fig. 1.8), based on a Zymark robot, was described in 1992 (76). This instrument positions several stations around a central robot arm. The machine is programmed to carry out multiple peptide syntheses using split-mix procedures and is designed to prepare exact equimolar mixtures of peptide mixtures for assay.

As directed work on solid-phase organic synthesis of small organic molecules, using more or less standard Merrifield-type chemistry, was reexamined and found to work well, the Parke-Davis group reported a semiautomated device for organic applications, now sold via Diversomer Technologies, Inc. (34). Recently, Advanced ChemTech (Louisville, KY) modified its peptide synthesis apparatus and began to sell an "organic synthesizer." The surge in interest in combinatorial libraries will undoubtedly prompt other entries in this field (77).

1.8 COMPUTATIONAL CHEMISTRY IN COMBINATORIAL CHEMISTRY: KEEPING UP WITH THE DATA

Computational tools for combinatorial chemistry include molecular spread sheet methods, databases, and software—all related to structure–activity relationship study and drug design. Biological results for a combinatorial library contain a lot more data to analyze than one had to deal with in the past (78,79).

In addition, chemists would like to be able to develop an intuition about structure–activity relationships and to explore what types of pharmacophores are useful in a particular assay. With so much data to sift, new tools are needed. Understanding the link between structure and the biological data is at the heart of medicinal chemistry (80). Many of the familiar tools for computer-aided modeling will probably be applied in the usual way, once combinatorial methods assist in the location of interesting leads.

Combinatorial libraries are usually represented by generic structures with a small number of differing R-group positions. For each R-group position there are lists of alternative structures. This results in a compound matrix spread sheet such as shown for the 1,4-benzodiazepine in Figure 1.4. A database representation of this matrix of compounds could, in principle, help the chemist keep track of the compounds and provide a framework for a combinatorial structure–activity relationship database. Several commercial sources are available for such software: The major molecular modeling companies such as Chemical Design (Oxon, England), Tripos (St. Louis, MO), and MDL (San Leandro, CA) all have entries in this field. Other newer software providers in this field include Daylight (Irvine, CA) and Synopsys (Leeds, England).

Chemical Design provides a three-dimensional combinatorial software package that allows mapping of pharmacophore patterns of collections of compounds in a library. For example, Figure 1.9 shows a pharmacophore plot of a benzodiazepam library. Each point in the box represents a library member with certain properties, and cluster points indicate similar types of compounds. Picking a point allows the user to display specific data such as the pharmacophore geometry. It often would be desirable to examine plots of assay results and then relate such groupings to the molecular structure of active compounds. Several software companies provide a software connection from such properties plots to a three-dimensional pharmacophore plot derived from the best "hit."

A second but important computation problem for combinatorial libraries relates to the general question of library design. It has been estimated that 10^{200} organic molecules can be constructed of molecular weight less than 850. Since it is not possible to prepare them all, how does one choose the best selection of building blocks that will provide the most diverse set of compounds? A report has appeared that proposes a computational measure of diversity and graphical plots to assist in the comparison of different types of libraries (81). The technique takes into account characteristics such as lipophilicity, shape and branching, chemical functionality, and specific binding features. Another related computational technique involves combinatorial growth of molecules that are complementary to the binding sites of enzymes (82).

Initially there was some feeling that combinatorial chemistry and computer modeling were somehow in competition. It is now clear that the combinatorial chemistry field poses many exciting new challenges and applications for modeling as it rapidly evolves over the next few years.

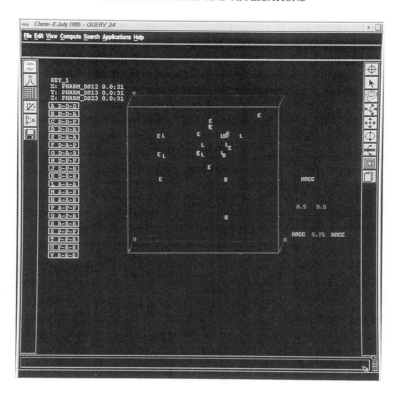

Figure 1.9 Pharmacophore plot for a benzodiazapam library. A single pharmacophore symbol has been picked from the plot and the corresponding pharmacophore geometry is displayed to the right of the plot.

1.9 OTHER APPROACHES AND APPLICATIONS

Although much of this introductory chapter has focused on solid-phase synthesis, solution-phase organic synthesis (see Chapter 5) can also be used for combinatorial chemistry. Carell and co-workers (83) have reported the use of a central core molecule with multiple reactive groups as a template for the construction of libraries. The essence of the principle is the use of either cubane or xanthene derivatives (Fig. 1.10) as tetrasubstituted core molecules for library construction. With only 19 building blocks, 11,191 compounds can be produced from the cubane core **A** and 65,341 different compounds can be produced with the xanthene core **B**. By iterative deletions of building blocks, and screening of sublibraries, an active (not necessarily the most active) compound can be identified (84).

A second strategy for the solution-phase synthesis of libraries was reported by Cheng and co-workers (85). A compound with multiple reaction sites, *N*-(*tert*-butyloxy)-carbonyl-iminodiacetic acid anhydride, was used to prepare collections

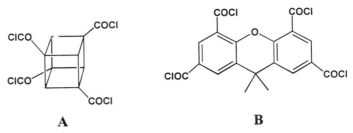

Figure 1.10   Combinatorial libraries can be prepared from cubane tetracarboxylic acid chloride **A** or xanthene tetracarboxylic acid chloride **B**.

of small nonpeptide organic molecules in solution by reaction with amines and carboxylic acids. The largest library was prepared from a $6 \times 8 \times 20$ matrix affording 1014 final compounds.

The solution-phase peptide synthesis methods pioneered by Mutter and Bayer (86) were recently applied to combinatorial library synthesis (87,88). Janda (87,88) has used PEG-supported chemistry, which allows homogeneous reactions to be carried out. By addition of diethyl ether, the polymer containing the desired product precipitates. Thus, some of the best advantages of both solid and solution chemistry are retained.

Finally, a recent perspective on the future of solution versus solid-phase synthesis was discussed in an article by Curran (89a). The principle of phase separation—that is, solid versus solution is compared with a novel technique of using saturated fluorocarbon phases in synthesis. Fluorocarbon phases are not misible with either water or organic solvents. This allows liquid–liquid extraction of reactants and products to be used in the same way as filtration for solid-phase synthesis. While little work has appeared in this area, it illustrates a subject for the future.

Combinatorial chemistry began as an application to the drug discovery process. As the field has developed, it has become clear that the technique of combinatorial libraries are applicable to the search for new useful properties of molecules in the broader sense. There have been a few reports that apply the library techniques described here to material science, catalyst design, metal chelation, and molecular recognition. Xiang and co-workers (89b) have deposited combinatorial arrays of inorganic salts to create a spatially defined thin film of potential superconducting composites. Sample arrays of 200×200 μm size can be made, which corresponds to 10,000 new materials per square inch. These arrays can be robotically tested for conductivity using a specially designed microprobe. A second report from the same group applied the technique to arrays of magnetoresistive materials (90). Hsieh-Wilson and co-workers have recently reviewed their work in this area (91).

Applications of combinatorial libraries to preparations of new catalysis was reported by Menger and co-workers (92) who prepared libraries of poly(allyl-amine)-based catalysts by reaction of the amine polymer with mixtures of functionalized carboxylic acids. This polymeric mixture was treated with various metal salts and examined for phosphatase catalyst activity in the hydrolysis of *bis-(p*-nitrophenyl)phosphate. It was possible to determine, in a scheme related to iterative or sublibrary synthesis, the best catalyst combinations.

Two reports have appeared concerning applications of combinatorial libraries to the discovery of optimal metal-binding ligands. The first method uses Still's encoded split synthesis to examine a collection of synthetic ionophores for Cu^{+2} and Co^{+2} (93). Up to 130,321 compounds can be prepared from a central tetra-aza-cyclododecane unit with three functionalized side arms containing mixtures of 19 amino acids. Because of the need for a bead-based assay, the process was limited to ions whose complexes were colored. When the collection of beads—one ligand per bead—was mixed with metal salt, blue-colored beads could be seen, harvested, and decoded to provide the structures of the best binders. Still also could conclude from these experiments that azamacrocycles were not a good scaffold for this type of assay. Another recent study (94) describes a combinatorial library of bipyridyl and crown ether derivatives. Metal-template-directed complexation was used to prepare a small mixture library in solution (94).

Lastly, although peptide and oligonucleotide combinatorial chemistry have not been stressed in this book, there are many biologically based techniques for combinatorial chemistry that may be of interest to organic chemists. One such system is called phage-display, which presents peptide sequences on the surface of a virus and holds promise for rapid studies of peptide architecture and lead discovery. A chapter describing these types of studies is included (Chapter 12) in this book so that organic chemists can have some understanding about these areas.

It is very unlikely that all the chemistry that can be applied to library synthesis is reported in this book. The phrase "combinatorial chemistry" may suggest to you organic libraries, peptides, oligonucleotides, arrays on chips, coding, or just plain rapid synthesis. I hope the reader realizes that this new frontier has plenty of work ahead for all fields of science and does not mean rejection of other methods. Combinatorial chemistry does not require us to ignore the great amount of knowledge of molecular structures that we have carefully built up over the past few decades. Instead, combinatorial chemistry should be considered an advanced tool to aid in the rapid discovery of molecules with desired properties. We hope that the subsequent chapters will stimulate you to apply your own creativity to this emerging area of intellectual pursuit.

REFERENCES

1. Geyson, H. M., Meloen, R. H., and Barteling, S. J. *Proc. Natl. Acad. Sci. U.S.A.* **91,** 3998–4002 (1984).
2. Furka, A., Sebestyen, M., and Dibo, G., *Abstr., 14th Congr. Biochem, Prague.* 1988, p. 47.
3. Merrifield, R. B., *J. Am. Chem. Soc.* **85,** 2149–54 (1963).
4. Houghten, R. A., *Proc. Natl. Acad. Sci, U.S.A.* **82,** 5131–5135 (1985).
5. Gorman, J. J., *Anal. Biochem.* **136,** 397–406 (1984).

6. Sweetnam, P. M., Price, C. H., and Ferkany, J. W., in *Burger's Medicinal Chemistry and Drug Discovery,* Vol. 1, M. E. Wolff (Ed.), Wiley, New York, 1995, pp. 697–731.

7. Danheiser, S. L., *Genetic Eng. News.* **13** (Nov. 15), 1 (1993).

8. Dooley, C. T. and Houghten, R. A., *Life Sci.* **52,** 1509–1517 (1993).

9. Houghten, R. A., *Curr. Biol.* **4,** 564–567 (1994).

10. Freier, S. M., Konings, D. A. M., Wyatt, J. R., and Ecker, D. J., *J. Med. Chem.* **38,** 344–352 (1995).

11. Hylands, P. J. and Nisbet, L. J., *Ann. Rep. Med. Chem.* **26,** 259–269 (1991).

12. Dower, W. J. and Fodor, S. P. A. *Ann. Rep. Med. Chem.* **26,** 271–280 (1991).

13. Pavia, M. R., Sawyer, T. K., and Moos, W. H., *Bioorganic Med. Chem. Lett.* **3,** 387–396 (1993).

14. Moos, W. H., Green, G. D., and Pavia, M. R., *Ann. Rep. Med. Chem.* **28,** 315–324 (1993).

15. Gallop, M. A., Barett, R. W., Dower, W. J., Fodor, S. P. A., and Gordon, E. M., *J. Med. Chem.* **37,** 1233 (1994).

16. Gordon, E. M., Barett, R. W., Dower, W. J., Fodor, S. P. A., and Gallop, M. A., *J. Med. Chem.* **37,** 1385 (1994).

17. Jung, G. and Beck-Sickinger, A. G., *Angew Chem. Int. Ed. Engl.* **31** 367–486 (1992).

18. Feldor, E. R., *Chimia* **48,** 531–541 (1994).

19. Liskamp, R. M. J., *Angew Chim., Int. Ed. Engl.* **33,** 633–636 (1994).

20. Janda, K. D., *Proc. Natl. Acad. Sci. U.S.A.* **91,** 10779–10785 (1994).

21. Baum, R. M., *Chem. Eng. News,* Feb. 7, 20–26 (1994).

22. Madden, D., Krchnak, V., and Lebl, M. *Perspectives Drug Discovery Design* **2,** 269–285 (1994).

23. Deai, M. C., Zuckermann, R. N., and Moos, W. H. *Drug Dev. Res.* **22,** 174 (1994).

24. Scott, J. K. and Craig, L. *Curr. Opin. Biotechnol.* **5,** 40 (1994).

25. Rohr, J., *Angew. Chim., Int. Ed. Engl.* **34,** 881–883 (1995).

26. (a) Terrett, N. K., Gardner, M., Gordon, D. W., Kobylecki, R. J., and Steele, J., *Tetrahedron* **51,** 8135–8173 (1995). (b) Thompson, L. A. and Ellman, J. A., *Chem. Rev.* **96,** 555 (1996).

27. *Molecular Diversity* (An Internet Journal), ESCOM Science Publishers, Leiden, the Netherlands.

28. Crowley, J. I. and Rapoport, H. *Acct. Chem. Res.* **9,** 135–144 (1976).

29. Leznoff, C. C., *Acct.. Chem. Res.* **11,** 327–333 (1978).

30. Neckers, D. C. *Chemtech* 108–116 (1978).

31. Frechet, J. M. J. *Tetrahedron* **37,** 663–683 (1981).

32. Hodge, P. and Sherrington, D. C. (Eds.), *Polymer-supported Reactions in Organic Synthesis,* Wiley-Interscience, Chichester, 1980.

33. Bunin, B. A. and Ellman, J. A., *J. Am. Chem. Soc.* **114,** 10997–10998 (1992).

34. DeWitt, S. H., Kiely, J. S., Stankovic, C. J., Schroeder, M. C., Cody, D. M. R., and Pavia M. R., *Proc. Natl. Acad. Sci. U.S.A.* **90,** 6909–6913 (1993).

35. Fruchtel, J. S. and Jung, G., *Angew. Chem. Int. Ed. Eng.* **35,** 17–42 (1996).

36. Yedida, V. and Leznoff, C. C., *Can J. Chem.* **58,** 1144 (1980).

37. Chen, C., Randall, L. A. A., Miller, R. B., Jones, D. A., and Kurth, M. J., *J. Am. Chem. Soc.* **116**, 2661–2662 (1994).

38. Kurth, M. J., Randall, L. A. A., Chen, C., Melander, C., and Miller, R. B., *J. Org. Chem.* **59**, 5862–5864 (1994).

39. Richter, L. S. and Gadek, T. R., *Tetrahedron Lett.* **35**, 4705 (1994).

40. Schore, N. E. and Najdi, S. D. J. J. *J. Am. Chem. Soc.* **112**, 441 (1990).

41. Farrall, M. J. and Frechet, J. M. J., *J. Org. Chem.* **41**, 3877–3882 (1976).

42. Deshpande, M. S., *Tetrahedron Lett.* **35**, 5613–5614 (1994).

43. Frenette, R., Friesen, R. W., *Tetrahedron Lett.* **35**, 9177–9180 (1994).

44. Backers, B. J. and Ellmann, J. A., *J. Am. Chem. Soc.* **116**, 11171 (1994).

45. Yu, K-L., Deshpande, M. S., and Vyas, D. M., *Tetrahedron Lett.* **35**, 8919–8922 (1994).

46. Frenette, R., and Friesen, R. W., *Tetrahedron Lett.* **35**, 9177–9180 (1994).

47. Hutchins, S. M., and Chapman, K. T., *Tetrahedron Lett.* **35**, 4055–4058 (1994).

48. Patek, M., Drake, B., and Lebl, M., *Tetrahedron Lett.* **35**, 2227–2230 (1994).

49. Boyce, R., Li, G., Nestler, P., Suenag, T., and Still, W. C., *J. Am. Chem. Soc.* **116**, 7955–7956 (1994).

50. Merrifield, R. B. "Life During the Golden Age of Peptide Chemistry," J. Seeman (Ed.), American Chemical Society, Washington, DC, 1993.

51. A. Guyot, in *Synthesis and Separations Using Functionalized Polymers,* D. C. Sherrington and P. Hodge (Eds.), Wiley, Chichester, 1988, pp. 1ff.

52. Bayer, E., and Rapp, W., *Chem. Pept. Prot* **3**, 3 (1986).

53. Anderson, R. C., Jarema, M. A., Stokes, J. P., and Shapiro, M., *J. Org. Chem.* **60**, 2650 (1995).

54. Anderson, R. C., Stokes, J. P., and Shapiro, M. J. *Tetrahedron Lett* **36**, 5311 (1995).

55. Look, G. C., Holmes, C. P., Chinn, J. P., and Gallop, M. A., *J. Org. Chem.* **59**, 7588–7590 (1994).

56. Youngquist, R. S., Fuentes, G. R., Lacey, M. P., and Keough, T., *Rapid Commun. Mass Spectrosc.* **8**, 77–81 (1994).

57. Egner, B. J., Langley, G. J., and Bradley, M., *J. Org. Chem.* **60**, 2652–2653 (1995).

58. Youngquist, R. S., Fuentes, G. R., Lacey, M. P., and Keough, T., *J. Am. Chem. Soc.* **117**, 3900–3906 (1995).

59. Brummel, C. L., Lee, I. N. W., Zhao, Y., Benkovic, S. J., and Winograd, N., *Science* **264**, 399–402 (1994).

60. Dollinger, G., Chiron Corporation. 1995 Medicinal Chemistry GRC and personal communication.

61. Lebl, M., Krchnak, V., Sepetov, N. F., Seligmann, B., Strop, P., and Felder, S., *Biopolymers* **37**, 177–198 (1995).

62. Brenner, S., and Lerner, R. A., *Proc. Natl. Acad. Sci. U.S.A.* **89**, 5381–5383 (1992).

63. Ohlmeyer, M. H. J., Swanson, R. N., Dillard, L. W., Reader, J. C., Asouline, G., Kobayashi, R., Wigler, M., and Still, W. C., *Proc. Natl. Acad. Sci. U.S.A.* **90**, 10922–10926 (1993).

64. Grinsrud, E. P., in *Detectors for Capillary Chromatography,* H. H. Hill and D. G. McMinn (Eds.), Wiley, New York, 1992, pp. 83–107.

65. Borchardt, A., and Still, W. C., *J. Am. Chem. Soc.* **116,** 373–374 (1994).

66. Baldwin, J. J., Burbaum, J. J., Henderson, I., and Ohlmeyer, M. H. J., *J. Am. Chem. Soc.* **117,** 5588–5589 (1995).

67. Still, W. C., *Acc. Chem. Res.* **29,** 155–163 (1996).

68. Kerr, J. M., Banville, S. C., and Zuckermann, R. N., *J. Am. Chem. Soc.* **115,** 2529 (1993).

69. Nicolaou, K. C., Xiao, X-Y., Parandoosh, Z., Senyei, A., and Nova, M. P., *Angew. Chem. Int. Ed. Engl.* **43,** 2289–2291 (1995).

70. Fodor, S. P. A., Read, J. L., Pirrung, M. C., Stryer, L., Lu, A. T., and Solas, D., *Science* **251,** 767–773 (1991).

71. Sundberg, S. A., Barrett, R. W., Pirrung, M., Lu, A. L., Kiangsoontra, B., and Holmes, C. P., *J. Am. Chem. Soc.* **117,** 12050–12057 (1995).

72. Holmes, C. P., Adams, C. L., Kochersperger, L. M., Mortensen, R. B., and Aldwin, L. A., *Biopolymers* **37,** 199–211 (1995).

73. Frank, R., *Tetrahedron* **42,** 9217–9232 (1992).

74. Frisbee, A. R., Nantz, M. H., Kramer, G. W., and Fuchs, P. L., *J. Am. Chem. Soc.* **106,** 7143–7145 (1984).

75. Kramer, G. W., and Fuchs, P. L., *Chemtech* 682–688 (1989).

76. Zuckerman, R. N., Kerr, J. M., Siani, M. A., and Banvile, S. C., *Int. J. Peptide Protein Res.* **40,** 497–506 (1992).

77. Glaser, V., *Genetic Eng.* **16,** 1 (1996).

78. Sullivan, M., *Today's Chemist* 19–26 (1994).

79. Krieger, J. H., *Chem. Eng. News,* 1996, February 12, 67.

80. Balbes, L. M., Mascarella, S. W., and Boyd, D. B., in *Reviews in Computational Chemistry,* Vol. V., K. B. Lipkowitz and D. B. Boyd (Eds.), VCH Publishers, New York, 1994.

81. Martin, E. J., Blaney, J. M., Siani, M. A., Spellmeyer, D. C., Wong, A. K., and Moos, W. H., *J. Med. Chem.* **38,** 1431–1436 (1995).

82. Bohacek, R. S., and McMartin, C., *J. Am. Chem. Soc.* **116,** 5560–5571 (1994).

83. Carell, T., Wintner, E. A., Bashir-Hashemi, A., and Rebek, Jr., J., *Angew Chem. Int. Ed. Eng.,* **33,** 2005–2007 (1994).

84. Carell, T., Wintner, E. A., and Rebek, Jr., J., *Angew Chem. Int. Ed. Eng.* **33,** 2061–2064 (1994).

85. Cheng, S., Comer, D. D., Williams, J. P., Myers, P. L., and Boger, D. L., *J. Am. Chem. Soc.* **118,** 2567–2573 (1996).

86. Mutter, M., and Bayer, E., in *The Peptides: Analysis, Synthesis and Biology,* Vol. 2, E. Gross and J. Meienhofer (Eds.), Academic, New York, pp. 285–332.

87. Han, H., Wolfe, M. M., Brenner, S., and Janda, K. D., *Proc. Natl. Acad. Sci. U.S.A.* **92,** 6419 (1995).

88. Han, H., and Janda, K. D., *J. Am. Chem. Soc.* **118,** 2539–2544 (1996).

89. (a) Curran, D. P. *Chemtracts* **9,** 75 (1996); (b) Xiang, X-D., Sun, X. D., Briceno, G., Lou, Y., Wang, K-A., Chang, H. Y., Wallace-Freedman, W. G., Chen, S-W., and Schultz, P. G., *Science* **268,** 1738–1740 (1995).

90. Briceno, G., Chang, H. Y., Sun, X. D., Schultz, P. G., and Xiang, X-D., *Science* **270,** 273 (1995).

91. Hsieh-Wilson, L. C., Xiang, X-D., and Schultz, P. G., *Accts. Chem. Res.* **29,** 164–170 (1996).

92. Menger, F. M., Eliseev, A. V., and Migulin, V. A., *J. Org. Chem.* **60,** 6666–6667 (1995).

93. Burger, M. T., and Still, W. C., *J. Org. Chem.* **60,** 7382–7383 (1995).

94. Goodman, M. S., Jubian, V., Linton, B., and Hamilton, A. D., *J. Am. Chem. Soc.* **117,** 11610–11611 (1995).

2

PARALLEL ORGANIC SYNTHESIS USING PARKE-DAVIS DIVERSOMER TECHNOLOGY

SHEILA HOBBS DEWITT AND ANTHONY W. CZARNIK
BioOrganic Chemistry Section, Department of Chemistry, Parke-Davis Pharmaceutical Research Division of Warner-Lambert Company, Ann Arbor, Michigan 48105

Combinatorial chemistry is the chemistry characterized by *divergent synthesis*, which makes possible the synthesis of larger numbers of samples than by linear or convergent synthesis. At its heart is an acceptance of the precept that our ability to predict some useful properties of molecules based on their structures is yet immature. Nevertheless, the discovery of molecules with useful properties can yield enormous value. It follows that the search for properties benefits by having access to many samples with different structures. This is the paradigm used by nature in situations where survival is the motivating force. Thus, one focus of combinatorial chemistry is the synthesis of large numbers (i.e., thousands and up) of compounds in amounts sufficient to test. This is referred to as *lead generation* and has been addressed using the split-mix approach described by Furka and adapted to small organic molecules by Pharmacopeia.

There is little sense in synthesizing more samples than can be tested, which in part explains why agrochemical and petrochemical companies have relied on screening methods longer than have pharmaceutical companies. Our relatively recent ability to prepare large amounts of biological macromolecules has enabled high-volume in vitro screens for small-molecule agonists and antagonists. This, in turn, has led to a plethora of available targets for drug discovery and a resulting plethora of interesting new structural leads with useful (often inhibitory) properties. Fine-tuning the property of interest as a function of structure is the process of *lead optimization* and most usefully requires the synthesis of smaller numbers of organic compounds but in greater amount (i.e., several milligrams). Both lead generation and lead optimization strategies have been based on the notion of divergent synthesis. The adaptation of the pioneering work of Geysen et al. (1) to the simultaneous synthesis of heterocycles was described early by Bunin and Ellman at Berkeley (2) and the BioOrganic Group at Parke-Davis (3). Contemporary efforts at UC-Davis, Chiron, Affymax, and Pfizer U.K. were reported in the literature soon afterward. It is now hard to imagine that the ideas of solid-phase organic synthesis and its logical extension to automated synthesis were only recently considered heretical. We will not try to review the field of combinatorial chemistry in this chapter; that is the overall purpose of this book. Instead, we will focus on describing the approach we have taken in the Chemistry Department at Parke-Davis and the reaction sequences to which it has been applied.

2.1   THE DIVERSOMER APPARATUS

Although it is certainly possible to run 40 reactions at one time in a single laboratory hood, in practice it would be a cumbersome exercise without some form of miniaturization, a method to physically manipulate all 40 reactions in a common unit and an ability to purify intermediates without resort to chromatography. The Geysen approach of synthesis on a rack of polypropylene rods (i.e., "pins") fulfills all three imperatives and indeed has been applied as a solution by Bunin and Ellman (2). In our setting, there is advantage in preparing more material than possible on the tip of such a pin. Furthermore, the compatibility of our desired chemistries with the plastic equipment proved to be limiting. The method of Houghton (4) in which polypeptide synthesis is accomplished on several hundred milligrams of resin beads seemed more appropriate for our needs. In the Houghton method, individual collections of beads are contained in tea bags in which chemical reactions can be accomplished directly. This approach serves polypeptide synthesis surprisingly well, but would be more limiting under the wide range of reaction conditions employed in organic synthesis. It is apparent that the ideal reactor would be constructed from rigid but porous glass, as the conditions employed by the synthetic chemist are already validated with glass vessels. The common gas dispersion tube (a PIN) serves this role well and became our group's reaction vessel of choice.

The design of an apparatus capable of organizing this set of PINs was likewise required. A functional prototype capable of organizing an eight-unit array is shown in Figure 2.1. Resin beads, from 100 to 800 mg depending on the size of the apparatus, reside in the fritted portion at the bottom of each PIN. The set of PINs is held in place by a block of chemically resistant material, normally Teflon. The fritted portions of the PINs can be inserted into glass reservoir vials, themselves organized by a reservoir block. This lower portion of the apparatus can be immersed in a heated or cooled ultrasound bath to provide both agitation and temperature control, thus increasing the range of reaction types that can be employed. Although a much more sophisticated design would provide for individual temperature control, we have chosen instead (and been successful in using) a single bath temperature in which the choice of temperature has been optimized before the array synthesis.

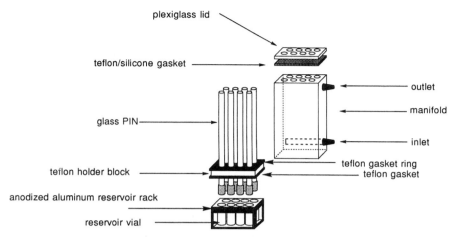

Figure 2.1 Eight-PIN synthesizer.

Above the holder block, a Plexiglass manifold is used to permit maintenance of an inert atmosphere. Reagents may be introduced to the PINs directly through an injectable gasket at the top. If a chilled, inert gas such as nitrogen or argon is passed through the gas inlet port, reflux conditions can be maintained as the reaction solvent condenses on the inner walls of individual PINs.

The eight-unit array pictured in Figure 2.1 is now available commercially (5). In practice it functions well with only a few caveats. First, the equalization of pressure between the dissolved reagents in the reaction vial and the resin in the filter is effectively achieved with three small release holes in the glass, above the filter but below the holder block. However, due to variations in resin mesh size, the copious washing of resin bound intermediates sometimes results in the loss of a small amount of resin through these holes. This is most often observed with solvents exhibiting high swelling capacity. Although dichloromethane is a serious culprit, use of other solvents largely avoids this problem. Second, the containment of volatile solvents at reflux (e.g., dichloromethane) over long periods of time is still imperfect. For this reason, we prefer to employ solvents with similar swelling properties but lower volatility. Third, gasket materials have finite lifetimes and must be replaced after long periods of solvent exposure, extremes in temperature, or repeated injection. This, however, is not unlike a chemist discarding a septum after repeated use.

Although the 8-unit array apparatus can be easily operated by a single chemist, the repetitive reagent and solvent dispersements required during use of the larger 40-unit array apparatus (not pictured) can easily lead to operator fatigue and error. There is an obvious value to employment of automated liquid sample handling techniques, among which valve-driven fluidic and motor-driven robotic approaches are the most obvious. Our group has focused on the application of robotic methods, largely because potential problems with multiple valving and tubing controls and general incompatibility with the wide range of corrosive, pyrophoric, flammable, and sensitive reagents employed in organic synthesis. An overview of methods for the automation of organic synthesis is available (6).

2.2   GENERAL ASPECTS OF SOLID-PHASE ORGANIC SYNTHESIS (SPOS)

The earliest literature reports describing multistep organic synthesis on a polymeric support (7,8) appeared soon after reports describing analogous polypeptide synthesis (9). In general, the idea is that an insoluble polymer bearing chemically reactive functional groups is "charged" (chemically functionalized) with a reagent that can serve as starting material for a multistep synthetic sequence. Schematically, this is depicted as addition of BB_1 in step one of Scheme 2.1. Subsequent chemical reactions then modify this starting material. Although Scheme 2.1 depicts this functionalization as linear, the actual mode of compound construction depends entirely on the sequence. The principle advantage of SPOS is the ability to remove excess reagent and solvent by way of simple washing. In the absence of such a time- and labor-saving device, parallel organic synthesis loses much of its time-saving potential.

Cleavage of the final product from the solid support prior to biological screening

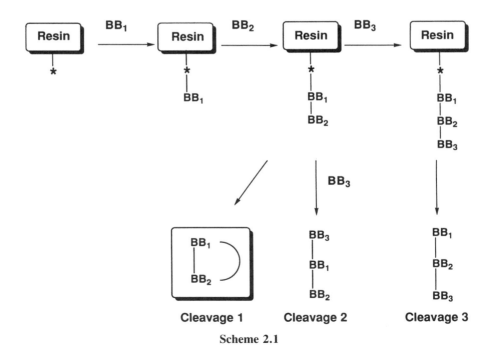

Scheme 2.1

is highly desirable, as many assays would be inhibited or completely untenable under heterogeneous conditions. Chemically, the removal can be viewed as resulting from several different cleavage strategies. Cleavage types 2 and 3 (Scheme 2.1) have been used effectively here and elsewhere. However, cleavage type 1 can bring unique advantage that makes it preferable when possible. Type 1 cleavage, or "cyclative cleavage," occurs when heating or reagent treatment induces a functionality on the growing product to "bite" into BB_1 with resulting breakage of the BB_1–polymer bond. When this occurs, the cyclized product is released from the resin for purification or direct assay. Because only those polymer sites that successfully reacted with BB_2 possess the (presumably) nucleophilic site required for cyclization, truncated sites are not expected to cleave from the support. In this way, some measure of purification can be achieved.

The obvious inability to purify intermediate resin-bound products is a major source of discontentment for organic chemists, and high-yielding schemes will prove valuable as they are discovered. Sequences that provide final products not requiring purification greatly facilitate rapid synthesis. However, practitioners in this field are finding that some valuable products are not sufficiently homogeneous for reliable assay and require purification. Indeed, a proton nuclear magnetic resonance (NMR) spectrum demonstrating homogeneity is not sufficient to guarantee a reliable biological assay. It is proving important to evaluate the activities of several reference compounds placed intentionally into an array synthesis. When required, parallel purification methods as well as quantitative analysis [to obtain quantitative structure-activity relationship (QSAR) information] will no doubt prove useful and will continue to be developed (10).

2.3   EXAMPLES OF REACTION SEQUENCES ACCOMPLISHED USING THE DIVERSOMER METHOD

All of the following recapitulations of synthetic schemes have been reported previously, as indicated by the identifying references. Some additional editorializing is included here given the wisdom of multiple successes and failures since the original reports. It is important to note that all of these syntheses afforded sufficient product amount for characterization using proton NMR and mass spectrometry of each successful reaction product. In general, resin-bound intermediates were characterized using gel phase ^{13}C-NMR spectroscopy (3a,11).

Members of the hydantoin class of compounds (e.g., Dilantin) are useful in controlling the symptoms of epilepsy, making targeted libraries of hydantoins of interest. Our hydantoin library synthesis, carried out with Ms. Donna Reynolds Cody, is shown in Scheme 2.2 (1). Any parallel synthesis benefits by starting with a set of reactions that work efficiently with a wide range of reagents. In this scheme, those reactions are: amine deprotection (step 1), reaction of an amine with an isocyanate to give a urea (step 2), and acid-catalyzed cyclization of the urea to give a hydantoin (step 3). Each of these reactions is known to be general and typically high yielding in solution, although one cannot predict how such reactions will

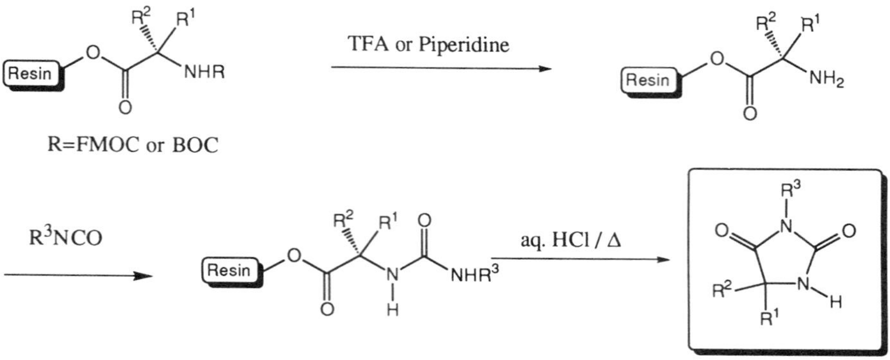

Scheme 2.2   Hydantoin library synthesis.

translate to chemistry on a solid support. Thus, one or two reactions are carried out on a solid-supported starting material before running a set of 40 compounds, to ensure that appropriate conditions can be found. The actual synthesis of hydantoins was carried out as follows. Eight resins containing different protected amino acids were each placed into five PINs, affording a total of 40 reaction vessels. Deprotection as shown in step 1 afforded the corresponding amino-acid-charged resins, now possessing free amine(—NH$_2$) groups. Each resin-bound amino acid was then reacted with five different isocyanates (step 2), to afford a total of 40 different ureas. In the final step, treatment of all PINs with 6M HCl and heat resulted in cyclative cleavage and release of the product hydantoins from the resin, which were dissolved individually in methanol, concentrated, and analyzed. Products and weight yields are shown in Table 2.1; it should be noted that we now determine mole yields instead using ^{1}H-NMR with an internal standard and/or quantitative high-pressure liquid chromatography (HPLC). The reader will note that one reaction (32) yielded no product. One accepts this deletion as the cost of making larger numbers of compounds; if the trend indicates it should be made, it will be synthesized individually. Each of the 39 product hydantoins in this library was then available for biological testing.

Benzodiazepines are well-known β-turn peptide mimetics, and structural variation leads to a wide range of biological activities. Our method for the synthesis of a combinatorial benzodiazepin array—accomplished by Mel Schroeder, Charles Stankovic, and John Kiely (all BioOrganic group members at the time)—is shown in Scheme 2.3 (1). Once again starting with lots of five different amino-acid-charged Merrifield resins, transimination using eight different benzophenone imines produced a set of 40 resin-bound imines. Cyclization of the aromatic amine onto the ester carbonyl group led to cyclative cleavage and release of the 40 benzodiazepine products in weight yields ranging from 9 to 63% (Table 2.2). These products were tested without purification for activity in their ability to displace radiolabeled fluoronitrazepam from bovine cortical membranes. The results, which have been reported previously (3a), demonstrate the same trends in activity that have been

TABLE 2.1 Benzodiazepines Generated in Array

Structure A   Structure B

Number	R^{1a}	R^{2a}	R^3	R^4	Yield[b] (mg)	Yield[b] (%)	IC-50[c] (nM)
1	Me	Ph	H	H	6.1	40	1,700
2	Me	Ph	Cl	H	9.6	56	200
3	Me	4-MeOPh	H	H	5.8	34	69,000
4	Me	Ph	NO2	H	4.9	28	91
5	Me	See structure B		H	9.6	63	29,000
6	Me	Ph	Cl	Me	3.2	18	160
7	Me	Chx	H	H	6.4	41	31,000
8	Me	2-Thn	H	H	7.4	47	5,500
9	H	Ph	H	H	9.4	44	1,100
10	H	Ph	Cl	H	13.7	55	19
11	H	4-MeOPh	H	H	5.5	23	33,000
12	H	Ph	NO2	H	8.0	31	16
13	H	See structure B		H	3.4	16	44,000
14	H	Ph	Cl	Me	5.2	20	21
15	H	Chx	H	H	7.0	32	6,100
16	H	2-Thn	H	H	8.8	41	940
17	Bn	Ph	H	H	8.6	52	19,000
18	Bn	Ph	Cl	H	8.8	46	1,800
19	Bn	4-MeOPh	H	H	7.3	41	>100 μM
20	Bn	Ph	NO2	H	4.9	26	2,400
21	Bn	See structure B		H	8.6	52	>100 μM
22	Bn	Ph	Cl	Me	2.5	13	5,000
23	Bn	Chx	H	H	6.5	39	>100 μM
24	Bn	2-Thn	H	H	8.4	48	47,000
25	3-MeInd	Ph	H	H	9.5	43	69,000
26	3-MeInd	Ph	Cl	H	8.0	33	16,000
27	3-MeInd	4-MeOPh	H	H	7.4	31	>100 μM
28	3-MeInd	Ph	NO2	H	5.8	23	12,000
29	3-MeInd	See structure B		H	5.2	23	>100 μM
30	3-MeInd	Ph	Cl	Me	2.5	10	14,000
31	3-MeInd	Chx	H	H	7.8	34	>100 μM
32	3-MeInd	2-Thn	H	H	9.2	40	71,000
33	iPr	Ph	H	H	7.1	31	>100 μM

TABLE 2.1   *(Continued)*

Number	R^{1a}	R^{2a}	R^3	R^4	Yield[b] (mg)	Yield[b] (%)	IC-50[c] (nM)
34	*i*Pr	Ph	Cl	H	7.0	28	>100 μM
35	*i*Pr	4-MeOPh	H	H	7.1	29	>100 μM
36	*i*Pr	Ph	NO2	H	2.2	9	>100 μM
37	*i*Pr	See structure B		H	6.4	29	>100 μM
38	*i*Pr	Ph	Cl	Me	3.0	11	82,000
39	*i*Pr	Chx	H	H	6.0	27	>100 μM
40	*i*Pr	2-Thn	H	H	8.4	37	>100 μM

[a]Benzyl (Bn), 3-methylindole (3-MeInd), 4-methoxyphenyl (4-MeOPh), cyclohexyl (Chx), 2-thienyl (2-Thn).
[b]Yields based on indicated loading of commercially available functionalized resins (0.50–0.89 meq/g).
[c]Approximate IC-50 values based on three-point fit. Values were also obtained for the commercially available Diazepam (1.46 nM), Nordiazepam (0.2 nM), and Nitrazeam (0.67 nM) corresponding to sample numbers 14, 10, and 12, respectively.

previously identified in this series. This important experiment indicated that the products of Diversomer syntheses could be used directly for property testing in at least one example. Our subsequent work has shown this to be the rule rather than the exception, although we have experienced the exceptions as well in our group.

A third array synthesis, that of benzisothiazolones, was accomplished by Mel Schroeder and is shown in Scheme 2.4 (12). Reaction of the chloromethyl Merrifield resin with 2-carboxythiophenol afforded the corresponding sulfide-linked starting material. BOP activation of the carboxylic acid group in the presence of 40 different amines/hydrazides yielded the corresponding amides. Oxidation of the sulfide linker to the corresponding sulfoxide provided an interesting problem. In solution, this oxidation can be accomplished using a stoichiometric amount of oxidant such that an undesirable overoxidation to the sulfone is avoided. In practice, it is not possible to control the stoichiometry of reagent–starting material in SPOS. In general, the ability to use a large excess of reagent and to remove it easily is considered an advantage of the SPOS method. In this case, it became necessary to find a kinetic solution to the overoxidation problem. Fortunately, sulfide oxidation is typically faster than sulfoxide oxidation. After surveying several potential oxidants, *N*-(phenylsulfonyl)-3-phenyloxaziridine was selected as the reagent of choice. Selective monooxidation was achieved by limiting the reaction time and removal of the reagent excess. Activation of the resulting sulfoxide-bound products with trichloroacetic anhydride led to the expected cyclative ring closure with release of the product benzisothiazolones in up to 60% yield. All yields were determined here by use of the NMR/internal standard method, which indicated that four of the reactions gave less than 1% yield. Several of these four gave, in fact, high crude weight yields, testifying to the desirability for quantitation.

We conducted a fourth multistep synthesis (in collaboration with Alasdair

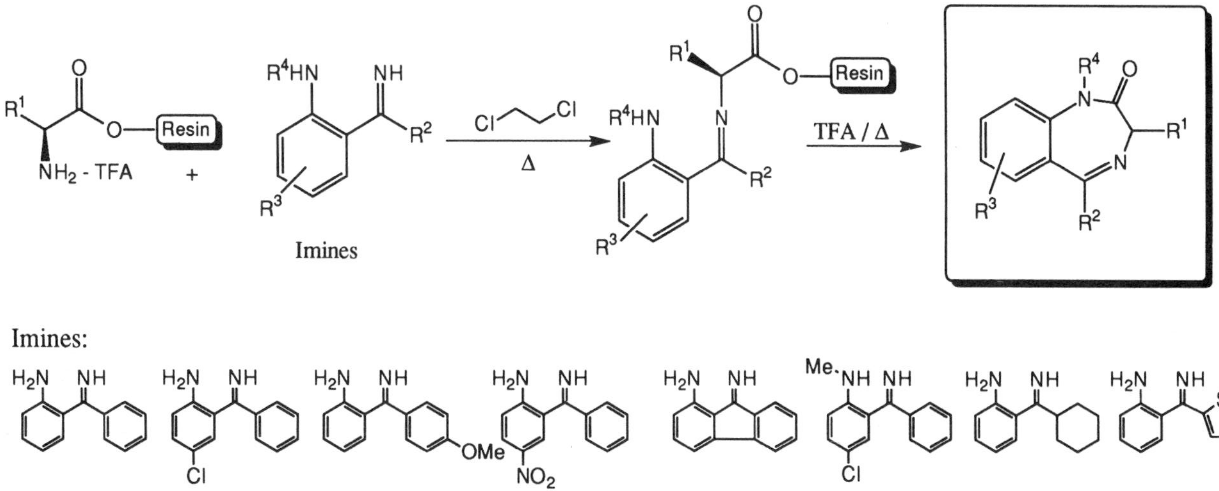

Scheme 2.3 Synthesis of a combinatorial benzodiazepin array.

TABLE 2.2   Hydantoins Generated in Array

Number	R¹	R²	R³	Yield[a] (mg)	Yield[a] (%)
1	H	Methyl	H	4.1	67
2	H	Benzyl	H	2.5	38
3	H	H	H	3.3	65
4	H	s-Butyl	H	3.1	42
5	H	i-Butyl	H	4.9	61
6	H	i-Propyl	H	4.9	58
7	H	2-Methylindole	H	5.0	35
8	Phenyl	Phenyl	H	1.4	5
9	H	Methyl	Butyl	1.6	17
10	H	Benzyl	Butyl	3.9	47
11	H	H	Butyl	1.0	13
12	H	s-Butyl	Butyl	5.3	48
13	H	i-Butyl	Butyl	0.7	7
14	H	i-Propyl	Butyl	0.9	8
15	H	2-Methylindole	Butyl	0.9	5
16	Phenyl	Phenyl	Butyl	1.6	5
17	H	Methyl	Allyl	0.3	4
18	H	Benzyl	Allyl	2.4	29
19	H	H	Allyl	3.7	48
20	H	s-Butyl	Allyl	3.6	36
21	H	i-Butyl	Allyl	5.0	54
22	H	i-Propyl	Allyl	1.6	14
23	H	2-Methylindole	Allyl	1.9	11
24	Phenyl	Phenyl	Allyl	2.1	7
25	H	Methyl	2-Trifluorotolyl	2.6	23
26	H	Benzyl	2-Trifluorotolyl	2.2	23
27	H	H	2-Trifluorotolyl	2.9	28
28	H	s-Butyl	2-Trifluorotolyl	5.7	46
29	H	i-Butyl	2-Trifluorotolyl	4.7	37
30	H	i-Propyl	2-Trifluorotolyl	4.9	33
31	H	2-Methylindole	2-Trifluorotolyl	3.0	15
32	Phenyl	Phenyl	2-Trifluorotolyl	0.0	0
33	H	Methyl	4-Methoxyphenyl	3.1	22
34	H	Benzyl	4-Methoxyphenyl	3.5	32
35	H	H	4-Methoxyphenyl	5.6	46
36	H	s-Butyl	4-Methoxyphenyl	11.5	81

TABLE 2.2 *(Continued)*

Number	R¹	R²	R³	Yield[a] (mg)	Yield[a] (%)
37	H	*i*-Butyl	4-Methoxyphenyl	3.2	21
38	H	*i*-Propyl	4-Methoxyphenyl	4.1	24
39	H	2-Methylindole	4-Methoxyphenyl	4.9	22
40	Phenyl	Phenyl	4-Methoxyphenyl	3.0	7

[a]Yields based on reported loading of commercially available functionalized resins (0.34–1.04 meq/g).

MacDonald and Robert Ramage, University of Edinburgh) of quinolones related to Ciprofloxacin, a broad-spectrum antibacterial agent (13). As shown in Scheme 2.5, transesterification of two ethyl benzoylacetates with Wang resin gave the corresponding resin-bound intermediates. Condensation with DMF acetal followed by displacement with a set of four primary amines afforded eight different resin-bound intermediates varying at R¹ and R² positions. Cyclization under basic conditions followed by displacement with a final set of seven amines afforded the resulting library of resin-bound quinolones. Type 3 cleavage from the resin yielded the free quinolones in yields of 7–90% (gravimetric yields). To the best of our knowledge, the quinolone synthesis described here represents the longest heterocyclic SPOS sequence yet described. The biological activity of these samples is not accurately determined using the unpurified products, and approaches to overcome this problem are currently in progress.

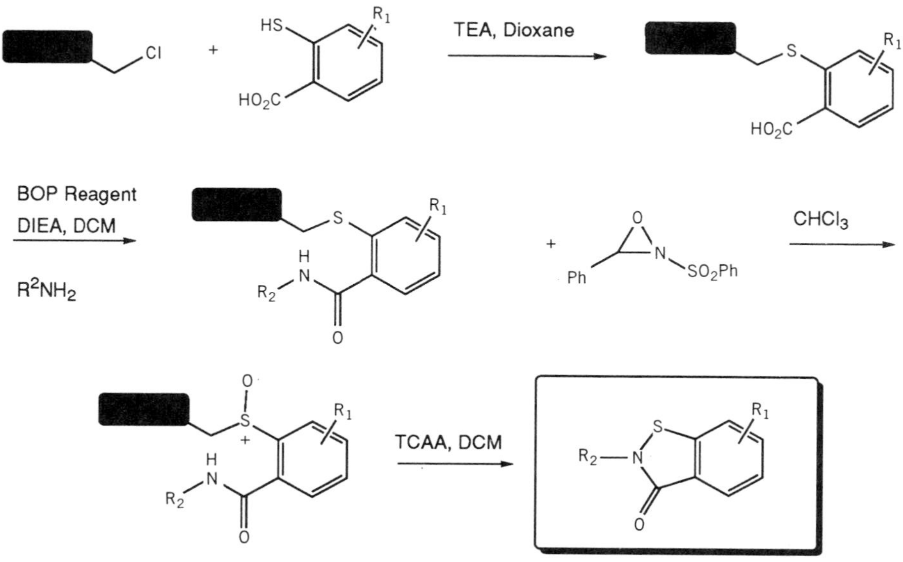

Scheme 2.4 Array synthesis of benzisothiazolones.

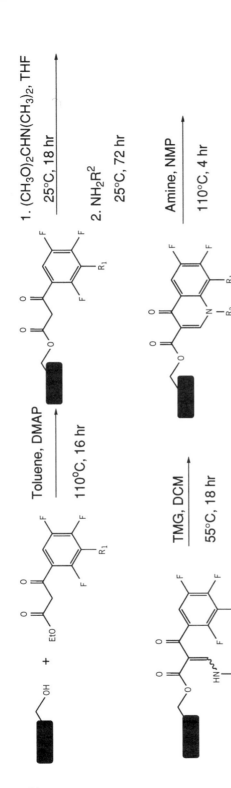

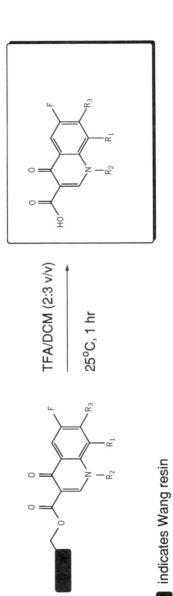

Scheme 2.5 Transesterification of two ethyl benzoylacetates.

2.4 SUMMARY AND CONCLUSIONS

It is apparent that multistep organic chemistry can be accomplished on a solid support in a way that facilitates the combinatorial synthesis of "druglike" molecules. Only 3 years ago, such a suggestion would have seemed preposterous to the practicing medicinal chemist. This is indeed a simple idea whose time has come.

The Diversomer method of combinatorial organic synthesis is not the preferred (or suggested) way of making very large libraries (i.e., thousands to millions) of compounds and was never intended as such. Such very high volume (VHV) synthesis is best accomplished to date using the split-mix method pioneered by Furka et al. (14) for the creation of peptide libraries. The VHV assay methods that must accompany the syntheses in order for them to be useful are being developed now. In the not-too-distant future, one of the productive avenues for drug discovery will be the identification of active structures based upon assay of bead-based libraries containing millions of components. When those "hits" are discovered, the practicing medicinal chemist will not have access to an archived library from which structural analogs can be requested. Even the initial SAR determination will require synthesis. Since the chemistry required to generate the library will have been developed previously for SPOS, the syntheses of focused libraries based on that chemistry should be straightforward. It is in this scenario, enablement of the chemist, that the Diversomer method will likely prove most useful.

REFERENCES

1. Geysen, H. M., Meloen, R. H., and Barteling, S. J., *Proc. Natl. Acad. Sci. USA* **82,** 5131 (1984).
2. Bunin, B. A., and Ellman, J. A., *J. Am. Chem. Soc.* **114,** 10997 (1992).
3. (a) DeWitt, S. H., Kiely, J. S., Stankovic, C. J., Schroeder, M. C., Cody, D. M. R., and Pavia, M. R., *Proc. Natl. Acad. Sci. USA* **90,** 6909 (1993); (b) DeWitt, S. H., Schroeder, M. C., Stankovic, C. J., Strode, J. E., and Czarnik, A. W., *Drug Devel. Res.* **33,** 116 (1994); (c) DeWitt, S. H., Kiely, J. K., Pavia, M. R., Stankovic, C. J., and Schroeder, M. C., US Patent 5,324,483 (1994).
4. Houghten, R. A., *Proc. Natl. Acad. Sci. USA* **82,** 5131 (1985).
5. available from ChemGlass, Inc., Vineland, NJ.
6. DeWitt, S. H., and Czarnik, A. W., *Curr. Opinion Biotechnol.* **6,** 640 (1995).
7. Crowley, J. I., and Rapoport, H., *Acc. Chem. Res.* **9,** 135 (1976).
8. (a) Leznoff, C. C., *Chem. Soc. Rev.* **3,** 65 (1974); (b) Leznoff, C. C., *Acc. Chem. Soc.* **11,** 327 (1978).
9. Merrifield, R. B., *J. Am. Chem. Soc.* **85,** 2149 (1963).
10. (a) MacDonald, A., Halim, N., Hobbs DeWitt, S., Hogan, E., Kieras, L., Ghosh, S., and Ramage, R., "Parallel Purification and Resin By-Products in Solid Phase Synthesis," paper presented at The Fourth International Symposium on Solid Phase Synthesis, Edinburgh, Scotland, September 12, 1995; (b) Halim, N., Hobbs DeWitt, S., Hogan, E., Kieras, L., Ghosh, S., MacDonald, A., and Ramage, R., "Parallel Purification and

Resin By-Products in Solid Phase Synthesis," Abs. ORGN 267, 209th American Chemical Society, National Meeting, Chicago, IL, August 23, 1995.

11. (a) Epton, R., Goddard, P., and Ivin, K. J., *Polymer* **21,** 1367 (1980); (b) Look, G. C., Holmes, C. P., Chinn, J. P., and Gallop, M. A., *J. Org. Chem.* **59,** 7588 (1994).

12. Schroeder, M. C., Kraker, A. J., Moore, C. W., Kiely, J. S., Hobbs DeWitt, S., and Czarnik, A. W., "DIVERSOMER™ Technology: The Synthesis of Benzisothiazolones as Epidermal Growth Factor Receptor Tyrosine Kinase Inhibitors," Abs. MEDI 239, 208th American Chemical Society National Meeting, Washington, DC, August 24, 1994.

13. MacDonald, A., Hobbs DeWitt, S., Hogan, E., and Ramage, R., "Synthesis of Quinolone Antibiotics by DIVERSOMER™ Technology. Innovation and Perspectives in Solid Phase Synthesis," R. Epton (Ed.), SPCC Ltd, Birmingham, AL, 1995, in press.

14. Furka, A., Sebestyen, F., Asgedom, M., and Dibo, G., *Int. J. Pept. Protein Res.* **37,** 487 (1991).

3

POLYMER-SUPPORTED SYNTHESIS OF ORGANIC COMPOUNDS AND LIBRARIES

MARK J. KURTH

Department of Chemistry, University of California, Davis, Davis, California 95616

Drug discovery demands for libraries of molecularly diverse compounds (1) have led to the development of numerous intriguing polymer-supported strategies for the synthesis of peptide (2) (combinatorial) and, to a lesser extent, small organic molecule (3) (analogous) collections. The synthetic advantages of polymer-supported chemistry include streamlined reaction manipulation and workup, increased ease of product isolation, and modified reaction selectivity. Unlike combinatorial peptide synthesis where polymer-supported reaction types are quite limited, extension of Merrifield's pioneering polypeptide work (4) to organic synthesis problems (5,6) has the potential to deliver analog libraries [analogous organic synthesis (3c)], which arise from and encompass an impressive array of reagent and chemical reaction diversity. In that context, interest in analogous synthesis commissions further development of polymer-based C—C bond-forming reactions, enantio- and diastereoselective methodologies, and small organic molecule library preparation. In this chapter, we survey our recent findings in these areas.

3.1 POLYMER-SUPPORTED SYNTHESIS OF 2,5-DISUBSTITUTED TETRAHYDROFURANS (THF)

Our first solid-phase synthesis efforts focused on implementing a multistep synthetic strategy to improve upon an α,ω-diene $\rightarrow$ cyclic ether solution-phase protocol previously reported from our laboratories (7). This process involved a five-step synthesis of 2,5-disubstituted tetrahydrofurans (cf. **1.2** in Fig. 3.1) via a tandem

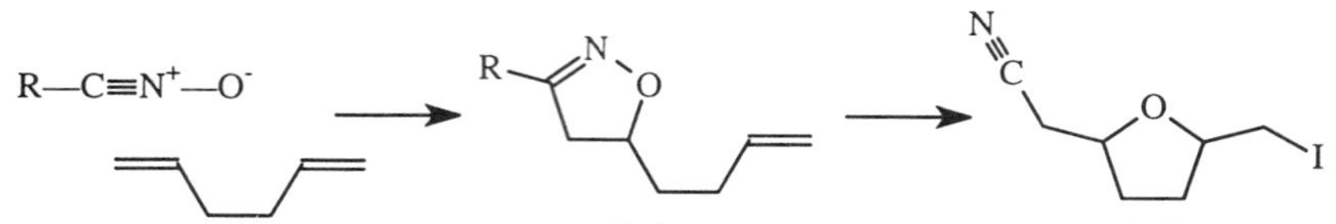

Figure 3.1   Cyclic ethers via a tandem 1,3-dipolar cycloaddition/electrophilic cyclization sequence.

1,3-dipolar cycloaddition/electrophilic cyclization sequence. This tandem process, outlined in Figure 3.1, suffers one major drawback when carried out under normal homogeneous conditions (8) in that it utilizes an α,ω-diene substrate in the 1,3-dipolar cycloaddition step and thus requires selective monoaddition of the nitrile oxide to this dipolarophile. However, in solution a second nitrile oxide is free to react with the remaining terminal alkene, leading to undesired bis-1,3-dipolar cycloaddition, which can be suppressed by using the diene in 10-fold excess.

To solve this problem, we considered potentially beneficial the partial isolation that might be achieved by covalent attachment of the nitrile oxide moiety to an insoluble polymer matrix. The terminal alkene remaining after isoxazole formation (i.e., C=C in **1.1**) would be less accessible to another polymer-bound nitrile oxide, which would then have a higher probability of reacting with remaining diene. The latter could then be used in smaller excess. An additional benefit of the polymer-supported method is that the iodocyclization reaction was envisioned to liberate exclusively the target cyclic ether.

The approach outlined in Figure 3.2 appeared especially attractive since the final

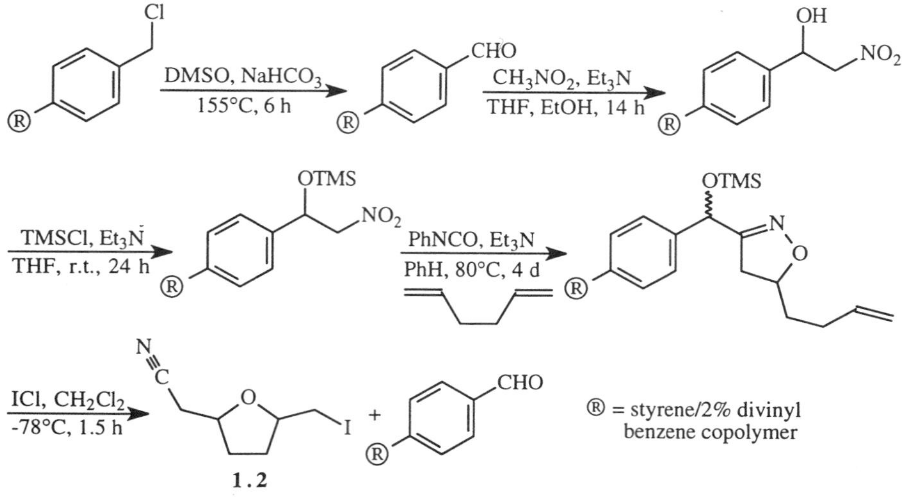

Figure 3.2   Benzaldehyde-based tandem 1,3-dipolar cycloaddition/electrophilic cyclization sequence.

cyclization step would regenerate the initial polymer-bound aldehyde for potential recycling. This chemistry was first investigated using conventional solution-phase methods (i.e., $\circledR$ = H) and employing a 10-fold excess of α,ω-diene in the critical cycloaddition step. 2-(Cyanomethyl)-5-(iodomethyl)tetrahydrofuran (**1.2**) was obtained as a 1:1.92 mixture of diastereomers in an 18% overall yield from benzaldehyde.

For our solid-phase studies, commercially available 2% crosslinked Merrifield polymer was oxidized to the corresponding aldehyde (9) and condensed with nitromethane to form polymer-bound 2-nitro-1-phenylethan-1-ol. In order to avoid dehydration to the corresponding β-nitrostyrene in the $-CH_2NO_2 \rightarrow -C\equiv N^+-O^-$ step, the hydroxyl moiety was protected as its trimethylsilyl ether. Subsequent phenylisocyanate-mediated dehydration of the nitroalkane moiety presumably generated the polymer-bound nitrile oxide, which then underwent 1,3-dipolar cycloaddition with 1,5-hexadiene (two- to threefold excess) to give the polymer-bound isoxazole. Polymer characterization at each step (oxidation, nitroaldol condensation, alcohol protection, and dehydrative 1,3-dipolar cycloaddition) in this sequence was accomplished by comparing the infrared (IR) spectrum of the functionalized polymer with that of the solution-phase analog.

Electrophilic cyclization of the isoxazole with iodine monochloride at $-78°C$ gave **1.2** and regenerated the polymer-bound aldehyde. Using three equivalents of 1,5-hexadiene, the overall yield was 0.26 mmol of **1.2** per gram of polymer. The overall yield using two equivalents of 1,5-hexadiene was 0.19 mmol of **1.2** per gram of polymer. When the polymer-bound aldehyde was recycled through this reaction scheme, **1.2** was obtained to the extent of 0.07–0.11 mmol per gram of polymer. In parallel with the solution phase chemistry, the cis–trans ratio for "polymer-prepared" **1.2** was 1:2.1.

Oxidation of the polymeric aldehyde to the corresponding carboxylic acid (MCPBA) followed by neutralization with cesium hydroxide and gravimetric analysis showed the degree of functionalization to be 0.65 ± 0.04 meq of aldehyde per gram of polymer. On this basis, the overall yield of the 2-(cyanomethyl)-5-(iodomethyl)tetrahydrofuran from polymer-bound aldehyde is calculated to be 40% using three equivalents of 1,5-hexadiene and 29% using two equivalents of 1,5-hexadiene. These yields were considerably higher than those of the solution-phase synthesis (18%). When recovered polymer-bound aldehyde was recycled through the sequence, the overall yield of **1.2** was 11–17%.

We have extended this 1,3-dipolar cycloaddition/electrophilic cyclization sequence to an *intramolecular* variant that yields cyclic ethers with four stereogenic centers (10). The intramolecular 1,3-dipolar cycloaddition of a nitrile oxide to a substituted double bond affords a novel heterocycle with excellent stereoselectivity. For example, Hassner and Murthy (11) have found that nitrile oxide **3.1** (Fig. 3.3) ($-R_1 = -CH_3$ or $-Ph$; $-R_2 = -H$) delivers heterocycle **3.2** (C_6-H trans to C_{3a}-H) selectively. These results have been rationalized by examining the stereochemistry of the resulting tetrahydrofuroisoxazoline (11) and by using product-based MM2 calculations (12). In related studies, we have found that moving the alkyl substituent from C_6 to C_4 (i.e., $-R_1 = -H$; $-R_2 = -CH_3$ or $-Ph$) results

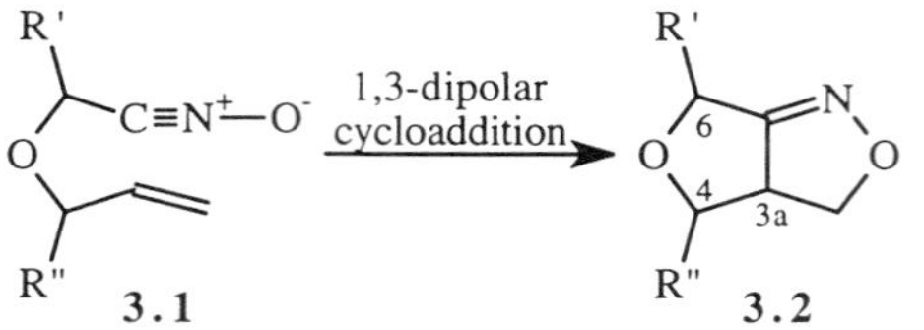

Figure 3.3   Stereocontrol elements in the intramolecular 1,3-dipolar cycloaddition reaction.

in complete diastereofacial selectivity; in each case, only the trans isomer (C_4-H trans to C_{3a}-H) was detected (13). Apparently a C_4 stereogenic center exerts greater control than a C_6 stereogenic center in these intramolecular 1,3-dipolar cycloadditions.

When the C=C of **3.1** is 1,2-disubstituted, the resulting heterocycle has an additional stereogenic center at C_3 which should be subject to control by manipulating the geometry of the now internal double bond. Using this strategy to incorporate a 3-butenyl group at C_3 (cf. **4.1** of Fig. 3.4) would set the stage for an electrophilic cyclization reaction to deliver cyclic ether **4.2** by concomitant unraveling of the tetrahydrofuroisoxazoline moiety.

This final transformation immolates the C_6 stereogenic center, exposes latent hydroxyl and cyano functional groups, and sets an additional stereogenic center in the cyclic ether. To be congruous with our solution phase studies, the polymer-supported studies reported here utilized an electron-donating group at C_6 (Ar = polymer-bound 4-benzyloxyphenyl) in order to help stabilize the positive charge that develops at this position in the electrophilic cyclization step.

Attachment of an electron-rich aryl group to the polymer support was accomplished by linking an anisaldehyde-like unit to Merrifield's resin. Thus, the phenoxide (4-hydroxybenzaldehyde + NaOH in DMSO) was added to chloromethylated polystyrene to provide polymer-supported (benzyloxy)benzaldehyde **5.1** (Fig. 3.5). Resin **5.1** exhibits a strong carbonyl IR absorbance at 1698 cm^{-1} and an aldehyde C—H stretch at 2725 cm^{-1}.

Two methods for the conversion of **5.1** to polymer-supported β-nitrostyrene **6.2** (Fig. 3.6) were investigated. The first method, a two-step process, was effected by nitroaldol condensation (CH$_3$NO$_2$, Et$_3$N) in a THF–ethanol mixed solvent to give polymer-supported nitroalcohol **6.1** (nitro IR absorbances at 1555 and 1375 cm^{-1}),

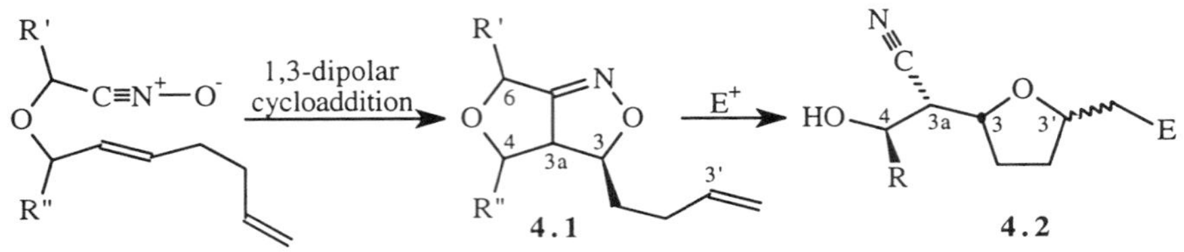

Figure 3.4   Intramolecular 1,3-dipolar cycloadditions: stereoselectivity with 1,2-disubstituted olefins.

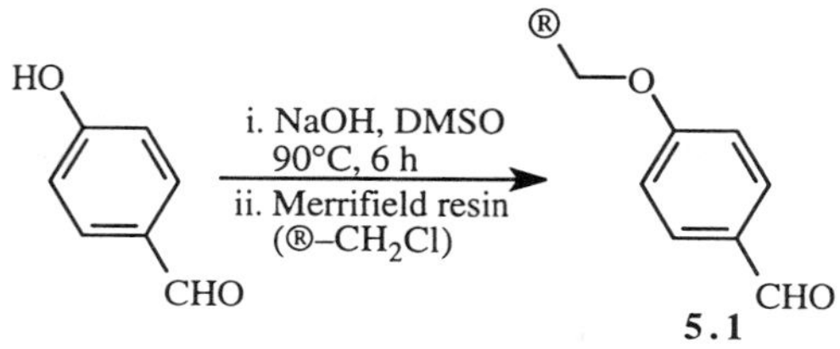

HO
i. NaOH, DMSO
90°C, 6 h
ii. Merrifield resin
(®–CH₂Cl)

CHO

®
O

CHO
5.1

Figure 3.5 Preparation of polymer-supported (benzyloxy)benzaldehyde.

which was then dehydrated to β-nitrostyrene **6.2** by sequential addition of methanesulfonyl chloride and triethylamine (14) (IR absorbances at 1340 and 1629 cm^{-1}). This two-step method is somewhat deficient in that a small carbonyl peak remains in the IR spectrum after the nitroaldol condensation, indicating that either the nitroaldol reaction does not go to completion or that dehydration is accompanied by some retro-aldol.

The second method employed nitromethane and glacial acetic acid with catalytic ammonium acetate (15) to effect nitroaldol and dehydration as a one-step process. While this solvent mixture does not appear to swell the polymer support, this one-step conversion delivered resin **6.2** that was spectroscopically identical to the product of the two-step method but with no remaining carbonyl present in the IR spectrum. This proved to be the preferred route to **6.2**.

Subsequent Michael addition of dienol alkoxides to **6.2** gave the polymer-supported nitroethers **7.1, 7.2,** and **7.3** (16). The progress of each addition reaction was monitored by Fourier transform–infrared (FT-IR). These Michael addition reactions must be quenched with acetic acid. When quenched with aqueous hydrochloric acid, the unconjugated nitro absorbances are weaker in intensity in the IR spectrum. This may reflect the fact that acetic acid is better able to permeate the polymer support than aqueous hydrochloric acid; if the nitronate anion is not properly quenched, it can undergo retro-Michael reaction to regenerate the nitrostyrene moiety.

Nitroethers **7.1–3** (Fig. 3.7) were then subjected to phenylisocyanate-mediated

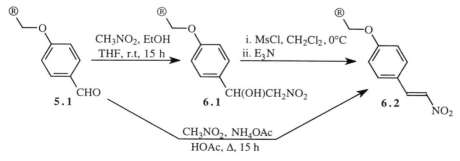

Figure 3.6 Preparation of polymer-supported β-nitrostyrene.

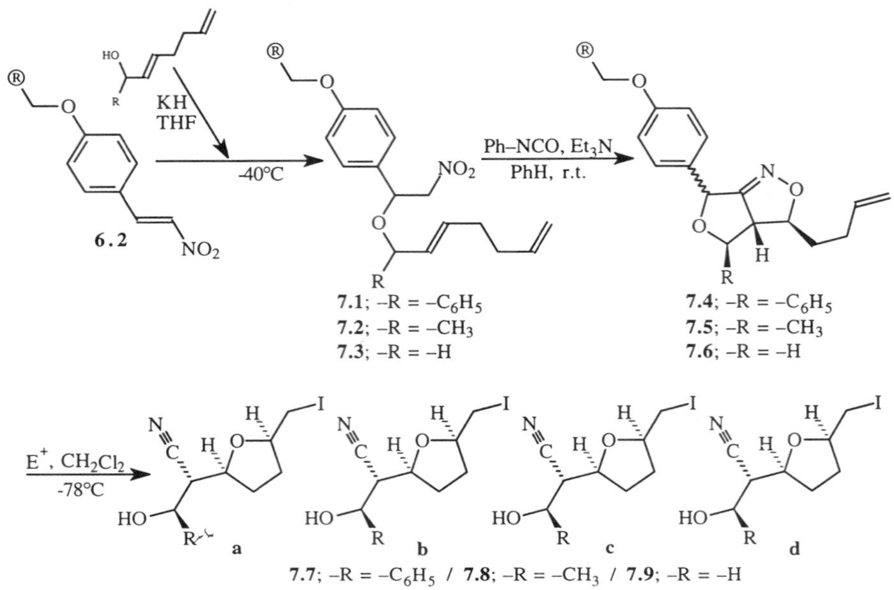

7.1; –R = –C$_6$H$_5$
7.2; –R = –CH$_3$
7.3; –R = –H

7.4; –R = –C$_6$H$_5$
7.5; –R = –CH$_3$
7.6; –R = –H

7.7; –R = –C$_6$H$_5$ / 7.8; –R = –CH$_3$ / 7.9; –R = –H

-R	cpd.	electrophile	yield (mmol/g P-S)	% yield[a]	a:b:c:d
-C$_6$H$_5$	7.7	ICl	0.069	46	[b]69:31:-:-
-C$_6$H$_5$	7.7	ICl	0.066	44	[b]69:31:-:-
-C$_6$H$_5$	7.7	IBr	0.071	47	[b]80:21:-:-
-C$_6$H$_5$	7.7	[d]IBr	0.065	43	[b]72:28:-:-
-C$_6$H$_5$	7.7	NIS	0.042	28	[b]72:28:-:-
-C$_6$H$_5$	7.7	[e]IBr	0.037	25	[b]82:18:-:-
-C$_6$H$_5$	7.7	[f]IBr	0.074	49	[b]80:20:-:-
-CH$_3$	7.8	ICl	0.052	35	[c]48:38:10:4
-CH$_3$	7.8	IBr	0.041	27	[c]62:18:11:9
-H	7.9	IBr	0.031	21	[b]80:20:-:-

[a]Calculated overall yield from **6.2** based on 0.15 meq. β-nitrostyrene/g of polymer.
[b]Ratio determined by ^{1}H NMR integration of H-1'. [c]Ratio determined by capillary GLC
of the crude reaction mixture. [d]Reaction solvent toluene. [e]Used 0.5 mmol dienol/g
polymer support. [f]Used 5 mmol dienol/g polymer support.

Figure 3.7 Polymer-supported synthesis of **7.7**, **7.8**, and **7.9**.

dehydration (17) to the polymer-supported nitrile oxide intermediates, which undergo concomitant intramolecular 1,3-dipolar cycloaddition to give the polymer-
supported tetrahydrofuroisoxazolines **7.4–6**. These reactions were monitored by a
decrease in the intensity of the unconjugated nitro absorbances in the IR spectrum
and, after 2 days, no further peak reduction was observed, and the reactions were

worked up. Electrophilic cyclization of the resulting heterocycles yielded solely the desired cyclic ethers. The overall yields from polymer-supported nitrostyrene **6.2** as well as the stereoselectivities of the electrophilic cyclization are given in Figure 3.7 and, as noted, the electrophile was varied to determine if the yield and cis–trans ratio (i.e., 2,5-relative stereochemistry) could be improved.

The best yield of tetrahydrofuran derivative **7.7** (47%) was obtained using iodine monobromide (18) in dichloromethane that gave a cis–trans ratio of 4:1. This yield is nearly identical to the 46% overall yield of **7.7** obtained in solution-phase studies. In these reactions, 2 mmol of dienol were used per gram of polymer-supported nitrostyrene in the Michael addition. When the number of equivalents was increased to 5 mmol of dienol per gram polymer support, the yield of **7.7** increased to 49%. When the number of equivalents was decreased to 0.5 mmol dienol per gram polymer support, the yield of **7.7** decreased to 25%. Iodine monobromide gave better cis–trans ratios throughout the R = —Ph, —CH$_3$, —H series, and there was essentially no difference in cis–trans ratios for iodine monochloride versus N-iodo-succinimide. When toluene was used instead of dichloromethane, the cis–trans product ratio decreased.

The electrophilic cyclization of **7.5** yielded cyclic ethers **7.8a–d** in a 35% overall yield, which may be compared to the 34% overall yield of **7.8** obtained in solution-phase studies. This cyclic ether ratio gives the diastereofacial selectivity of the nitrile oxide in the 1,3-dipolar cycloaddition; it can be seen that the selectivity is about 5:1 α:β, a ratio comparable to the 4.6:1 α:β selectivity observed in solution phase. Cis–trans product ratios in the cyclizations of these compounds are also interesting as the C$_4$-α tetrahydrofuroisoxazoline gives cis–trans ratios of 1.3:1 for ICl and 3.4:1 for IBr. On the other hand, the C$_4$-β tetrahydrofuroisoxazoline gives cis–trans ratios of 2.5:1 for ICl and 1.2:1 for IBr. These are comparable to the stereoselectivities seen in solution-phase studies. These data indicate that the relative stereochemistry at C$_4$ partially directs the cis—trans selectivity in the electrophilic cyclization. The envelope of the furan ring in the heterocycle presumably shifts to minimize a C$_4$–C$_3$ pseudodiaxial interaction, thus moderating the energies of the corresponding transition states. The relative energies of *endo* versus *exo* electrophilic attack are probably closer, resulting in a lower cis–trans ratio of the cyclic ethers. The overall yield for the polymer-supported synthesis of cyclic ether **7.9** was 21%, as compared to the solution-phase synthesis, which gave **7.9** in an overall yield of 29%.

A variety of electrophiles were investigated for the cyclization of **7.4** to determine if the electrophile exerted any effect on the cis–trans ratio of the cyclic ethers. These included PdCl$_2$, phenyl sulfuryl chloride, phenyl selenyl bromide, phenyl selenyl chloride, Nicholas' cation, and mercuric chloride. Unfortunately, none of these electrophiles affected the cyclization. The crude material obtained from these reactions, although not fully characterized, showed no nitrile absorbances in their IR spectra, indicating that no cyclization had taken place.

The separation and isolation benefits associated with polymer-supported synthesis are demonstrated by the collated ^{1}H nuclear magnetic resonance (NMR) presented in Figure 3.8. The bottom ^{1}H-NMR spectrum is the crude product obtained

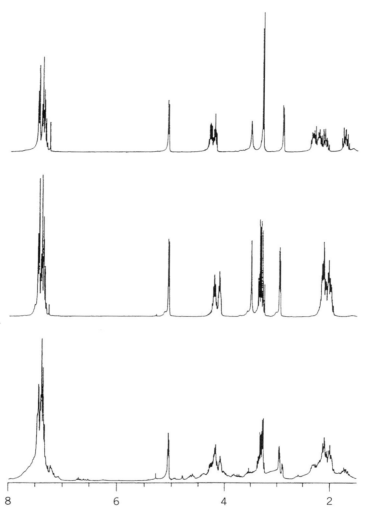

Figure 3.8 ¹H NMR spectra of crude **7.7** (bottom), pure **7.7a** (middle), and pure **7.7b** (top).

by simple filtration from the resin and subsequent solvent evaporation. The top two spectra are the chromatographically separated cis (**7.7a**; middle) and trans (**7.7b**; top) diastereomers. Examination of these spectra demonstrates that each peak in the crude ¹H-NMR spectrum (the result of five solid-phase synthetic steps) can be accounted for in the spectra of the two purified stereoisomers.

Cyclic ethers were also formed from Merrifield's peptide resin without an electron-donating aryl group (i.e., starting with polymer-supported nitroolefin **9.1**; Fig. 3.9). The yields and stereoselectivities for these reactions are presented in Figure 3.9 and are very similar to those obtained starting with polymer-supported aldehyde **5.1**

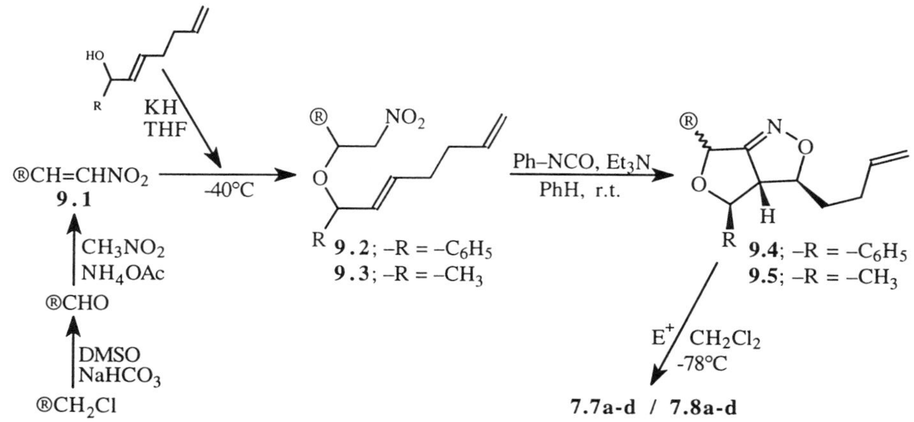

-R	cpd.	electrophile	yield (mmol/g P-S)	% yield[a]	a:b:c:d
-Ph	7.7	IBr	0.074	49	[b]81:19:-:-
-CH₃	7.8	ICl	0.070	47	[c]54:32:8:6
-CH₃	7.8	IBr	0.038	25	[c]65:15:11:9

[a]Calculated overall yield from **9.1** based on 0.15 meq. β-nitrostyrene/g of polymer. [b]Ratio determined by ¹H NMR integration of H-1'. [c]Ratio determined by capillary GLC of the crude reaction mixture.

Figure 3.9 Yield and stereoselectivity of cyclic ethers starting from **9.1** (®CH=CHNO₂)

(Fig. 3.5). The electron-donating aryl group in **5.1** increases the yield of the electrophilic cyclization reaction, but the tetrahydrofuroisoxazoline intermediate appears to be less stable. These effects appear to offset one another resulting in comparable overall yields from **5.1** and **9.1**.

To determine the overall yield of cyclic ether formation for comparison with the conventional solution-phase sequence, the degree of functionalization of the polymer-supported β-nitrostyrene (**6.2**; Fig. 3.10) was quantified. This was accomplished by reducing the β-nitrostyrene with lithium aluminum hydride in refluxing ether to give polymer-supported primary amine **10.1** (19). A quantitative ninhydrin

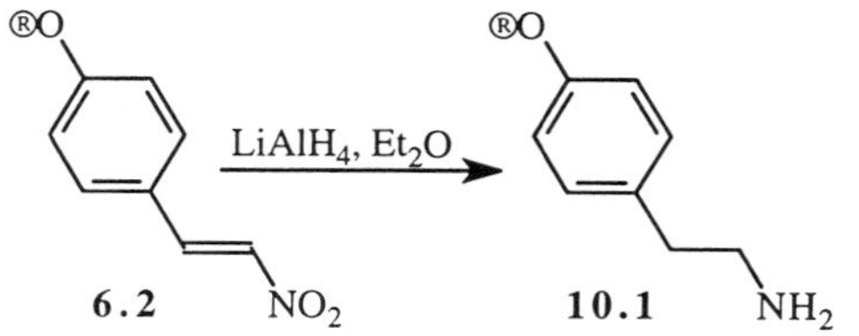

Figure 3.10 —NO₂ → —NH₂ Interconversion: a quantitative ninhydrin test.

test for amines gave a value of 0.15 meq/g polymer support as the degree of functionalization of the polymer supported primary amine (20).

Cis and trans stereochemical assignments for the 2,5-disubstituted cyclic ethers proved to be nontrivial. Although separable by high-pressure liquid chromatography (HPLC), NOE studies on all of the diastereomers in a variety of solvents proved unrevealing. This situation may be due to the terminal hydroxyl hydrogen bonding with the cyclic ether oxygen, resulting in a six-membered ring. In the resulting conformation, the ring protons at C2 and C5 are quite distant from one another in both the cis and trans diastereomers.

The solution to this dilemma involved a combination of x-ray crystallographic and ^{1}H-NMR chemical shift data. Although phenyl-substituted tetrahydrofurans **7.7a** and **7.7b** were crystalline, the crystals proved to be unsuitable for x-ray crystallography. Therefore, the iodomethyl group of each diastereomer (**7.7a** and **7.7b**) was reduced by tributyltin hydride, yielding **11.1** and **11.2**, respectively (Fig. 3.11) (21). These reduced compounds were also crystalline, and an unambiguous stereochemical assignment for **11.2** was made by single crystal X-ray diffraction analysis. The crystal structure (Fig. 3.12) shows that the *minor* diastereomer has a 2,5-trans configuration.

Since the only unambiguous stereochemical assignment available was from tetrahydrofuran **11.2**, a spectroscopic correlation was necessary to assign the correct stereochemistry for the other diastereomeric cyclic ethers. This was possible by comparing of the ring —CH$_2$CH$_2$—^{1}H-NMR signals of the various compounds. These signals appear as two multiplets, each with an integration of 2H, for all major diastereomers. In contrast, all minor diastereomers show three or four different multiplet signals for these same ring methylene protons. Another important benchmark is the signal multiplicity for the iodomethyl group. In minor diastereomers, this methylene appears as an apparent doublet, while in major diastereomers each methylene proton appears as a doublet of doublets. Chromatographic similarities are also evident, with each minor diastereomers elutings before the corresponding major diastereomer in HPLC (SiO$_2$) separations.

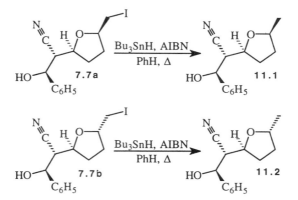

Figure 3.11 Cyclic ether de-iodination with tributyltin hydride.

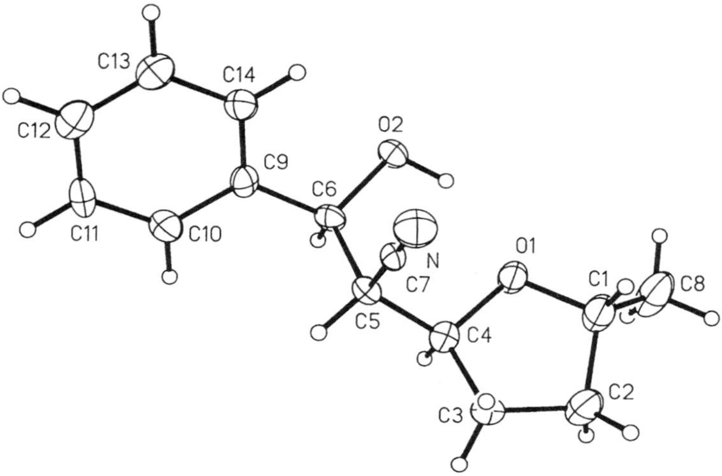

Figure 3.12　X-ray crystal structure of **11.2.**

3.2　POLYMER-SUPPORTED ENANTIOSELECTIVE SYNTHESIS

Our efforts to develop an effective *sequent auxliary* (i.e., a chiral auxiliary that is used to mediate two sequential diastereoselective steps) for amide alkylation (6e,22,23) and subsequent heterocyclization (24,25) reactions led to C_2-symmetric auxiliary **13.1** (Fig. 3.13) for solution-phase reactions. As illustrated in Figure 3.13, this mediates diastereoselective C—C bond formation in step 1 and diastereoselective heterocyclization in step 2. The resulting iodolactone (**13.2**) is obtained optically pure in excellent overall yield (6e,23,26).

These solution-phase studies, coupled with the documented advantages of polymer-bound auxiliaries (27), led us to consider resin-bound auxiliary **13.3** as a promising candidate for a three-step enantioselective process consisting of N-acylation, Cα-alkylation, and subsequent iodolactonization to deliver optically pure 3,5-disubstituted-γ-butyrolactone **13.2**. The pyrrolidine-based auxiliary required to launch this study, trans-(2R,5R)-(N-propionyl)-2,5-bis(hydroxymethyl)pyrrolidine (**14.1**) (Fig. 3.14), is readily available from 1,2:5,6-di-O-isopropylidene-D-mannitol by adaptation of chemistry developed by Marzi and Misiti (28). Taking advantage of the kinetic site isolation afforded by polymer attachment (29), a THF solution of the potassium alkoxide of pyrrolidine **14.1** was coupled to DMF swollen Merrifield's resin containing catalytic 18-crown-6. Incubation of this mixture at 90°C for 5 days followed by filtration and thorough washing of the resulting resin delivered **14.2** as evidenced by the appearance of FT-IR (KBr) bands for the resulting hydroxyl and amide moieties (1647 and 3440 cm^{-1}, respectively).

We next attempted Cα-alkylation of polymer-bound amide **14.2**. Unfortunately, FT-IR analysis indicated that the desired Cα-alkylation process was complicated by competing alkoxide alkylation, so **14.2** was first converted to "C_2-symmetric" pyr-

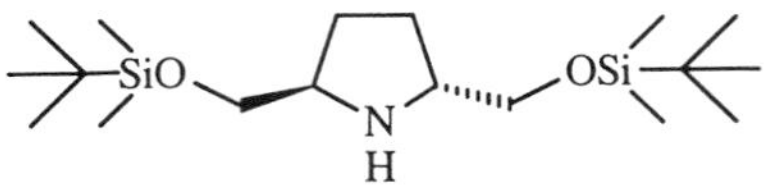

Figure 3.13 Sequent auxiliary for enantioselective preparation of iodolactones.

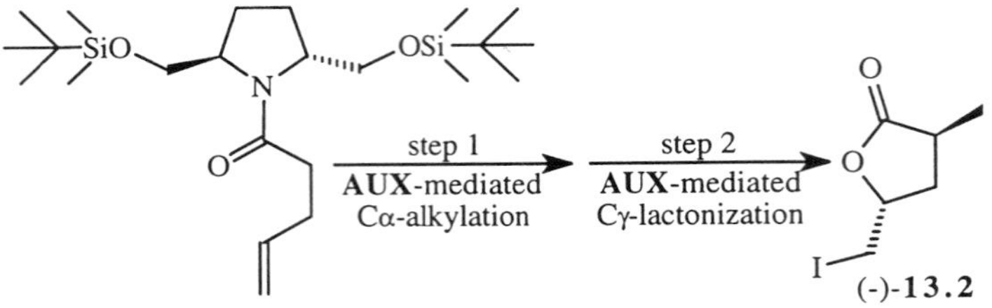

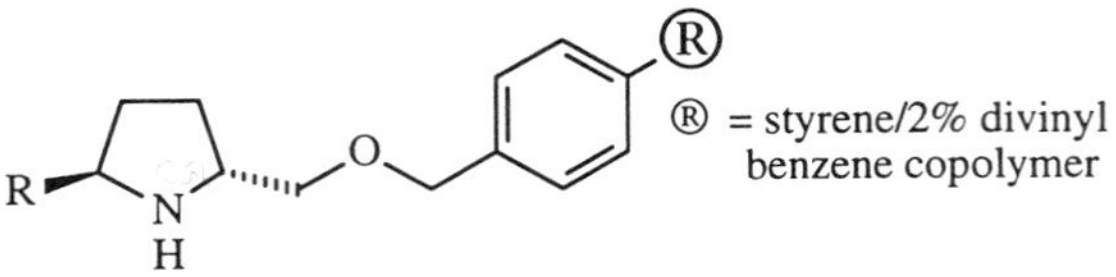

rolidine **14.3** (1-methyl-2-pyrrolidone swollen resin treated with sodium hydride and benzyl bromide; 100°C, 2 d; disappearance of the 3440 cm^{-1} FT-IR band).

Treating THF swollen resin **14.3** with lithium diisopropylamide (2 eq, 0°C, 30 min) presumably gives the highly favored Z-enolate, which upon treatment with allyl iodide (3 eq; 0°C → r.t., 24 h), produced Cα-alkylated resin **14.4**. While the stereoselectivity of this transformation could not be established while the substrate was still polymer bound, final iodolactone ratios (vide infra) established this Cα-alkylation selectivity to be 93.5:6.5.

Iodolactonization of **14.4** was effected by treating a THF/H$_2$O (1.5:1) suspension of this resin with iodine for 3 days at room temperature. Filtration and ether washing of the resin delivered only γ-butyrolactones (−)/**13.2** and (+)−13.2 (93.5:6.5 ratio; 34% overall yield from **14.1**); no trace of the corresponding cis-3,5-disubstituted lactones were detected by capillary gas chromatography (GC) analysis of the crude reaction mixture. These lactone product ratios establish the polymer-supported selectivity of both the alkylation (>14:1) and electrophilic cyclization (>99:1) steps. When contrasted with the L-prolinol derived auxiliary **13.4**, C$_2$-symmetric pyrrolidine **13.3** is a great deal more selective in both the Cα-alkylation step (2:1 selectivity with **13.4**) and, surprisingly, the iodolactonization step (92:8 selectivity with **13.4**) (6e).

Transformation **14.4** → **13.2** also liberates chiral resin **13.3** as evidenced by disappearance of the FT-IR amide band at 1647 cm^{-1}. The resin-bound chiral auxiliary is trivial to isolate by simple filtration of the crude reaction mixture, and we were pleased to find that reuse of resin **13.3** is eminently practical. Thus,

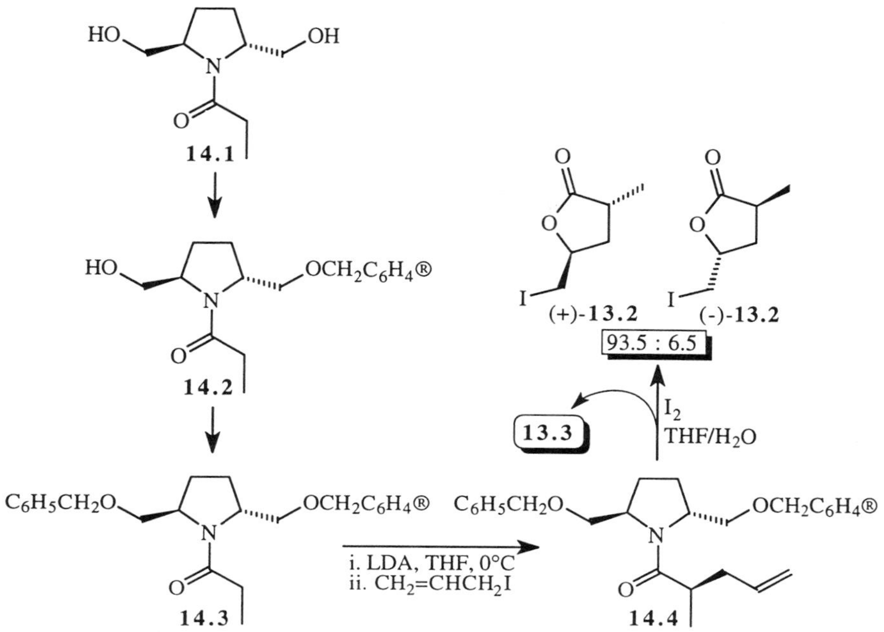

Figure 3.14 Polymer-bound Sequent Chiral Auxiliaries.

swelling recovered **13.3** [washed sequentially with DMF, H_2O, CH_3OH, dioxane, acetone, THF, and Et_2O; dried overnight under vacuum (0.8 torr)] in THF and treating the resulting resin with 4-pentenoyl chloride and triethylamine (2 eq each; r.t., 2 d) delivers the 4-pentenoylamide ($C=O$ FT-IR absorbance at 1639 cm^{-1}). Subsequent enolate formation (2 eq LDA, THF, 0°C) followed by Cα-alkylation with methyl iodide (3 eq) gives the Cα-alkylated resin. Although we anticipated that the product of this alkylation would be the Cα stereoisomer of resin **14.4**, we were indeed gratified to find that iodolactonization (I_2, THF:H_2O :: 1.5:1, r.t., 3d) delivered γ-butyrolactone $(-)/$**13.2** as the major product [90.3:9.7::$(-)/$**13.2**:$(+)/$ **13.2**]. The reduced enantioselectivity (from 87% ee to 81% ee) most probably reflects the reduced steric requirements of methyl versus allyl iodide in the alkylation step (30). Again, the cis-lactones were not detected in the crude reaction mixture. It is also interesting to note that the nor-methyl lactone, which would arise by electrophilic cyclization of the unalkylated 4-pentenoylamide, was not detected in the crude iodolactonization reaction mixture. Apparently, polymersupported Cα-alkylation is an efficient process. Finally, resin **13.3** can again be recovered by filtration and washing [washed sequentially with DMF, H_2O, CH_3OH, dioxane, acetone, THF, and Et_2O; dried overnight under vacuum (0.8 torr)]. If care has been taken to avoid mechanical damage to the resin, this chiral auxiliary can be repeatedly reused with no loss of chemical yield or stereoselectivity.

In summary, we find that polymer-supported C_2-symmetric pyrrolidine **13.3** is an effective sequent chiral auxiliary that is easily recovered and reused. The three-step process outlined above affords an excellent route to chiral, trans-2,5-disubstituted-γ-butyrolactones and, perhaps more importantly, commissions further developments in polymer-supported asymmetric synthesis.

3.3 POLYMER-SUPPORTED SYNTHESIS OF SMALL MOLECULE LIBRARIES

These solid-phase studies plus the recent interest in the preparation of large libraries of molecularly diverse compounds for deployment in various screening protocols led us to explore small molecule combinatorial chemistry. Indeed, the recent development of a number of intriguing polymer-supported synthetic strategies for library preparation has been reported (1). This renaissance in compound screening of combinatorial libraries has, for the most part,* focused on chemically synthesized peptide libraries where the diversity is constrained to amide and protecting group chemistries (2).

Intrigued by the potential of rational synthesis applied to organic (nonpeptide, nonoligosaccharide, and nonnucleotide) molecule libraries, we set out to validate a number of the key issues inherent in "analogous" (i.e., solid-phase split-mix) organic synthesis† as such technology would combine the potentially limitless diversity of synthetic organic reactions and reagents with the innate advantages that small organic molecules bring to the discovery of bioavailable therapeutic agents. Our first efforts in this area addressed a number of the chemical questions relevant to preparing small organic molecule libraries by targeting the analogous organic synthesis of nine β-mercaptoketones **15.6** (Fig. 3.15).

These nine substrates were selected for this investigation for three reasons. First, solid-phase split-mix synthesis of these β-mercaptoketones would serve to illustrate the potentially tremendous *reaction* versatility of analogous organic synthesis. Constructing a library of β-mercaptoketones **15.6** by this strategy requires adapting solution-phase protection, oxidation, Horner–Emmons condensation, Michael addition, and deprotection reaction protocols to solid-phase split-mix chemistry. Second, solid-phase split-mix synthesis of these β-mercaptoketones demonstrates the vast *reagent* selection potential that can be brought to bear in analogous organic synthesis. Readily available ylide and thiolate reagents make this point in this example. Finally, targeting a limited (i.e., nine compound) library in this demonstration project allowed us to hold the components of this library to the normal

---

*A "diversomer" approach where nonpeptide/nonoligosaccharide/nonnucleotide targets are simultaneously, but separately, synthesized on a solid support in an array format has recently been reported; see Ref. 3b. The potential of solid-phase synthesis in the preparation of small organic molecule libraries has been discussed; see Ref. 3a.

†We propose the term "analogous organic synthesis" to set small molecule diversity apart from peptide/oligosaccharide/nucleotide diversity (e.g., these strategies being refered to as "combinatorial synthesis") as well as to convey the notion that the resulting "analog libraries" arise from and encompass *both* reagent and chemical reaction diversity.

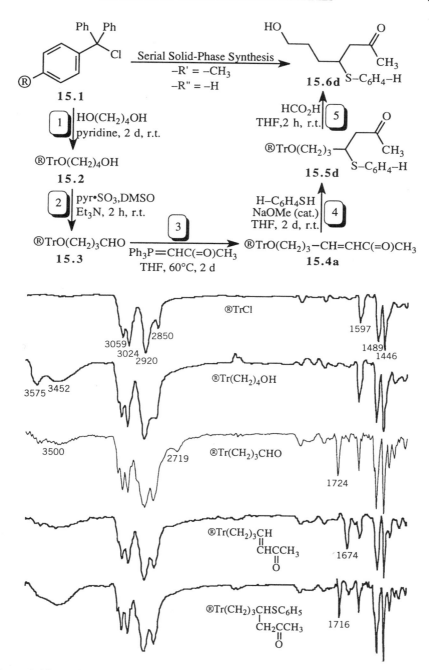

Figure 3.15 Serial solid-phase synthesis of β-mercaptoketone **15.6d.** It is noteworthy that each transformation in this scheme can be monitored by KBr pellet FT-IR analysis of the polymer.

structural characterization (^{1}H- and ^{13}C-NMR, LR- and HR-MS) standards of organic chemistry.

The chemistry targeted for this study was first explored as a solid-phase serial synthesis to establish the validity of each synthetic step. 1,4-Butanediol was attached to the polystyrene support (® = polystyrene/2% divinyl benzene copolymer) by trityl ether (31) mono-protection in pyridine. Polymer-based kinetic site isolation (3a,29) with 3.4 eq of diol effectively minimizes bis-protection. Workup consisted of isolating the resin by filtration, washing with dry pyridine and anhydrous ether, and ether Soxhlet extraction overnight. Drying under vacuum gave resin **15.2** (FT-IR absorption peaks at 3575 and 3452cm^{-1}). The free hydroxyl of resin **15.2** was converted to the corresponding aldehyde (**15.3**) by a sulfur trioxide–pyridine mediated oxidation (32).* Horner–Emmons condensation of THF-swollen resin **15.3** with 1-triphenylphosphoranylidene-2-propanone delivered enone **15.4** and set the stage for Michael addition of aryl thiolate. Treating resin **15.4** with thiophenol and a catalytic amount of sodium methoxide delivered Michael adduct **15.5,** which, upon trityl ether solvolysis with formic acid, delivered the targeted formate ester **15.6d.**

The next objective was to adapt this chemistry to a split-mix organic synthesis method (2b,33). To showcase this approach, it was decided that polymer-bound aldehyde **15.3** would be divided into equal portions in three separate flasks and subsequently condensed with three different ylide reagents. The ylides selected for conversion **15.3** → **15.4** were the —R' = —Me/^{t}Bu/Ph analogs of Ph$_3$P=CHC(=O)R' and, after the separation–reaction–recombination sequence [split-mix method; represented in Fig. 3.16 as "{→}"], a resin mixture was obtained that consisted of beads of **15.4a,** beads of **15.4b,** and beads of **15.4c.**

This mixture of beads was again equally divided into three flasks, the resin swollen with THF, and each flask treated with a Michael donor; flask 1 received thiophenol, flask 2 received p-thiocresol, and flask 3 received 4-chlorothiophenol. Prior to recombining the contents of each flask (i.e., each sublibrary), small samples of resin were removed and incubated with a THF–HCO$_2$H mixture (1:1) to liberate the small molecule products. The THF–HCO$_2$H solution was withdrawn from the beads, evaporated, and the residue taken up in benzene and analyzed by capillary GC. We were pleased to find that each sublibrary mixture showed essentially only the targeted products (i.e., mixtures of the free alcohol and formate esters from **15.6d–f, 15.6g–i,** and **15.6j–l;** see Figures 3.17, 3.18, and 3.19, respectively, and note that these chromatograms illustrate that the desired products are obtained in excellent purity), which were fully characterized by ^{1}H- and ^{13}C-NMR, HR-MS, and low-resolution GC mass spectroscopy (GC-MS).*

At this point, we were intrigued with the question of whether compound identity could be determined on a per bead basis. This question posed the challenge of

---

*While oxalyl chloride/Et$_3$N/DMSO conditions resulted in acid-catalyzed deprotection of the trityl moiety, sulfur trioxide pyridine complex gave very satisfactory results.
*The use of GC to characterize the products of a combinatorial synthesis has recently been reported; see Ref. 2h.

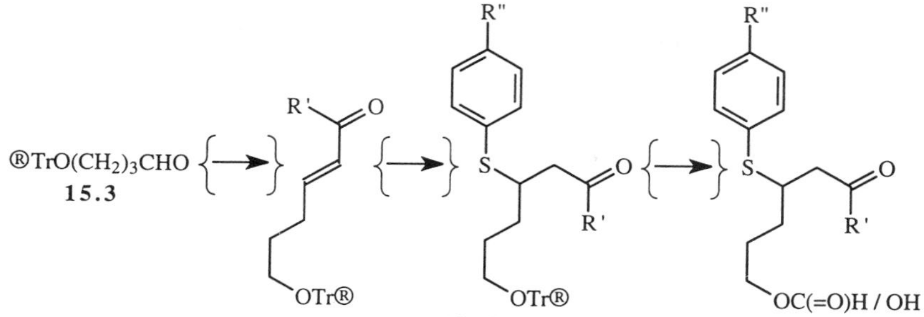

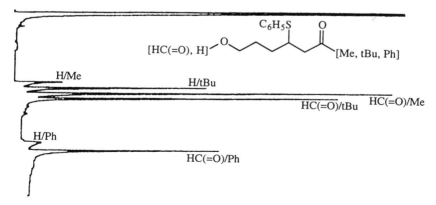

®TrO(CH₂)₃CHO
15.3

15.4a; R' = Me
15.4b; R' = *t*-Bu
15.4c; R' = Ph

15.5d; R' = Me, R" = H
15.5e; R' = *t*-Bu, R" = H
15.5f; R' = Ph, R" = H
15.5g; R' = Me, R" = Me
15.5h; R' = *t*-Bu, R" = Me
15.5i; R' = Ph, R" = Me
15.5j; R' = Me, R" = Cl
15.5k; R' = *t*-Bu, R" = Cl
15.5l; R' = Ph, R" = Cl

15.6d; R' = Me, R" = H
15.6e; R' = *t*-Bu, R" = H
15.6f; R' = Ph, R" = H
15.6g; R' = Me, R" = Me
15.6h; R' = *t*-Bu, R" = Me
15.6i; R' = Ph, R" = Me
15.6j; R' = Me, R" = Cl
15.6k; R' = *t*-Bu, R" = Cl
15.6l; R' = Ph, R" = Cl

Figure 3.16   Analogous solid-phase synthesis of β-mercaptoketone **15.6d–l.**

demonstrating the feasibility of characterizing product mixtures complicated by: (i) diversity of synthetic subunits (potentially far exceeding that encountered in peptide synthesis), (ii) the small amounts of material available ($\approx 10^{-10}$ mol/bead), and (iii) the potential for heterogeneity among modified polymer beads. Clean sample preparation and handling techniques coupled with sensitive GC-MS protocols were employed for this purpose. Because common substructures often yield characteristic mass spectral peaks, potential undesired side reactions as well as optimization of the analogous organic synthesis could be addressed by searching for the presence of these peaks by GC-MS.

To address this issue of per bead analysis, a single bead (200–400 mesh) was

Figure 3.17   Capillary GC analysis of crude **15.6d–f.**

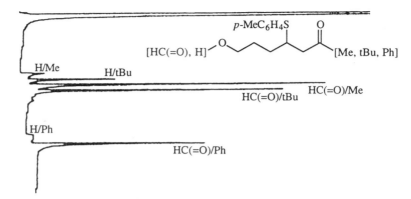

Figure 3.18 Capillary GC analysis of crude **15.6g–i.**

isolated with the aid of a microscope and placed in a glass melting point tube (1 mm diameter). Incubation with THF/HCO$_2$H (10 μL, overnight) followed by evaporation, residue dissolution in hexane (2 μL), and GC-MS analysis easily detected that single bead's formate ester product **15.6.** Nine random single-bead analyses of our nine-compound analog library (pooled resins **15.5**) detected the formates of **15.6d** (detected in three analyses), **15.6e, 15.6g, 15.6h, 15.6k** (detected in two analyses), and **15.6l.** Clearly, single-bead analysis of 200–400 mesh resin is straightforward, with the only difficulty being mechanical issues related to handling a single small bead (≈100 μm diameter). A representative single-bead GC-MS trace is depicted in Figure 3.20.

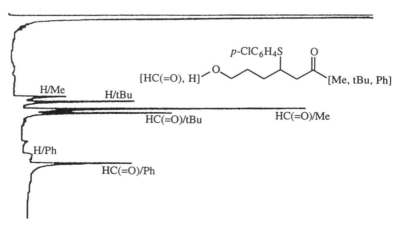

Figure 3.19 Capillary GC analysis of crude **15.6j–l.**

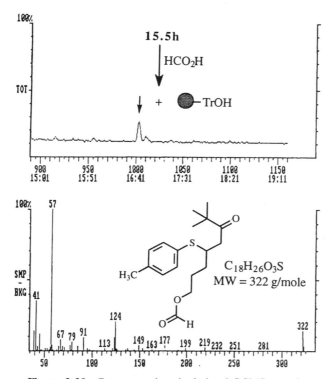

Figure 3.20   Representative single-bead GCMS experiment.

As a final demonstration of the reliability of analogous organic synthesis, a separate 800-mg sample of each resin sublibrary of **15.5** was incubated with THF–HCO_2H and the THF-soluble residues purified by preparative thin-layer chromatography. An ultraviolet active band was observed for each formate ester, which was subsequently isolated and fully characterized. By this process, flask 1 delivered the formate ester derivatives **15.6d–f** in 27, 11, and 25% (respectively) overall isolated yield based on 1.57 mmol trityl chloride/g resin (flask 2 gave **15.6g–i** in 24/17/19%; flask 3 gave **15.6j–l** in 24/7/20%).

These results demonstrate that analogous organic synthesis using simple and universally available laboratory technology can deliver organic compound analog libraries that appear suitable for both resin-bound and resin-free bioassays. This demonstration project utilized a two (number of linear synthetic steps) by three (number of flasks used per step) matrix and reliably delivered the nine targeted substrates. It is noteworthy that an "analogous organic synthesis" matrix where X_{i-n} denotes the number of flasks in analogous steps i through n leads to an analog library of $X_i X_{ii} X_{iii} \ldots X_n$ compounds. Hence, analogous organic synthesis can result in analog libraries of great diversity.

3.4 POLYMER-SUPPORTED SYNTHESIS AND DECONVOLUTIVE ASSAYING OF SMALL MOLECULE LIBRARIES

With these results in hand, the stage was set to employ analogous organic synthesis to prepare assay-targeted libraries. To this end, a two-part demonstration project was undertaken that utilized analogous synthesis to deliver a 27-analog library, which was subsequently evaluated for antioxidative efficiency in a resin-free (ferric thiocyanate assay) deconvolutive assay.

Figure 3.21 provides an overview of part one; our analog synthesis plan. The solid-phase synthesis was envisioned to proceed from commercial Merrifield's peptide resin (® = chloromethylated styrene/2% divinyl benzene copolymer; ≈1 meq Cl/g) to resin library **L2** by two analogous synthetic steps consisting of esterification and aldol condensation. Subsequent reduction of resin library **L2** would liberate the target, 1,3-propanediol library (**L3**) from the polymeric matrix. Part two employs a resin-free deconvolution assay strategy (i.e., a strategy wherein the lead compound in a library is "discovered" by successive analysis of the analog library and its predecessor sublibraries) to evaluate the antioxidative efficiency of analogs **L3** (34).

The chemistry targeted for the synthesis of library **L3** was first explored as a solid-phase serial synthesis to establish the validity of each synthetic step (Fig. 3.22). For step 1, THF-swollen Merrifield resin (®PhCH$_2$Cl) was treated with sodium hydrocinnamate at reflux to effect carboxylate O-alkylation (35). Following filtration and solvent wash, the resulting resin was again swollen in THF, cooled to −78%C, and treated with commercial lithium diisopropylamide (Aldrich; 2.0M in heptane–THF–ethylbenzene, 90 min). A THF–anhydrous zinc chloride solution was added (30 min, 0°C; the presumed zinc-enolate minimizes retro-aldolization) followed by p-anisaldehyde (30 min, 0°C). Addition of saturated aqueous ammonium chloride followed by filtration and solvent wash gave the resin-bound aldol product. Since lithium aluminum hydride reduction resulted in significant retro-aldolization, diisobutylaluminum hydride (DIBAL-H) was selected for this ester reduction and the diol depicted in Figure 3.22 was obtained in a 7:5 ratio of threo to erythro products in 26% overall isolated yield from Merrifield resin. It is noteworthy that polymer-supported reactions can be monitored by KBr pellet FT-IR analysis of the polymer (36).

Following the synthetic steps outlined in Figure 3.21, a 3 × 9 matrix analogous synthesis delivered the 27-analog library shown in Figure 3.23. Analogous step 1 involved the split-vessel O-alkylation of sodium acetate, methoxyacetate, and

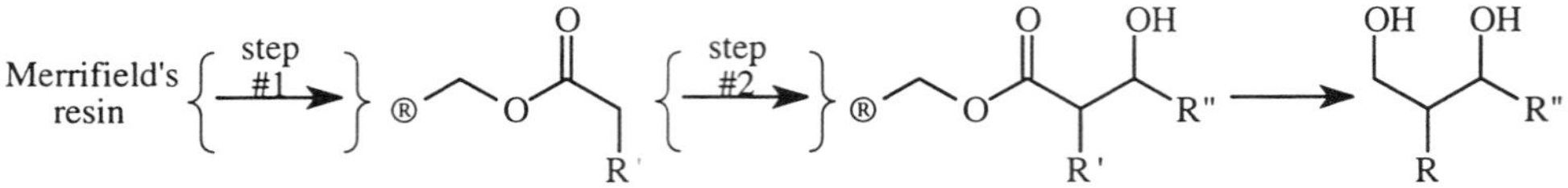

Figure 3.21 Planned library synthesis of 1,3-diols.

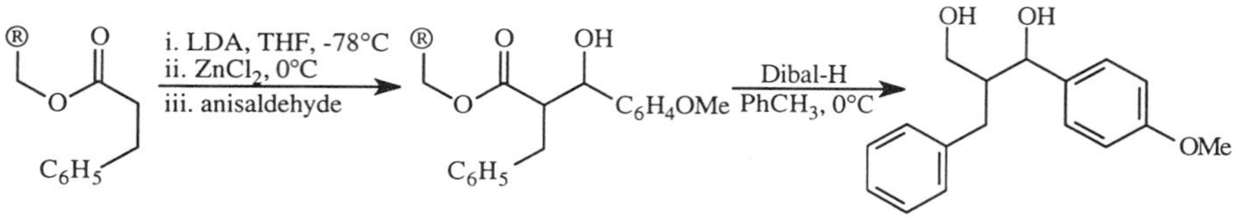

Figure 3.22   Solid-phase serial synthesis of 1,3-diols.

hydrocinnamate with the chloromethyl moiety of Merrifield resin. The resulting resins were combined and mixed to give solid-phase pool **L1** (—R^1 = —H\—OMe\—CH$_2$Ph), which was then equally partitioned into nine flasks for analogous step 2. Lithium diisopropylamide effected enolate formation, which was directly followed by metal exchange (ZnCl$_2$) and aldol condensation with a series of seven aryl aldehydes (sublibraries **SL•1–7**) and two aryl ketones (sublibraries **SL•8** and **SL•9**). FT-IR analysis was employed to establish that each sublibrary condensation had been achieved.

At this juncture, a portion of each three-product sublibrary was mixed to give solid-phase pool **L2,** which was subjected to diisobutylaluminum hydride reduction to liberate the propanediol derivatives. The resulting mixture was subjected to preparative thin-layer chromatography (TLC; hexane:EtOAc::50:50 eluent) and a broad band (i.e., everything excluding baseline and solvent front) was eluted to give the targeted 27-analog library **L3.** In a series of separate operations, a second portion of each three-product sublibrary was submitted to this reduction/preparative TLC procedure (appropriate hexane:EtOAc eluent selected to give a diol band with $R_f \approx 0.2$–0.6) and afforded the nine three-compound sublibraries (**SL•1–9**). All nine sublibraries were analyzed by low-resolution GC-MS to verify that each targeted propanediol derivative was present in the relevant sublibrary and, therefore, in whole library **L3.**

The ferric thiocyanate method (37), a colorimetric assay that measures the amount of linoleic acid hydroperoxide in an emulsion system, was used in a deconvolutive assay of our antioxidant analog library and sublibraries. Briefly, after incubating an analog pool (library or sublibrary) for a period of 3 days, an aliquot of the sample solution was mixed with ammonium thiocyanate plus iron(II) chloride, and the 490-nm absorbance of the resulting red color was determined as a measure of the degree of oxidation present. We have developed this assay in a 96-well format, yielding a rapid, reliable method for screening that maximizes sensitivity versus antioxidant sample size.

A schematic view of this deconvolution approach is presented in Figure 3.24. Step A, ferric thiocyanate assay of antioxidant library **L3,** established that this pool of 27 compounds afforded meaningful antioxidative efficiency (inhibition of color development) and thus warranted ferric thiocyanate assay of each sublibrary (step B). As illustrated in the bar graph (Fig. 3.24), the nine sublibraries **SL•1–9** afforded disparate antioxidative efficiency with sublibrary **SL•6** (compounds **SL•6a** (38), **SL•6b,** and **SL•6c**) producing the least color development in quantitative studies. The three analogs of this lead sublibrary were then prepared serially from the

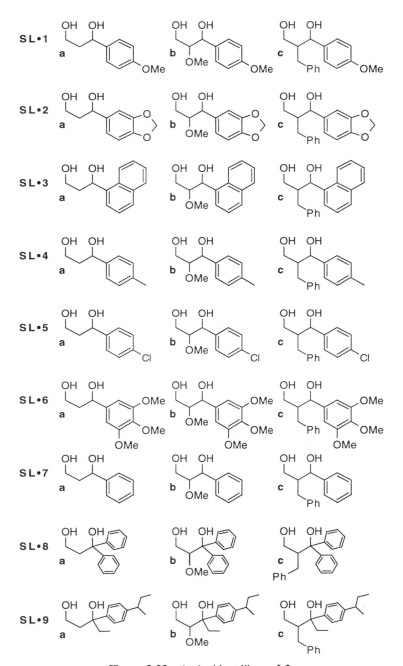

Figure 3.23 Antioxidant library **L3**.

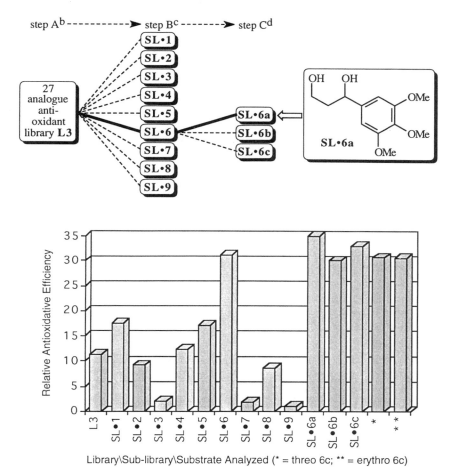

Figure 3.24 Deconvolutive assay to determine antioxidative efficiency. Efficiency expressed as a ratio to sub-library **SL•9** where maximum oxidation occurred. Step A: 1350 μg of library **L3**/mL.

acetate, methoxyacetate, and hydrocinnamate resins and submitted for individual analysis (step C; **SL•6b** and **SL•6c** were ≈1:1 mixtures of diastereomers). The ferric thiocyanate assay results in step C indicate that all three trimethoxy analogs have comparable antioxidative efficiency.* Furthermore, the threo and erythro isomers of **SL•6c** respond similarly in this assay.

   In conclusion, these results demonstrate that analogous synthesis coupled with a resin-free deconvolution assay can lead to the discovery of compounds with targeted activity. This demonstration project utilized analogous synthesis to reliably deliver

---

*Water solubility data: **SL•6a** and **SL•6b** are infinitely miscible with water and **SL•6c**'s water solubility is 3 mg/mL.

27 targeted analogs that were then evaluated for antioxidative efficiency in a resin-free ferric thiocyanate assay. Analogous synthesis studies coupled with resin-bound assays are currently in progress and will be reported shortly.

ACKNOWLEDGMENT

The author is grateful to U.C. Davis collaborators Xenia Beebe, Neil Schore, Hong-sik Moon, Chixu Chen, Lisa Randall Ahlberg, Christian Melander, and Bryan Miller, Takasago Institute for Interdisciplinary Science collaborators Kelly McAlister, Gary Reitz, and Carter Green as well as to the National Science Foundation (Grant CHE-9406891), the U.C. Cancer Research Coordination Committee (Grant 3-504001), and the Petroleum Research Fund of the American Chemical Society for the financial support of this research. Fellowship support was obtained for Chixu Chen through a DOW Polymer Science Fellowship and for Xenia Beebe from the U.C.-Davis Research Mentorship Program as well as the UC Graduate Research Award Program.

REFERENCES

1. (a) Jung, G., and Beck-Sickinger, A. G., *Angew. Chem. Int. Ed. Engl.* **31,** 367–383 (1992); (b) Pavia, M. R., Sawyer, T. K., and Moos, W. H., *Bioorg. Med. Chem. Lett.* **3,** 387–396 (1993).

2. (a) Fodor, S. P. A., Read, J. L., Pirrung, M. C., Stryer, L., Lu, A. T., and Solas, D., *Science* **251,** 767–773 (1991); (b) Lam, K. S., Salmon, S. E., Hersh, E. M., Hruby, V. J., Kazmiersky, W. M., and Knapp, R. J., *Nature* **354,** 82–84 (1991); (c) Houghten, R. A., Pinilla, C., Blondelle, S. E., Appel, J. R., Dooley, C. T., and Cuervo, J. H., *Nature* **354,** 84–86 (1991); (d) Zuckermann, R. N., Kerr, J. M., Siani, M. A., Banville, S. C., and Santi, D. V., *Proc. Natl. Acad. Sci U.S.A.* **89,** 4505–4509 (1992); (e) Nikolaiev, V., Stierandova, A., Krchnak, V., Seligmann, B., Lam, K. S., Salmon, S. E., and Lebl, M., *Peptide Res.* **6,** 161–170 (1993); (f) Kerr, J. M., Banville, S. C., Zuckermann, R. N., *J. Am. Chem. Soc.* **115,** 2529–2531 (1993); (g) Nielsen, J., Brenner, S., and Janda, K. D., *J. Am. Chem. Soc.* **115,** 9812–9813 (1993); (h) Ohlmeyer, M. H. J., Swanson, R. N., Dillard, L. W., Reader, J. C., Asouline, G., Kobayashi, R., Wigler, M., and Still, W. C., *Proc. Natl. Acad. Sci. USA* **90,** 10922–10926 (1993); (i) Borchardt, A., and Still, W. C., *J. Am. Chem. Soc.* **116,** 373–374 (1994).

3. (a) Bunin, B. A., and Ellman, J. A., *J. Am. Chem. Soc.* **114,** 10997–10998 (1992); (b) DeWitt, S. H., Kiely, J. S., Stankovic, C. J., Schroeder, M. C., Cody, D. M. R., and Pavia, M. R., *Proc. Natl. Acad. Sci U.S.A.* **90,** 6909–6913 (1993); (c) Chen, C., Randall, L. A. A., Miller, R. B., Jones, D. A., and Kurth, M. J., *J. Am. Chem. Soc.* **116,** 2661–2662 (1994).

4. Merrifield, R. B., *J. Am. Chem. Soc.* **85,** 2149–2154 (1963).

5. (a) Hodge, P., in *Polymer-Supported Reactions in Organic Synthesis,* P. Hodge and D. C. Sherrington (Eds.), Wiley-Interscience, Chichester, 1980, Chapter 2; (b) Pittman, C. U., Jr., In ibid., Chapter 5; (c) Bergbreiter, D. E., in *Polymeric Reagents and Catalysts,* W. T. Ford (Ed.), *ACS Symp Ser.* **308,** 17 (1986); (d) Hodge, P., in *Synthesis and Separations Using Functional Polymers,* D. C. Sherrington and P. Hodge (Eds.),

Wiley: Chichester, 1988, Chapter 2; (e) Hodge, P., in *Innovation and Perspectives in Solid Phase Synthesis,* R. Epton (Ed.), Collected Papers, First International Symposium, 1989, Oxford SPCC (UK) Ltd., Birmingham.

6. (a) Schore, N. E., and Najdi, S. D., *J. Am. Chem. Soc.* **112,** 441–442 (1990); (b) Gerlach, M., Jördens, F., Kuhn, H., Neumann, W. P., and Peterseim, M., *J. Org. Chem.* **56,** 5971–5972 (1991); (c) Blanton, J. R., and Salley, J. M., *J. Org. Chem.* **56,** 490–491 (1991); (d) Beebe, X., Schore, N. E., and Kurth, M. J., *J. Am. Chem. Soc.* **114,** 10061–10062 (1992); (e) Moon, H.-S., Schore, N. E., and Kurth, M. J., *J. Org. Chem.* **57,** 6088–6089 (1992).

7. Kurth, M. J., and Rodriguez, M. J., *J. Am. Chem. Soc.* **109,** 7577 (1987).

8. Kurth, M. J., Rodriguez, M. J., and Olmstead, M. M., *J. Org. Chem.* **55,** 283 (1990).

9. Ayres, J. T., and Mann, C. K., *J. Polym. Sci. Polym. Lett. Ed.* **3,** 505 (1965).

10. Beebe, X., Chiappari, C. L., Kurth, M. J., and Schore, N. E., *J. Org. Chem.* **58,** 7320 (1993).

11. (a) Murthy, K. S. K., and Hassner, A., *Israel J. Chem.* **31,** 239 (1991); (b) Dehaen, W., and Hassner, A., *Tetrahedron Lett.* **31,** 743 (1990); (c) Hassner, A., and Dehaen, W., *Chem. Ber.* **124,** 1181 (1991); (d) Hassner, A., and Dehaen, W., *J. Org. Chem.* **55,** 5505 (1990); (e) Padwa, A., Chiacchio, U., Dean, D. C., Schoffstall, A. M., Hassner, A., and Murthy, K. S. K., *Tetrahedron Lett.* **29,** 4169 (1988).

12. Hassner, A., Murthy, K. S. K., Padwa, A., Chiacchio, U., Dean, D. C., and Schoffstall, A. M., *J. Org. Chem.* **54,** 5277 (1989).

13. Kim, H. R., Kim, H. J., Duffy, J. L., Olmstead, M. M., Ruhlandt-Senge, K., and Kurth, M. J., *Tetrahedron Lett.* **32,** 4259 (1991).

14. Tanaka, T., Hazato, A., Bannai, K., Okamura, N., Sugiura, S., Manabe, K., Toru, T., Kurozumi, S., Suzuki, M., Kawagishi, T., and Noyori, R., *Tetrahedron* **43,** 813 (1987).

15. Gairaurd, C. B., and Lappin, G. R., *J. Org. Chem.* **18,** 1 (1953).

16. Duffy, J. L., Kurth, J. A., and Kurth, M. J., *Tetrahedron Lett.* **34,** 1259 (1993).

17. (a) Curran, D. P., Scanga, S. A., and Fenk, C. J., *J. Org. Chem.* **49,** 3474 (1984); (b) Mukaiyama, T., and Hoshino, T., *J. Am. Chem. Soc.* **62,** 5339 (1960).

18. Duan, J. J. W., and Smith, A. B., *J. Org. Chem.* **58,** 3703 (1993).

19. Colvin, E. W., Beck, A. K., and Seebach, D., *Helv. Chim. Acta* **64,** 2264 (1981).

20. (a) Sarin, V. K., Kent, S. B. H., Tam, J. P., and Merrifield, R. B., *Anal. Biochem.* **117,** 147 (1981); (b) Kaiser, E., Colescott, R. L., Bossinger, C. D., and Cook, P. I., *Anal. Biochem.* **34,** 595 (1970).

21. (a) Gagnaire, D., and Monzeglio, P., *Bull. Soc. Chim. Fr.* 474 (1965); (b) Katagiri, K., Tori, K., and Kimura, Y., *J. Med. Chem.* **10,** 1149 (1967).

22. (a) Sonnet, P. E., and Heath, R. R., *J. Org. Chem.* **45,** 3137 (1980); (b) Evans, D. A., and Takacs, J. M., *Tetrahedron Lett.* **21,** 4233 (1980); (c) Mori, K., and Ito, T., *Tetrahedron* **39,** 2303 (1980); (d) Kawanami, Y., Ito, Y., Kitagawa, T., Taniguchi, Y., Katsuki, T., and Yamaguchi, M., *Tetrahedron Lett.* **25,** 857 (1984); (e) Ito, Y., Katsuki, T., Yamaguchi, M., ibid., 6015; (f) Enomoto, M., Ito, Y., Katsuki, T., and Yamaguchi, M., *Tetrahedron Lett.* **26,** 1343 (1985); (g) Schultz, A., Sundararaman, P., Macielag, M., Lavieri, F. P., and Welch, M., ibid., 4575; (h) Ito, Y., Katsuki, T., and Yamaguchi, M., ibid., 4643; (i) Hanamoto, T., Katsuki, T., and Yamaguchi, M., *Tetrahedron Lett.* **27,** 2463 (1986); (j) Uchikawa, M., Hanomoto, T., Katsuki, T., and

Yamaguchi, M., ibid., 4577; (k) Evans, D. A., Dow, R. L., Shih, T. L., Takacs, J. M., and Zahler, R., *J. Am. Chem. Soc.*, **112,** 5290 (1990).

23. Najdi, S. D., Reichlin, D., and Kurth, M. J., *J. Org. Chem.* **55,** 6241 (1990).

24. Bartlett, P. A., in *Asymmetric Synthesis,* Vol. 3, J. D. Morrison (Ed.), Academic, Orlando, 1983, pp. 411–454.

25. (a) Tamaru, Y., Mizutani, M., Furukawa, Y., Kawamura, S., Yoshida, Z., Yanagi, K., and Minobe, M., *J. Am. Chem. Soc.* **106,** 1079 (1984); (b) Hart, D. J., Huang, H. C., Krishnamurthy, R., and Schwartz, T., *J. Am. Chem. Soc.* **111,** 7507 (1989); (c) Fuji, K., Node, M., Naniwa, Y., and Kawabata, T., *Tetrahedron Lett.* **31,** 3175 (1990).

26. Najdi, S., and Kurth, M. J., *Tetrahedron Lett.* **31,** 3279–3282 (1990).

27. Aglietto, M., Chiellini, E., D'Antone, S., Ruggeri, G., and Solaro, R., *Pure Appl. Chem.* **60,** 415–430 (1988).

28. Marzi, M., and Misiti, D., *Tetrahedron Lett.* **30,** 6075–6076 (1989).

29. Crowley, J. I., and Rapoport, H., *Acc. Chem. Res.* **9,** 135–144 (1996).

30. (a) Evans, D. A., Bartroli, J., and Shih, T. L., *J. Am. Chem. Soc.* **103,** 2127–2129 (1981); (b) Evans, D. A., Ennis, M. D., and Mathre, D. J., *J. Am. Chem. Soc.* **104,** 1737–1739 (1982).

31. (a) Frechet, J. M. J., and Nuyens, L. J., *Can. J. Chem.* **54,** 926–934 (1978); (b) Fyles, T. M., Leznoff, C. C., and Weatherston, J., *Can. J. Chem.* **56,** 1031–1041 (1978).

32. Parikh, J. R., and von E. Doering, W., *J. Am. Chem. Soc.* **89,** 5505–5507 (1967).

33. Furka, A., Sebestyen, F., Asgedom, M., and Dibo, G., *Int. J. Pept. Prot. Res.* **37,** 487–493 (1991).

34. (a) Larson, R., *Phytochemistry* **27,** 969–978 (1988); (b) Culvelier, M.-E., Richard, H., and Berset, C., *Biosci. Biotech. Biochem.* **56,** 324–325 (1992).

35. (a) Wang, S. S., *J. Org. Chem.* **40,** 1235–1239 (1975); (b) Stewart, J. M., and Young, J. D., *Solid Phase Peptide Synthesis,* 2nd ed., Pierce Chemical Co., Rockford, IL, 1984, p. 55.

36. Frechet, J. M., and Schuerch, C., *J. Am. Chem. Soc.* **93,** 492–496 (1971).

37. (a): Osawa, T., and Namiki, M., *Agric. Biol. Chem.* **45,** 735–739 (1981); (b) Nakatani, N., and Inatani, R., *Agric. Biol. Chem.* **47,** 353–358 (1983); (c) Imai, S., Morikiyo, M., Furihata, K., Hayakawa, Y., and Seto, H., *Agric. Biol. Chem.* **54,** 2367–2371 (1990).

38. Pearl, I. A., and Gratzl, J., *J. Org. Chem.* **27,** 2111–2114 (1962).

4

MACRO BEADS AS MICROREACTORS: NEW SOLID-PHASE SYNTHESIS METHOLOGY

WOLFGANG E. RAPP

Rapp Polymere GmbH, Ernst Simon Str. 9, D 72072 Tübingen, Germany

4.1 INTRODUCTION

Since the introduction of solid-phase peptide synthesis (SPPS) on low-crosslinked polystyrene by R. B. Merrifield in 1962 (1–4) this method was developed and applied in many other fields, for example, oligonucleotide synthesis (5–7), catalysis (8–16), biotechnology for immobilization of enzymes (17–28), and for polymeric reagents (29–34). A new very rapidly growing field is the use of solid-phase chemistry in combinatorial chemistry and libraries. Beside the well-established resins, mainly dominated by low-crosslinked polystyrene, there is a need for new tailored polymeric supports in the expanding fields of applications in organic solid-phase chemistry.

In the beginning of solid-phase chemistry, 5 and 2% crosslinked polystyrene supports were used for many applications. Nowadays polystyrene resins crosslinked with 1% divinyl benzene (DVB) is the mostly used resin. In addition to the classical support of 1% crosslinked chloromethylated polystyrene, originally introduced by Merrifield, a variety of other polymeric supports have been developed and are in use. From the chemical and physicochemical architecture of the resins, there are in principle two main groups of resins in use: gelatinous resins and macroporous resins.

In contrast to the gelatinous resins, macroporous supports of group 2 consist of a very rigid nonswellable backbone. The backbone could be either Kieselgur, glass [e.g., controlled pore glass (CPG), which is used in oligonucleotide synthesis] or highly crosslinked polystyrene. In contrast to the swellable resins the macroporous resins show a permanent porosity and no swelling is necessary. Dependent on the manufacturing process, the supports have a beaded shape (CPG polystyrene) or irregular shape similar to Kieselgur and polystyrene (Polyhipe). Composite supports consist of such a macroporous rigid skeleton that is either Kieselgur (Pepsyn resin) or polystyrene (Polyhipe) (35,36). Low-crosslinked polyacrylamide is then poly-merized within the pores to form a gel phase where the synthesis takes place. The rigid skeleton protects the soft gelatinous part of the resin. Nevertheless tremendous swelling differences of the gelatinous part of the support, dependent on solvent, destroys the rigid skeleton and produces fines that cause difficulties by the filtration processes. Typical capacities are in the range of 0.1–0.5 mmol/g. The structure of the composite resins is illustrated in Figure 4.1. These resins are pressure stable but mechanically very fragile, and their use is strictly restricted to flow-through systems.

Group 1 comprises the well-known 1% crosslinked polystyrene resins and the crosslinked polyacrylamides introduced by Sheppard (37), as well as the ultrahigh loaded core Q resins (38), which are also polyacrylamide-type resins. Typical ca-pacities of these resins are in the range of 0.1–1.5 mmol/g, with core Q up to 5 mmol/g. However, this high loaded resin never became very important. All these gelatinous resins are available with beaded shape, having a particle size distribution typically in the range of 200–400 mesh (73–37 μm) or 100–200 mesh (150–75 μm). But with the development of combinatorial chemistry, there is a need for more distinct particle sizes and well-characterized resins.

All gel-type resins are low-crosslinked supports and have to swell in the reactions solvent in order to build up and expand their polymeric network. The reactive groups are located along the polymeric strains that form the network. The swelling process exposes the reactive sites and makes them accessible to the reactants. The polymeric network is very soft and flexible. Therefore the use of the swollen beads is mostly restricted to batch processes. It is important to notice that on gelatinous resins up to 99% of the reactive sides are located inside the bead and only 0.1–1%

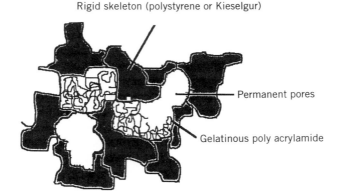

Figure 4.1 Macroporous composite resins.

on the outer surface shell. In all polymer-supported reactions the polymeric support represents the reaction space where the chemical reaction takes place. Using polymer beads for synthesis, the total polymeric reaction space, represented by a certain amount of beads, is divided into small individual reaction compartments represented by each bead. Therefore, resin parameters such as crosslinking, swelling properties, mass transport, phase transition phenomens, bead size, and particle size distribution have to be taken into account as each individual bead represents the reaction space.

The liquid-phase method (39–43) was developed as an alternative approach to the solid-phase method of Merrifield. In general, soluble and functionalized polyethylene glycol (PEG) of molecular masses between 3000 and 20,000 daltons are used in the liquid-phase method. PEG is very compatible to many solvents and with biopolymers such as peptides and proteins. To assemble a peptide or nucleotide the couplings are done in homogeneous solution on the polymer as shown by Mutter and Bayer (44). Kinetic investigations have shown that the coupling rates are in the same order as low-molecular-mass amino acid esters (45). Diffusion phenomena play no role in this technique, which is a major advantage over the solid-phase technique. PEG often solubilizes even insoluble substrates. One practical advantage of the peptide–PEG conjugates is their easy use for instrumental analysis, for example, recording of circular dichroism spectra for conformational analysis of the growing peptide chain. Instead of simple filtration, as used in solid-phase chemistry, membrane filtration or crystallization is applied to separate the polymer-bound product from the low-molecular-mass molecules. However, the main disadvantages of liquid-phase technique are the time-consuming workup operations such as membrane filtration or crystallization and the impossibility of automatization.

To benefit from the advantages of both the liquid-phase technique and the solid-phase technique PEG chains are grafted onto low-crosslinked polystyrene (PS) beads [TentaGel resins (46–51)]. This hybrid-type resin combines the advantages of gelatinous resins (group 1) and macroporous resins (group 2) in addition of the advantages of liquid-phase chemistry. The graft copolymers allow solid-phase chemistry under liquid-phase conditions. The grafted resin can be characterized as a hybrid-type resin.

4.2 PROPERTIES OF PS–PEG TENTACLE POLYMERS

The simplest immobilization procedure is to couple PEG via one of its terminal hydroxyl groups to chloromethylated PS according to the classical ether synthesis (52,53) or to use other bifunctional PEGs for coupling onto the solid support (54). However, when long-chain PEGs (>800 daltons) are used, the yields of this approach are unsatisfactory. Moreover, the homobifunctional PEGs react to a large extent at both ends to give cyclic PEGs and additional crosslinking. Consequently, the number of free functions will be reduced, which results in lower capacity of the graft copolymer. We have found that by means of anionic graft copolymerization setting up the PEG step by step directly on the matrix, PEG chains of molecular masses up to 20 kilodaltons have been immobilized on functionalized crosslinked polystyrenes (55–60). Graft copolymers with PEG chains of about 3000 daltons proved to be optimal in respect to kinetic rates, mobility, swelling, and resin capacity. These graft copolymers are pressure stable and can be used in batch processes as well as under continuous-flow conditions. Figure 4.2 illustrates schematically the architecture of the tentacle polymer. Because of a PEG content up to 70% w/w, the properties of these polymers are highly dominated by the properties of PEG and no longer by the PS matrix. This is especially shown by the very consistent, and from the solvent nearly independent, swelling of the graft copolymer in comparison to 1% crosslinked polystyrene.

Table 4.1 summarizes the swelling volumes of TentaGel resins in comparison to PS. The dry volume of TentaGel is approximately 1.7 mL/g and for PS 1.6 mL/g. For measuring the swelling volume, 1 g of resin is swollen in the solvent for 24 h.

The PEG–graft copolymer swells in all solvents that dissolve PEG and, on the other hand, swelling is negligible in solvents that do not dissolve PEG, for example, aliphatic hydrocarbons and diethyl ether. This broad range of usable good swelling solvents allows the use of TentaGel resins in almost every solvent system. Thus, after a reaction (e.g., in toluene) one can use a solvent gradient, (e.g., from toluene via dioxane to aqueous systems) and then go back from this hydrophilic system via a gradient to pure organic solvent systems [e.g., from water via dioxane, tetrahydrofuran (THF), or ethanol to methylene chloride].

The reactive sites, which are located at the end of the PEG spacers, behave kinetically like in solution. This could be demonstrated by kinetic measurements where the coupling constants of the Boc-Gly-ONp active ester to both low-molecular-

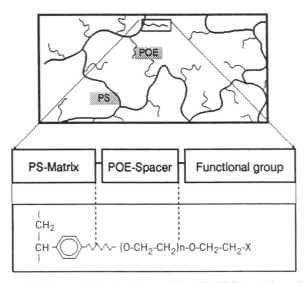

Figure 4.2   Chemical architecture of the PS–PEG tentacle resin.

TABLE 4.1 Swelling Volume of 1 g PS (1% Crosslinked) and 1 g TentaGel Resins in Different Solvents (mL/g)[a]

Solvent	Water	MeOH	EtOH	CH_2Cl_2	Toluene	DMF	MeCN	THF	Dioxane	Ether
Polystyrene 1% DVB	—	1.6	1.68	8.3	8.5	5.6	3.2	8.8	7.8	4.0
TentaGel S resins 0.25–0.3 mmol/g	4.25	4.25	2.1	5.1	5.3	5.4	5.1	5.8	6.2	1.9
TentaGel HL resins, 0.5–0.6 mmol/g	3.1	3.6	3.5	5.7	4.1	4.6	3.9	4.2	4.8	2.4

[a]Dry volume PS: 1.6 mL/g; dry volume TentaGel: 1.7 mL/g; TentaGel S resin: S = standard, TentaGel HL resin: HL = high loaded.

mass compounds and graft copolymer are in the same order of magnitude (61). Because of the flexibility and the good solvation properties of the PEG tentacles, polymer reactions can be performed on the solid support under quasihomogeneous conditions.

The ^{13}C nuclear magnetic resonance (NMR) relaxation time measurements (T_1) also indicate the high flexibility of the PEG spacers and the reactive sites at the end of the spacer. Figure 4.3 illustrates the conditions when the resin is swollen and the PEG spacers well solvated (Fig. 4.3b) or not swollen (Fig. 4.3a). In the nonswollen or incomplete swollen state of the resin, the NMR signals of the PEG spacers are rather broad, as known from solid-state NMR studies. When the resin is swollen, the PEG tentacles are well solvated and highly flexible, which results in high T_1 values. The NMR signals show a very narrow linewidth, which is comparable to that of soluble small molecules. This physicochemical property of the resin allows the use of ^{13}C-NMR and magic angle spinning (MAS) ^{1}H-NMR spectroscopic techniques for investigations and for analysis of resin-bound molecules and resin functionality (60–63). Recently Kiefer has shown that with the graft copolymers in comparison to other resins the highest spectral quality is obtained and the narrowest line width (64). As an example, palmitic acid was coupled to the amino-functionalized resin, and the derivatized resin was investigated by ^{13}C-NMR spectroscopy under various conditions. Figure 4.4 shows the ^{13}C-NMR spectrum of a sample of resin (100 mg), which is swollen in CDCl$_3$ and measured in a 5-mm tube (Fig. 4.4a). Because of the high flexibility and good solvation of the PEG spacer and the attached palmitic acid, rather sharp signals were recorded for the carbon resonance and a good signal-to-noise ratio is obtained. The same investigation was done using deuterated water (D$_2$O) as a solvent (Fig. 4.4b). Again, the PEG spacer

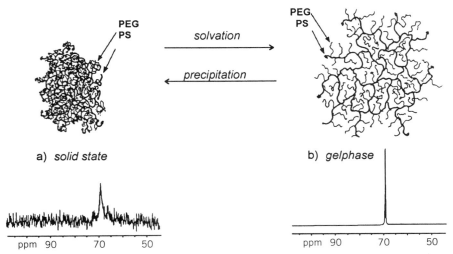

Figure 4.3 NMR monitoring of solvation: (*Top*) Tentacle resin in solid-state and solvated: (*Bottom*) corresponding gel-phase ^{13}C-NMR of the PEG tentacles.

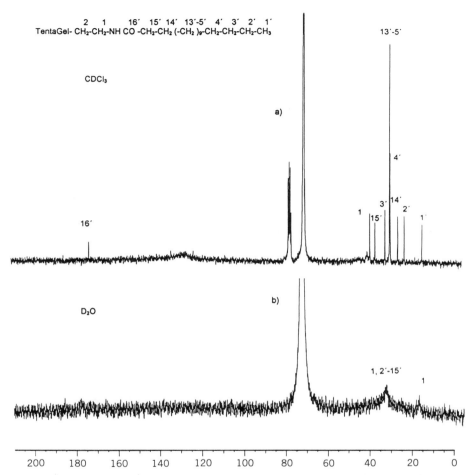

Figure 4.4 Solvent-dependent mobility monitored by gel-phase ^{13}C-NMR of TentaGel-immobilized palmitic acid.

shows a sharp resonance signal whereas the signals of the palmitic acid are rather broad. This is readily explained since PEG is well solvated in chloroform and in water, whereas the palmitic acid is only well solvated in CDCl$_3$ and not in the aqueous systems. This results in sharp signals for CDCl$_3$ (highly flexible, well solvated) and broad signals for the water system (not solvated, restricted mobility). As a result of these investigations, it is necessary to take care of both the resin and the attached molecule and to choose a good solvent for both of them to have them solvated and to get informative NMR spectra. On the other hand this very simple NMR investigation allows the selection of an optimal solvent system for the reaction on solid phase. Good solvation of the immobilized molecule is necessary for successful synthesis. In Table 4.2 chemical shifts for some TentaGel derivatives are summarized.

Look et al. (62) have used ^{13}C-enriched molecules as an internal standard on the TentaGel resin to follow the chemical shift of the ^{13}C-enriched centers during a synthesis sequence on the resin. This technique allows one to use fast ^{13}C-NMR analysis for monitoring gel-phase reactions. Recently Fitch et al. (63) have used the MAS technique to obtain ^{1}H-NMR spectra from the gel-phase resin, for analysis of the functionalities and molecules immobilized on the TentaGel matrix. All these NMR techniques yield analytical information of resin-bound molecules and analytical data are available during a reaction sequence directly on the resin.

As mentioned earlier, particle size and particle size distributions are of major importance and have to be taken into account during organic chemistry on solid supports. In all polymer-supported reactions there must be a mass transport of the activated compound from the surrounding solvent to the reactive sites located inside the resin bead. The driving force for mass transport is diffusion, and diffusion is dependent on path length. By correlation of the size fraction with the mass fraction of a given size distribution and assuming a size range within 20–60 μm, whereas 80% of the beads were represented in the main fraction, and a 10% fraction with smaller beads and a 10% fraction of larger beads, the 10% size fraction of the larger beads represents 29% of the total mass of all three fractions. Suppose there is an equal distribution of the reactive groups on the mass fraction; this 10% size fraction of larger beads contains also 29% of the reactive groups. Assuming that the kinetic rate is much faster than the diffusion, and the diffusion rate is dependent on particle size, the largest beads control the overall reaction time. Only monosized beads show an ideal homogeneous distribution of reactive sites within all beads. Using monosized beads, there are identical reaction conditions on each bead at each time. Beside diffusion, sorption properties also influence the overall reaction rates. Sorption is dependent on crosslinking, swelling properties, solvent, and polarity of the resin. The degree of sorption of reagents in the bead is rather important and influences the kinetic rates to a great extend. To drive the reaction to completion, normally a huge excess of reagents in the fluid medium is used. However, for the

TABLE 4.2 Chemical Shifts in Gel-Phase ^{13}C-NMR for TentaGel Derivatives

X	OH	Br	SH	NH$_2$	N(CH$_3$)$_2$	Boc-NH CH$_2$COO
CH$_2$-X	61.9	30.9	31.6	42.5	59.3	64.2
[CH$_2$-CH$_2$-O]$_n$	71.0	70.9	70.8	71.1	71	70.4
N—CH$_3$					46.1	
Boc CH$_3$—C—O—C— (with CH$_3$, CH$_3$, O groups)						28.2

Solvent: CDCC$_3$.

effective reaction rates (65–68) the concentration of reactants within the beads is decisive and is expressed by the partition coefficient k determined in acetonitrile for PS beads with $k = 1.11$ kg/L^{-1} and for TentaGel $k = 1.58$ kg/L^{-1}.

A partition coefficient $k > 1$ indicates higher concentration inside the bead in comparison to the surrounding liquid medium. With increasing the PEG content on the graft copolymer, resulting in lowering the PS contents (w/w), the partition co-efficient increases. PEG–graft copolymers having different PEG molecular masses re-sult in different ratios of PEG to PS. The sorption and partition coefficients of Boc-Gly-ONP active esters were measured by standard procedures, developed by Hori et al. (67,68). A comparison of sorption curves of the dye Oracett blue 2 R on polystyrene beads, (1% divinyl benzene 44 μm particle size) and PS–PEG graft copolymers (88 μm particle size, 75% w/w PEG) is shown in Figure 4.5. Although the particle size is doubled compared to the originally used PS matrix, the sorption increases by a factor of 4 accompanied by an increase of the sorption capacity.

Setting up a chemical library or peptide library by the "one bead one compound" approach (69,70), it is essential to know the number of beads available within a certain amount of resin as well as the capacity of single beads. Table 4.3 summa-rizes some particle sizes and correlates them to the corresponding capacity of one bead. The calculations are based on a typical loading of TentaGel beads, which is in the range of 0.25–0.3 mmol/g. For example, a pentamer peptide library, containing all 20 natural amino acids, ends up in $20^5 = 3.2 \times 10^6$ individual peptides.

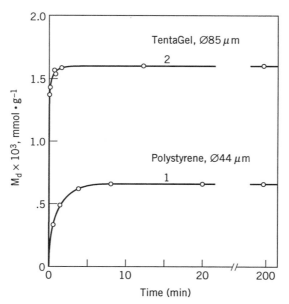

Figure 4.5 Sorption of oracet blue 2 dye in acetronitrile (1.3×10^{-4} mol/L, 25°C). Polymer/solvent 1:120 (w/w). Curve 1 represents 1% crosslinked polystyrene whereas curve 2 shows the corresponding PS–PEG graft copolymer.

TABLE 4.3 Correlation of Particle Size, Number of Beads per Gram Resin and Capacity per Single Bead[a]

Resin	Size (μm)	Beads/g	Capacity/Bead
TentaGel NH$_2$	750	4.62×10^3	65 nmol
TentaGel NH$_2$	500	1.5×10^4	19 nmol
TentaGel NH$_2$	300	6.4×10^4	4 nmol
TentaGel NH$_2$	200	2.15×10^5	1.3 nmol
TentaGel NH$_2$	130	8.87×10^5	280–330 pmol
TentaGel NH$_2$	90	2.86×10^6	80–100 pmol
TentaGel M NH$_2$	35	4.55×10^7	5.5 pmol
TentaGel M NH$_2$	20	2.4×10^8	1.0 pmol
TentaGel M NH$_2$	10	1.95×10^9	0.13 pmol

[a]Calculation of single-bead capacity is based on a capacity of 0.25–0.3 mmol/g resin.

Therefore a minimum of 3.2 million beads are necessary. For 3.2 million beads there is a need for 1.6 mg of 10-μm resin, 70 mg of 35-μm resin, 1.1 g of 90-μm resin, and about 700 g of 750-μm beads. For analytical characterization at least 5 pmol of resin-bound peptide are needed for sequencing on a bead (71). To estimate the optimum resin quantity for the library that can be handled economically, one has to take into account the bead sizes and bead capacities. Table 4.4 summarizes some available tentacle derivatives for use in chemical synthesis, combinatorial chemistry, and libraries.

Physicochemical properties such as mechanical stability, pressure stability, and equal swelling volumes in different solvents as well as high kinetic rates (60,61) allow the use of the TentaGel resins in all commercial synthesizers [e.g., continuous flow (CF) (59), vortexing, shaking, gas bubbling, or multiple synthesizers]. Our investigations show that the overall reaction rate is influenced by the method of mixing (and therefore the synthesizer). There is no difference in kinetic rates by shaking, gas bubbling, or even no mixing (72), whereas vortexing (ABI 431, 433) and flow-through systems (MilliGen 9050) have an impact on overall kinetic rates. Vortexing and optimized flow-through systems show remarkable higher coupling rates compared to other mixing methods.

Because of the heterogeneous nature of the reaction in solid-phase synthesis resin parameters such as polarity, particle size, solvation, mass transport, and diffusion are of prime importance in all polymer-supported reactions (73). The driving force for mass transport is diffusion, and diffusion is dependent on path length. All solid supports normally used in solid-phase chemistry show a more or less broad particle size distribution. Particle sizes of PS, polyacrylamide, and TentaGel resins are in the range of 50–200 μm; Kieselgur/polyamide and Polyhipe are in the range of 500–1000 μm. Therefore mass transport and reaction rates are individual parameters for each particle, whereas the overall reaction time is controlled by the largest bead. To overcome these problems we have developed small monosized microbeads having 10, 20, and 35 μm particle size (74).

TABLE 4.4 Functionalized Graft Copolymer Resins for Combinatorial Organic Synthesis

Resin	Functionality
TentaGel OH	$\sim$O—CH$_2$—CH$_2$—OH
TentaGel Br	$\sim$O—CH$_2$—CH$_2$—Br
TentaGel NH$_2$	$\sim$O—CH$_2$—CH$_2$—NH$_2$
TentaGel COOH	$\sim$NH—CO—CH$_2$—CH$_2$—COOH
TentaGel SH	$\sim$NH—CO—(CH$_2$)$_n$—SH
TentaGel COOSu	
TentaGel CHO	$\sim$NH—CO—(CH$_2$)$_n$—CHO
TentaGel NHNHBoc	$\sim$NH—CO—CH$_2$—CH$_2$—CO—NH—NH—Boc
TentaGel AC	
TentaGel Trt	
TentaGel PHB	
TentaGel HMB	
TentaGel RAM	

The monosized nature of the beads divides the total reaction space (represented by all beads) in identical small reaction compartments having identical reaction dimensions. The monosized nature and the uniform architecture allow one to optimize the reaction conditions to a great extend because of identical reaction conditions for each individual bead. In contrast to 90-μm particles, where, for example, the release of the Fmoc group and the wash out was finished within 2.5 min, the time can be reduced to 80 s by using 25-μm particles at 45°C. This time corresponds to the kinetic rate of the Fmoc deprotection. There is no longer any contribution of the mass transport to the overall reaction rate. From this investigation it is very highly recommended to use particles with a very narrow size distribution.

4.3 MACROBEADS AS POLYMERIC MICROREACTORS IN COMBINATORIAL CHEMISTRY

The generation of molecular diversity either by synthesis of peptide libraries or the use of combinatorial chemistry methods require resins that are compatible to a broad range of organic reaction conditions, which include various solvent systems, for example, very polar and even aqueous solvent systems. Aqueous buffer systems are used for resin-bound biological assays and screening. Based on the "split synthesis technique" for generating libraries originally introduced by Furka et al. (69) and further developed by Salmon et al. (70), a number of peptide libraries have been synthesized and screened on TentaGel beads of various particle sizes (76–93).

Whereas in peptide chemistry only a restricted number of solvents are in use [NNdimethylformamide, dichloromethane, 1-methyl-2-pyrrolidone (DMF, DCM, NMP) or mixtures thereof], organic chemistry requires the whole range of solvents. With the development of combinatorial organic chemistry on solid supports, TentaGel resins are used extensively in this approach for screening reactions and creating small molecule nonpeptide libraries as well as tagging and encoding techniques (36,63,64,94–112). Fenniri et al. (96) described a technique for an encoded cassette for the highly sensitive detection of the success of chemical reactions on TentaGel. They synthesized a peptide on the resin by Fmoc strategy followed by DNA synthesis. Enzymatic treatment in aqueous solution cleaves off the peptide–DNA complex, which was then exposed to polymer chain reaction (PCR). Virgilio and Ellman (95) described the synthesis of β-turn mimetics on solid supports that involved a reduction of a disulfide bond in aqueous solvent mixtures. A clean reduction without side reactions was only found by using TentaGel supports. These two selected examples may demonstrate the importance of resin compatibility to different synthesis conditions.

Nevertheless many applications suffer from the restricted amount of substance available on one single bead. Several attempts were made to overcome this disadvantage, either by increasing the degree of substitution on the bead or by lysine branching (81). Both attempts suffer from extremely slow reaction rates, incomplete reactions, intermolecular interactions within one bead, and slow release from the support.

Dependent on particle size and the swelling volume in a given solvent, a polymer bead can only take up a restricted amount of solvent, and therefore a limited amount of reactants. The maximum amount of the take-up of a dissolved reagent is only dependent on the expansion of the bead in the solution and the concentration of the reactant. Table 4.5 correlates swelling to the maximum take-up. Assuming that the expanding volume (dry bead to a swollen state) is completely covered by a 0.5 molar reactant solution, PS in acetonitrile shows a 2.5 less concentration to equimolarity, whereas only by using very good solvents equimolarity or an excess of reagent can be achieved. Resins that are compatible to a broad range of solvent do not show this adverse effect. This also has impact on the synthesis. In automated systems, normally the reactants are added at a constant concentration but in different solvents. Changing of swelling influences the ratio of reactive sites on the bead, which is constant, to the amount of reactants available in the bead dependent on swelling.

Our goal was therefore to increase the amount of substance per bead by increasing the particle size and not the concentration of substance within the bead. Based on PS–PEG graft copolymers (TentaGel), macrobeads with unusually high particle sizes of 300–800 μm were developed. This increase of particle size raises the capacity/bead by a factor of 100–1000 up to 100 nmol whereas the beads used so far have diameters of 90–130 μm and 50–200 pmol capacity. The amount of product obtained from one of these smaller beads by sequential cleavage is not sufficient for unequivocal analytical investigations and simultaneous application to bioassays. Dependent on particle sizes, capacities of 10–100 nmol/bead have been detected by quantitative Fmoc determination from single macrobeads. Each bead is characterized by measuring its size and capacity (Table 4.6). As the reaction volume and concentration of each single bead is now defined, the beads can be used as *polymeric microreactors.*

The use of polymeric microreactors as new tools in combinatorial chemistry, bioassays, and structural characterization of diverse molecules is described here. In many bioassays high-molecular-weight biopolymers are used for screening a library. Due to the gelatinous nature of TentaGel resins, biopolymers (enzymes, receptors, etc.) cannot penetrate into the resin and therefore interact only with the outer surface of the bead. Of the reactive sites 98–99% are located inside the bead and only 1–2% are accessible on the outer surface for interaction with large molecules. Vágner et al. (82) have described an enzymatic shaving method to modify the bead surface. Polymeric reagents are used to distinguish between the outer surface of the bead and the internal reaction volume. The reactive sides on the surface and within the beads are orthogonally protected by Fmoc and Boc. The orthogonal protecting groups were selectively cleaved by using either polymeric acids or bases followed by modification of the reactive sides inside the beads with two orthogonal handles: acid-labile handle AC (4-hydroxymethyl-3-methoxy-phenoxyacetic acid) or RAM (Rink Amide, *p*-[(R,S)-α-(9H-fluoren-9-yl)-methoxyformamido]-2,4dimethoxy benzyl]-phenoxy-acetic acid) and the base-labile *p*-hydroxymethylbenzoic acid (HMB) to create a multifunctional microreactor (Fig. 4.6). Dependent on particle size, the accessible sides on the surface are in the range of 0.1–1 nmol. This amount of reactive sites

TABLE 4.5 Correlation of Swelling to Maximum Take-up of Reactants

	Polystyrene				Tentacle Copolymer			
Solvent	Size (μm)	ΔV (10^{-3} μL)	Take-up 0.5 M solution (pmol)	Capacity/bead (pmol)	Size (μm)	ΔV (10^{-3} μL)	Take-up (pmol)	Capacity/bead (pmol)
Dry	55			100	90			100
MeOH	55			100	122.4	0.581	290	100
CH$_3$CN	69	0.085	42	100				
DMF	84	0.223	111	100	139.5	1.039	519	100
Toluene								
CH$_2$CL$_2$	97	0.477	195	100	139.5	1.039	519	100
THF								

TABLE 4.6 Capacity of Selected Macro Beads

Bead size (μm)	458	459	494	547	564	590	675	777	860
Found (nmol)	21	20	25	26	32	38	50	61	93
Volume (nL)	50	50	63	86	94	101	161	245	332
Conc. dry bead (mol)	0.42	0.42	0.39	0.3	0.34	0.36	0.31	0.25	0.28

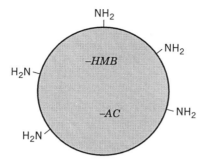

HMB = 4-Hydroxymethyl-benzoyl
AC = 4-Hydroxymethyl-3-methoxy-phenoxyacetyl

Figure 4.6   Trifunctional polymeric microreactor.

allows screening with bioassays, sequencing, mass spectrometry, or high-pressure liquid chromatography (HPLC) investigations. We have sequenced peptides down to the 5-pmol level on a single 30-μm microparticle, and with peptides attached only on the outer surface of 90- and 640-μm particles. A reasonable signal–noise ratio was obtained with a minimum amount of 2–4 pmol peptide/bead (71). The result of this investigation is that on a 30-μm bead the whole amount of peptide is necessary for analysis and identification whereas on particles of >90 μm only the peptide content of the surface is sufficient for sequencing. The capacity per bead and the number of beads per gram resin are strongly dependent on the bead size. Figure 4.7 correlates particle size, capacity per bead, and the number of beads per gram. The amount of 10-

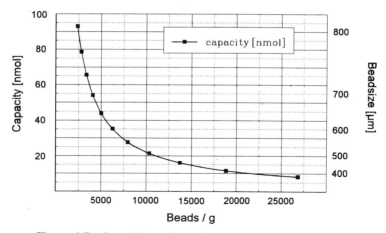

Figure 4.7   Correlation of capacity and number of beads/g resin.

to 90-nmol substance inside the 300- to 800-μm macrobeads allows multiple sequential release with reasonable amounts of substance from one single bead. The released compounds from 90- or 130-μm particles typically yield 1–3 μM solutions (100–300 pmol/100 μL) compared to 1–5 mM solutions (2–10 nmol/200 μL) obtained by five sequential releasing steps on 300 to 800-μm beads. Thus assay sensitivity increases by a factor of 100–1000.

Based on the described polymer, three peptide libraries are synthesized on trifunctional macrobeads: acid-labile amide handle RAM and base-labile HMB are located inside the bead, and amino functions are on the surface (113). Subsequent synthesis of the libraries XXYFKN, PXXFKN, PEXFKN by the split synthesis technique (69,70) results in a trifunctional peptide resin with acid-cleavable peptides, base-cleavable peptides, and noncleavable peptides on the outer surface. Trifluoracetic acid (TFA) treatment deprotects the peptides and creates a soluble peptide library that is screened by a solution assay and a resin bound library.

Sixty beads of the polymer-bound hexapeptide amide library PEXFKN-resin were investigated by an enzyme linked immuno assay (ELISA) and fluorescence assays. Peptide beads were filled in filter tubes (1–8 per vessel); and after washing steps they were incubated with the Mab SN 20, which binds to the HIV 1-Nef protein epitope PEYFKN. Staining of antigen beads was achieved by peroxidase-conjugated antimouse antibody and enzyme substrate tetramethylbenzidine. Blue-colored beads were selected manually by a pair of tweezers. Basic treatment of the selected beads released the peptide from HMB linker. The soluble peptide from each bead was then characterized and identified by HPLC, mass spectroscopy (MS), and amino acid analysis (AAA). Five beads were selected, and the following sequences identified by sequencing of the surface bound peptide: $3 \times$ PEEFKN-NH$_2$, $1 \times$ PEGFKN-NH$_2$ and $1 \times$ PEYFKN-NH$_2$. The amount of peptide immobilized on the surface of a single macrobead is also sufficient for a quantitative ELISA.

Mab SN 20 incubated beads XXYFKN were investigated for interaction with a tetramethylrhodamine-labeled antimouse antibody. ELISA positive beads were detected by confocal laser microscopy, and beads showing surface fluorescence were selected. The peptide sequence was determined following the same procedure as shown above. Competition of peptides mixtures with the biotinylated antigen N-α-biotinyl-N-α-Ac-PEYFKN-Ahx-Ahx-Lys for binding to the Mab SN 20 was achieved with soluble peptide mixtures AC-XXYFKN-NH$_2$, Ac-PXXFKN-NH$_2$, and Ac-PEXFKN-NH$_2$. Streptavidin-coated ELISA plates were incubated with increasing concentrations of acetylated hexapeptide amide mixtures and dose-dependent (0.5 μm–0.5 mg) competition was obtained. Both the solution assay and the resin-bound ELISA indicate that Tyr-3 is not essential for binding, as expected up to now.

For investigations of peptide–oligonucleotide interactions the C-terminal sequence KSGKPKVX$_1$X$_2$A (X_1 = K,L,G,Y,F and X_2 = R,L,G,E,F) of the Hlc histone was synthesized as a sublibrary (114,115). The sublibrary was constructed on trifunctional macrobeads (NH$_2$ on surface, AC and HMB inside) as described above (Fig. 4.6). Acid treatment deprotects the peptides and cleaves off approximately 50% of the peptide. This procedure results in a soluble and a resin-bound peptide library within one synthesis run.

In natural systems histones interact with the DNA. To screen the oligonucleotide interaction with the modified histone sequences, 25 beads of the polymer-bound peptide library were incubated with the fluorescence-labeled oligonucleotide 5′-CAC TCG TTA G-FZ-3′ (Fig. 4.8). To differentiate between the strength of the interaction, single beads were incubated with increasing concentrations of aqueous NaCl. Negative beads or beads with reduced intensity are selected. Release of the peptide by basic treatment, followed by HPLC and MS analysis, identifies the peptides. Hydrophobic amino acids show weak to medium interactions, whereas Tyr always shows strong interaction. Substitution of aromatic amino acid Tyr by the aromatic Phe amino acid results in a weak interaction. This indicates that the activated aromatic system of Tyr interacts with the oligonucleotide by additional mechanism, for example, π-π and charge-transfer interactions (Table 4.7).

In combinatorial chemistry there are in principle two distinct approaches for the construction of libraries: the split-and-pool procedure as described above or by a spatially addressable technique where the compounds are synthesized individually by parallel and often semiautomated synthesis techniques. Reaction screening and optimization are here performed on dozens of individual parallel reactions.

The reduction in reaction volume to the size of one single bead allows one to minimize the amount of required solvents as well as the amount of expensive building blocks to the nanomolar range (114). Combinatorial chemistry methods were applied for the synthesis of a set of hydantoins (Fig. 4.9) on single beads in glass capillaries having 10 cm length and 2.6 mm internal diameter (Fig. 4.10). Even when applying a 100-fold excess of building block, up to 500 reactions can be done with 1 mmol of building block. Typical reaction conditions are: 1–4 single beads are placed in the capillary. The Fmoc-amino acid is hooked to the acid-labile

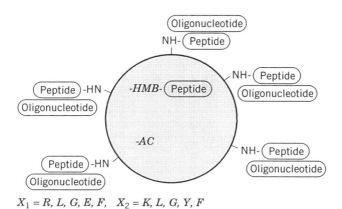

$X_1 = R, L, G, E, F, \quad X_2 = K, L, G, Y, F$

Figure 4.8 Scheme of peptide/oligonucleotide interaction on the resin bound histone sublibrary KSGKPKVX$_1$X$_2$A after acid treatment.

TABLE 4.7 Stability of the Fluorescence-labeled Resin-bound Complex KSGKPKVX$_1$X$_2$A/5'-CACTCGTTAG-FZ-3' Dependent on Increasing Concentrations of NaCl Solution[a]

Histone Sequence KSGKPKVX$_1$X$_2$A	Fluorescence after Wash with 0.2M NaCl Solution			Fluorescence after Wash with 0.5M NaCl Solution			Fluorescence after Wash with 1M NaCl Solution		
	w	m	s	w	m	s	w	m	s
KSGKPKVTKA			XX			XX			XX
KSGKPKVRKA			XX			XX			XX
KSGKPKVRLA			XX	XX			XX		
KSGKPKVRGA			XX			XX		XX	
KSGKPKVRYA			XX			XX			XX
KSGKPKVRFA		XX			XX		XX		
KSGKPKVLKA			XX			XX			XX
KSGKPKVLLA			XX			XX			XX
KSGKPKVLGA	XX	XX		XX	XX		XX	XX	
KSGKPKVLYA		XX			XX			XX	
KSGKPKVLFA			XX			XX		XX	

KSGKPKVGKA			XX			XX			XX
KSGKPKVGLA	XX	XX		XX	XX		XX	XX	
KSGKPKVGGA			XX			XX			XX
KSGKPKVGYA			XX			XX			XX
KSGKPKVGFA	XX	XX		XX	XX		XX	XX	
KSGKPKVEKA		XX			XX			XX	
KSGKPKVELA	XX			XX			XX		
KSGKPKVEGA			XX			XX			XX
KSGKPKVEYA			XX			XX			XX
KSGKPKVEFA			XX		XX			XX	
KSGKPKVFKA			XX			XX			XX
KSGKPKVFLA			XX			XX		XX	
KSGKPKVFGA	XX	XX		XX	XX		XX	XX	
KSGKPKVFYA			XX			XX			XX
KSGKPKVFFA	XX			XX			XX		

[a]w = weak, m = medium, and s = strong.

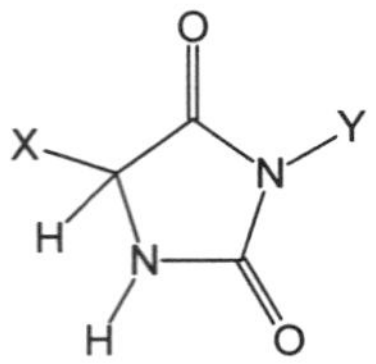

Figure 4.9 Hydantoin.

AC handle; 20 μL of a 1*M* isocyanate solution in DMF is transferred into the capillary, and the reaction is performed for 3 h without using protecting gas for prevention of moisture. Cleavage and condensation were done simultaneously by treatment with 6*M* HCl in water at 100°C for 45 min or by 4*M* HCl in THF at room temperature for 120 min (Fig. 4.9, Table 4.8). The formation of each resin-bound compound was controlled during synthesis and identified on each single bead by gel-phase ¹H-NMR (Fig. 4.11) and Fourier transform–infrared (FT-IR) using the ATR (attenuated total reflectance, Fig. 4.12) technique or photoacoustic spectroscopy (PAS, Fig. 4.13). Photoacoustic spectroscopy is a very powerful technique because it is absolutely free of any damage to the bead. In contrast to the ATR technique, where the IR beam can penetrate into the bead for ~1–2 μm, by photoacoustic spectroscopy technique the IR beam penetrates 30–40 μm into the resin bead resulting in more intensive resonance signal. After release and cyclization of the hydantoins from each single bead, the compounds were analyzed and

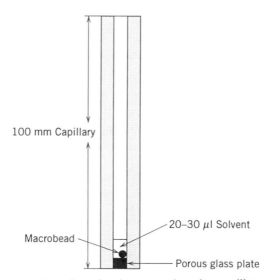

Figure 4.10   Single beaded polymeric microreactor in a glass capillary of 2.6 mm diameter.

TABLE 4.8 Set of Hydantoins Synthesized on Individual TentaGel Micro Reactors

Compound	X	Y
Hydantoin 1	Benzyl	Phenyl
Hydantoin 2	Benzyl	Propyl
Hydantoin 3	Benzyl	Phenylethyl
Hydantoin 4	H	Phenyl
Hydantoin 5	H	Propyl
Hydantoin 6	H	Phenylethyl
Hydantoin 7	Isopropyl	Phenyl
Hydantoin 8	Isopropyl	Propyl
Hydantoin 10	Isopropyl	Phenylethyl

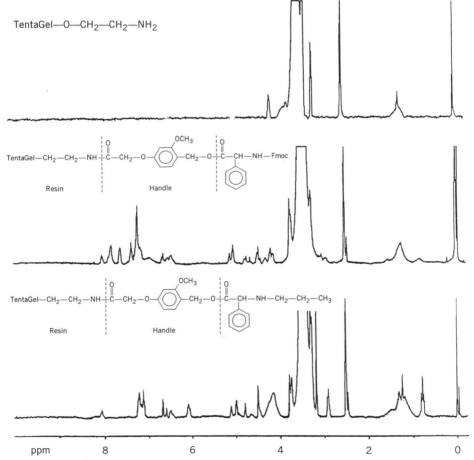

Figure 4.11 Reaction sequence followed by gel-phase MAS ^{1}H-NMR of one single bead. Conditions: Bruker NMR spectrometer A6-300, rotor 4 mm (modified), spinning frequence: 2000 Hz, solvent CDCl$_3$, scans 256.

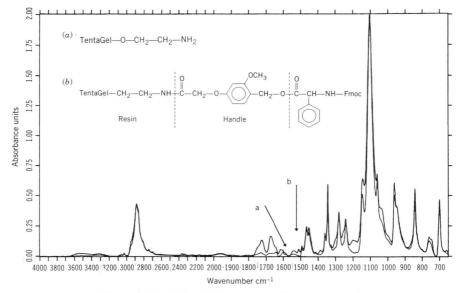

Figure 4.12 ATR FT-IR spectrum from single bead.

characterized by HPLC (Fig. 4.14a), gas chromatography-mass spectroscopy (GC-MS) (Fig. 4.14b), and ion cyclotron resonance (ICR) spectrometry. ICR spectroscopy is a high-resolution MS technique that allows the detection of masses with extremely high accuracy (Fig. 4.15, calculated: 267.113 m/z, found 267.107 m/z).

One of the key steps in all combinatorial approaches is chemical analysis and

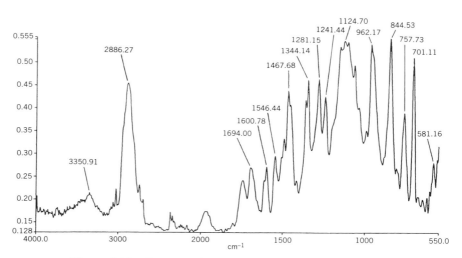

Figure 4.13 Photoacoustic FT-IR spectrum from two beads.

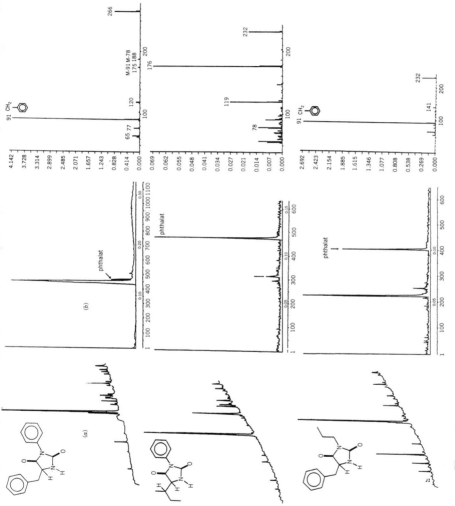

Figure 4.14 (a) HPLC and (b) GC-MS of crude hydantoins synthesized on single beads (phthalat impurities from sealings).

87

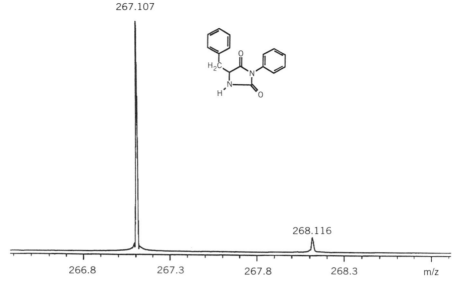

Figure 4.15   High-resolution ICR mass spectrum.

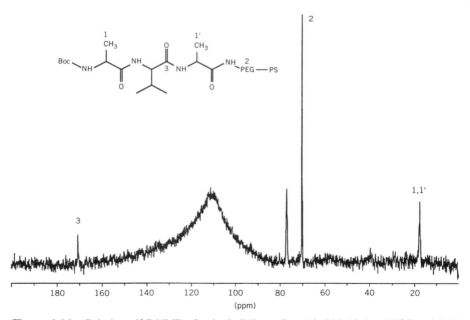

Figure 4.16   Gel-phase ^{13}C-NMR of a single 740-μm Boc-Ala-Val-Ala bead [^{13}C-enriched alanine (CH$_3$) and valine (CO)]. Conditions: Bruker 600 MHz, scans 5920, solvent CDCl$_3$, temp. 298 K.

structural identification of "hits" within a library. Identification by indirect methods such as tagging or encoding has been proposed. An alternative way may be the direct identification of the ligand on the resin by the combination of different spectroscopic methods, for example, gel-phase proton NMR on single beads as shown in Figure 4.11, FT-IR spectroscopy on single beads (101), as well as MAS ^{13}C-NMR spectroscopy. As an example a ^{13}C-enriched tripeptide was synthesized on macrobeads and one bead was analyzed by MAS ^{13}C-NMR spectroscopy. A standard tube was simply modified by introducing Teflon plugs to fix the bead at the right position in magnetic field. Figure 4.16 shows the resulting NMR spectrum. The broad peak at 140–90 ppm is caused by the Teflon plugs.

ACKNOWLEDGMENTS

The author greatly acknowledges the NMR group of K. Albert, G. Schlotterbeck, and M. Pursch, University of Tübingen, for their NMR work. He also thanks G. Nicholson, University of Tübingen, J. Metzger, University of Stuttgart, and G. Baykut, Bruker for the mass spectroscopy as well as A. Rau, Perkin-Elmer, for photoacoustic measurement.

REFERENCES

1. Merrifield, R. B., *Fed. Proc., Fed. Am. Soc. Exp. Biol.* **21,** 412 (1962).

2. Merrifield, R. B., *J. Am. Chem. Soc.* **85,** 2149 (1963).

3. Marshall, G. R., and Merrifield, R. B., in *Biochemical Aspects of Reactions on Solid Supports,* Academic, New York, 1971.

4. Barny, G., and Merrifield, R. B., *The Peptides,* Vol. 2, Academic, New York, 1980.

5. Letsinger, R. L., Finnan, J. L., Heavner, G. A., and Lunsford, W. B., *J. Am. Chem. Soc.* **97,** 3278 (1975).

6. Uhlmann, E., and Peyman, A., *Chem. Rev.* **90,** 543 (1990).

7. Engels, J. W., and Uhlmann, E. *Angew. Chemie Int. Ed. Engl.* **28,** 716 (1989).

8. Grubbs, R. H., and Kroll, L. C., *J. Am. Chem. Soc.* **93,** 3062 (1971).

9. Pittmann Jr., C. U., and Smith, L. R., *J. Am. Chem. Soc.* **97** 1749 (1975).

10. Pittmann Jr., C. U., Smith, L. R., and Hanes, R. M. *J. Am. Chem. Soc.* **97,** 742 (1975).

11. Grubbs, R. H., *Chem. Techn.,* **7**(8), 512 (1977).

12. Chaurin, Y., Commerenc, D., and Dawens, F., *Prog. Polym. Sci.* **5,** 95 (1977).

13. Kubanov, V. A., and Smetanyuk, V. J., *Makromol. Chem. Phys.,* Suppl. **5,** 121 (1981).

14. Manecke, G., and Storck, W., *Angew. Chem.* **90,** 682 (1978).

15. Pittmann Jr., C. U., in *Comprehensive Organometallic Chemistry,* Vol. 8, G. Wilkinson (Ed.), Pergamon, Oxford, 1982, p. 553.

16. Kaneko, M., and Tsuchida, E., *Macromol. Rev.* **16,** 397 (1981).

17. Orth, H. D., and Brummer, W., *Angew. Chem.* **84,** 314 (1972).

18. Weetall, H. H., *Chemiker Zeitung* **97,** 611 (1973).

19. Manecke, G., *Chimia* **28,** 467 (1974).

20. Chibata, J., in *Immobilized Enzymes,* Wiley, New York, 1978, pp. 9–142.

21. Manecke, G., Ehrenthal, E., and Schlünsen, J., in *Characterization of Immobilized Biocatalysts,* K. Buchholz (Ed.), Schön u. Wetzel GmbH, Frankfurt, 1979, pp. 49–109.

22. Scharma, B. P., Baily, L. F., and Messing, R. A., *Angew. Chem.* **94,** 836 (1982).

23. Goldstein, L., and Manecke, G., in *Applied Biochemistry and Bioengeneering,* L. S. Wingard Jr., E. Katchalski-Kutzir, and L. Goldstein (Eds.), Academic, New York, 1976, pp. 23–110.

24. J. F. Kennedy, in *Solid Phase Biochemistry, Analytical and Synthetic Aspects,* W. H. Scouten (Ed.), Wiley, New York, 1983, pp. 257–361.

25. Poralla, K., Biotechnol., Presentation at Hauptversammlung MNU, 74th, pp. 21 ff. (1983).

26. Rosevear, A., *J. Chem. Technol. Biotechnol.* **34B**(3), 127 (1984).

27. Attiyat, A. S., and Christian, G. D., *Am. Biotechnol. Lab.* **2**(2), 12–16 (1984).

28. Fyles, T. M., and Lenzoff, C. C., *Can. J. Chem.* **54,** 935 (1975).

29. Crosby, G. A., Weinshenker, N. M., and Uh, H. S., *J. Am. Chem. Soc.* **97,** 2232 (1974).

30. Weinshenker, N. M., and Shen, C. M., *Terahedron Lett.,* (32), 3285 (1972).

31. Daly, W. H. *Makromol. Chem. Suppl.* **180,** 3 (1979).

32. Overberger, C. G., and Sannes, K. N., *Angew. Chem.* **86,** 139 (1974).

33. Akelah, A., and Sherrington, D. C., *Polymer* **24,** 1369 (1983).

34. Atherton, E., and Sheppard, R. C., in *Peptides 1974,* Y. Wolman (Ed.), Halsted, New York, 1975, pp. 123–127.

35. Small, P. W., and Sherrington, D. C., *J. Chem. Soc. Chem. Commun.,* 1589–1591 (1989).

36. Bayer, E., Hemmasi, B., Albert, K., Rapp, W., and Dengler, M., in *Peptides: Structure and Function,* V. J. Hruby and D.ˇH. Rich (Eds.), Pierce Chemical Company, Rockford, Ill., 1983, pp. 87–89.

37. Butwell, F. G. W., Haws, E. J., and Epton, R., *Macromol. Chem. Macromol. Symp.* **19,** 69–77 (1986).

38. Atherton, E., Brown, E., and Sheppard, R. C., *J. Chem. Soc. Chem. Commun.,* **21,** 1151–1152 (1981).

39. Mutter, M., Hagenmaier, H., and Bayer, E., *Angew. Chem.* **83,** 883 (1991).

40. Bayer, E., and Mutter, M. *Nature (London)* **237,** 512 (1971).

41. Mutter, M., and Bayer, E., in *The Peptides,* Vol. 2, Academic, E. Gross and J. Meienhofer (Eds.), New York, 1970, p. 285.

42. Mutter, M., Uhmann, R., and Bayer, E., *Liebigs Ann. Chem.,* **2,** 901 (1975).

43. Bayer, E., Mutter, M., Uhmann, R., Polster, J., and Mauser, H., *J. Am. Chem. Soc.* **96,** 7333 (1974).

44. Mutter, M., and Bayer, E., *Angew. Chem. Int. Ed. Engl.* **13,** 149 (1974).

45. Warshavsky, A., Kaliv, R., Doshe, A., Berkovitz, H., and Patchornik, A., *J. Am. Chem. Soc.* **101,** 4249 (1979).

46. Bayer, E., and Rapp, W., in *Chemistry of Peptides and Proteins,* Vol. 3, W. Voelter,

E. Bayer, Yu. A. Ovchinnikov, and V. T. Ivanov (Eds.), Walter de Gruyter, Berlin, 1986, pp. 3–8.

47. Bayer, E., and Rapp, W., *Dtsch. Offen.* DE 3,500,180, C.A. **106,** p. 50859 (1985).

48. Bayer, E., *Angew. Chem. Int. Ed. Engl.* **30,** 113 (1991).

49. Bayer, E., and Rapp, W., in *Poly(Ethylene Glycol) Chemistry: Biotechnical and Biomedical Application*, M. Harris (Ed.), Plenum, New York, 1992, pp. 325–345.

50. TentaGel, registered trademark of Rapp Polymere GmbH, Tübingen.

51. Bayer, E., *Nachr. Chem. Techn.* **20,** 495 (1972).

52. Tsuchida, E., Nishide, H., Shimidazu, N., Yamada, A., and Keneko, M., *Makromol. Chem. Rapid Comm.* **2,** 621 (1981).

53. Zalipsky, S., Albericio, M., and Barany, G., in *Peptides, Chemistry and Biology*, C. Deber, V. J. Hruby, and K. D. Kopple (Eds.), Proceedings of the Ninth American Peptide Symposium, Pierce Chemical Company, Rockford, Ill., 1985, pp. 257–260.

54. Bayer, E., Hemmasi, B., Albert, K., Rapp, W., and Dengler, M., in *Peptides: Structures and Function*, V. J. Hruby and D. H. Rich (Eds.), Pierce Chemical Company, Rockford, Ill., 1983, p. 87.

55. Bayer, E., and Rapp, W., German Patent DOS 3 714 258, 1988.

56. Bayer, E., Dengler, M., and Hemmasi, B., *Int. J. Pept. Protein Res.* **25,** 178 (1985).

57. Bayer, E., and Rapp, W., in *Chemistry of Peptides and Proteins*, W. Voelter, E. Bayer, Y. A. Ovchinnikov, and V. I. Ivanov (Eds.), Walter de Gruyter, Berlin, 1986, p. 3.

58. Bayer, E., Hellstern, H., and Eckstein, H., *Z. Naturforsch.* **42c.,** 455 (1987).

59. Rapp, W., Zhang, L., Häbich, R., and Bayer, E., in *Peptides 1988*, Proceedings of the 20th European Peptide Symposium, G. Jung and E. Bayer (Eds.), Walter de Gruyter, Berlin, 1989, p. 199.

60. Rapp, W., Ph.D Thesis, 1985, University of Tüebingen.

61. Bayer, E., Albert, K., Willisch, H., Rapp, W., and Hemmasi, B., *Macromolecules* **23,** 1937 (1990).

62. Look, G. C., Holmes, C. P., Chinn, J. P., and Gallap, M. A., *J. Org. Chem.* **59,** 7588–7590 (1994).

63. Fitch, W. L., Detre, G., and Holmes, C. P., *J. Org. Chem.* **59,** 7955–7956 (1994).

64. Kiefer, P. A., *J. Org. Chem.* **61,** 1558 (1996).

65. Rudinger, J., and Buetzer, P., in *Peptides 1974*, J. Wolman (Ed.), Wiley, New York, 1975, p. 211.

66. Bayer, E., and Rapp, W., in *Poly(Ethyleneglycol) Chemistry: Biotechnical and Biomedical Application*, M. Harris (Ed.), Plenum, New York, 1992, pp. 325–344.

67. Hori, T., Rapp, W., and Bayer, E., *Proceedings of the 30th Symposium on Chemistry of Dying*, Osaka, Japan, 1988, p. 42.

68. Hori, T., Rapp, W., and Bayer, E., unpublished results, University of Tüebingen.

69. (a) Furka, A., Sebestyén, M., Asgedom, M., Dibó, G., *Int. J. Pept. Prot. Res.*, **37,** 487 (1991); (b) Furka, A., Sebestyén, M., Asgedom, M., Dibó, G., 14th Int. Cong. of Biochem., Prague, 1988.

70. Salmon, S. E., Hersh, E. M., Hruby, V. J., Kazncierski, W. M., and Knapp, R. J., *Nature* **354,** 82–84 (1991).

71. Rapp, W., and Gnau, V., unpublished results, University of Tüebingen.

72. Rapp, W., unpublished results, University of Tüebingen.

73. Rapp, W., and Bayer, E., in: *Innovations and Perspectives in Solid Phase Synthesis, Peptides, Polypeptides and Oligonucleotides,* R. Epton (Ed.), Intercept, Andover, 1992, p. 259.

74. Rapp, W., Fritz, H., and Bayer, E., in *Peptides, Chemistry and Biology,* J. A. Smith and J. E. Rivier (Eds.), Proceedings of the Twelfth American Peptide Symposium, ESCOM Science Publishers B.V., Leiden, 1992, p. 529.

75. Bayer, E., and Goldammer, C., in *Peptides, Chemistry and Biology,* J. A. Smith and J. E. Rivier (Eds.), Proceedings of the Twelfth American Peptide Symposium, ESCOM Science Publishers B.V., Leiden, 1992, p. 589.

76. Lebl, M., Krchñák, V. Sepetov, N. F., Seligmann, B., and Felder, S., *Biopolymers* (Peptide Sience) **37,** 177–198 (1995).

77. Salmon, S. E., Lam, K. S., Lebl, M., Kandola, A., Khattri, P. S., Wade, S., Pátek, M., Kocis, P., Krchñák, V., Thorpe, D., and Felder, S., *Proc. Natl. Acad. Sci. USA* (*Chem.*) **90,** 11708–11712 (1993).

78. Lebl, M., Krchñák, V., Salmon, S. E., and Lam, K. S., *Methods: A Companion to Methods in Enzymology* **6,** 381–387 (1994).

79. Lam, K. S., Zhao, Z., Wade, S., Krchñák, V., and Lebl, M., *Drug. Devel. Res.* **33,** 157–160 (1994).

80. Nikolaiev, V., Stierandová, A., Krchñák, V., Seligmann, B., Lam, K. S., Salmon, S. E., and Lebl, M., *Peptide Res.* **6,** 161–170 (1993).

81. Lebl, M., Pátek, M., Kocis, P., Krchñák, V., Hruby, V., Salmon, S. E., and Lam, K. S., *Int. J. Pept. Prot. Res.* **41,** 201–203 (1993).

82. Vágner, J., Krchñák V., Sepetov, N. F., Strop, P., Lam, K. S., Barany, G., and Lebl, M., in *Innovation and Perspectives in Solid Phase Synthesis and Related Technologies,* R. Epton (Ed.), collected papers, Third International Symposium, Mayflower Worldwide Ltd., Birmingham, 1994, p. 347.

83. Lebl, M., Krchñák, V., Sepetov, N. F., Nikolaiev, V., Stierandová, A., Safar, P., Seligmann, B., Strop, P., Lam, K. S., and Salmon, S. E., in *Innovation and Perspectives in Solid Phase Synthesis and Related Technologies,* R. Epton (Ed.), collected papers, Third International Symposium, Mayflower Worldwide Ltd., Birmingham, 1994, p. 233.

84. Lebl, M., Krchñák, V., Safar, P., Stierandová, A., Sepetov, N. F., Kocis, P., and Lam, K. S., *Techn. Protein Chem.* **5,** 541–548 (1994).

85. Nikolaiev, V., Stierandová, A., Krchñák, V., Seligmann, B., Lam, K. S., Salmon, S. E., and Lebl, M., *Peptide Res.* **6,** 161–170 (1993).

86. Lebl, M., Pátek, M., Kocis, P., Krchñák, V., Hruby, V., Salmon, S. E., and Lam, K. S., *Int. J. Peptide Protein Res.* **41,** 201–203 (1993).

87. Kocis, P., Krchñák, V., and Lebl, M., *Tetrahedron Lett.* **34,** 7251–7252 (1993).

88. Salmon, S. E., Lam, K. S., Lebl, M., Kandola, A., Khattri, P. S., Wade, S., Pátek, M., Kocis, P., Krchñák V., Thorpe, D., and Felder, S., *Proc. Natl. Acad. Sci. USA* (*Chem.*) **90,** 11708–11712 (1993).

89. Torneiro, M., and Still, W. C., *J. Am. Chem. Soc.* **117,** 5887–5888 (1995).

90. Wennemers, H., and Still, W. C., *Tetrahedron Lett.* **35,** 6413–6416 (1994).

91. Youngquist, R. S., Fuentes, G. R., Lacey, M. P., and Keough, T., *J. Am. Chem. Soc.* **117,** 3900–3906 (1995).

92. Wenschuh, H., Beyermann, M., Rothemund, S., Carpino, L. A., and Bienert, M., *Tetrahedron Lett.* **36,** 1247–1250 (1995).

93. Youngquist, R. S., Fuentes, G. R., Lacey, M. P., and Keough, T., *J. Am. Chem. Soc.* **117,** 3900–3906 (1995).

94. Baldwin, J. J., Burbaum, J. J., Henderson, I., and Ohlmeyer, M. H. J., *J. Am. Chem. Soc,* **117,** 5589 (1995).

95. Virgilo, A. A., and Ellman, J. A., *J. Am. Chem. Soc.* **116,** 11580–11581 (1994).

96. Fenniri, H., Janda, K. D., and Lerner, R. A., *Proc. Natl. Acad. Sci, USA (Chem.)* **92,** 2278–2282 (1995).

97. Forman, F. W., and Sucholeiki, I., *J. Org. Chem.* **60,** 523–528 (1995).

98. Look, G. C., Murphy, M. M., Campbell, D. A., and Gallop, M. A., *Tetrahedron Lett.* **36,** 2937–3940 (1995).

99. Rano, T. A., and Chapman, K. T., *Tetrahedron Lett.* **36,** 3789–3792 (1995).

100. Krchňák, V., Flegelová, Z., Weichsel, A. S., and Lebl, M., *Tetrahedron Lett.* **36,** 6193–6196 (1995).

101. Yan, B., Kumaravel, G., Anjaria, H., Wu, A., Petter, R. C., Jewell Jr., C. F., and Wareing, J. R., *J. Org. Chem.* **60,** 5736–5738 (1995).

102. Hauske, J. R., and Dorff, P., *Tetrahedron Lett.* **36,** 1589–1592 (1995).

103. Pátek, M., Drake, B., and Lebl, M., *Tetrahedron Lett.* **36,** 2227–2230 (1995).

104. Sucholeiki, I., *Tetrahedron Lett.* **35,** 7307–7310 (1994).

105. Pátek, M., Drake, B., and Lebl, M., *Tetrahedron Lett.* **35,** 9169–9172 (1994).

106. Nielsen, J., Brenner, S., and Janda, K. D., in *Proceedings of the 14th American Peptide Symposium,* P. T. P. Kaumaya and R. S. Hodges (Eds.), Columbus, OH 1995, pp. 92–93.

107. Forman, F. W., and Sucholeiki, I., *J. Org. Chem.* **60,** 523–528 (1995).

108. Baldwin, J. J., Burbaum, J. J., Henderson, I., and Ohlmeyer, M. H. J., *J. Am. Chem. Soc.* **117,** 5588–5589 (1995).

109. Campbell, D. A., Bermak, J. C., Burkoth, T. S., and Patel, D. V., *J. Am. Chem. Soc.* **117,** 5381–5382 (1995).

110. Murphy, M. M., Schullek, J. R., Gordon, E. M., and Gallop, M. A., *J. Am. Chem. Soc.* **117,** 7029–7030 (1995).

111. Nicolaou, K. C., Xiao, X., Parandoosh, Z., Senyei, A., and Nova, M. P., *Angew. Chem., Int. Ed. Engl.* **107,** 2476–2479 (1995).

112. Burbaum, J. J., Ohlmeyer, M. H. J., Reader, J. C., Henderson, I., Dillard, L. W., Li, G., Randle, T. L., Sigal, N. H., Chelsky, D., and Baldwin, J. J., *Proc. Natl. Acad. Sci. USA (Pharmacology)* **92,** 6027–6031 (1995).

113. Rapp, W., Zhang, L., Müller, C., Zühl, F., Wiesmüller, K. H., Jung, G., and Bayer, E., in *Innovations and Perspectives in Solid Phase Synthesis, Peptides, Proteins and Nucleic Acids,* Proceedings of the 3rd International Symposium 1993, R. Epton (Ed.), Mayflower Worldwide, Birmingham, 1994, p. 197.

114. Rapp, W., Maier, M., Schlotterbeck, G., Pursch, M., Albert, K., and Bayer, E., in *Peptides, Chemistry and Biology,* Proceedings of the 14th American Peptide Symposium, P. T. P. Kaumaya and R. S. Hodges (Eds.), Columbus, OH 1995.

5

COMBINATORIAL LIBRARIES IN SOLUTION: POLYFUNCTIONALIZED CORE MOLECULES

EDWARD A. WINTNER AND JULIUS REBEK, JR.

Skaggs Institute for Chemical Biology, The Scripps Research Institute, La Jolla, California 92037

5.1 INTRODUCTION

The screening of organic substances to discover lead compounds of pharmaceutical interest has traditionally involved the testing of individual compounds of high purity. Compounds are synthesized and assayed one at a time, a process that, though successful, is labor intensive. The advent of techniques of combinatorial chemistry offers the means to generate a large number of different chemicals simultaneously, allowing rapid access to vast numbers of new chemical entities. Modern analytical methods allow the screening of such combinatorial libraries to select those species in the generated pool that possess desirable properties (1). The first attempts at combinatorial synthesis involved peptides and include the "pin method" devised by Geysen et al. (2) and the "tea bag" procedure invented in the Houghten group (3). Both techniques allow the preparation of up to 300 individual peptides at the same time. With the introduction of the "split-bead technology" of Furka et al. (4,5), the parallel synthesis of peptides was increased dramatically to several million compounds in a library of molecules supported on polymer beads. As a result, the limiting factor in the successful screening of peptide libraries has become the characterization of active species; the amount of any individual compound present in a library of millions is too minute for its structure to be determined using conventional spectrometric methods (6) [see, however, methods of structure determination by coding schemes, i.e., molecular tags (7)].

Peptides, however, have several drawbacks as drug candidates, most notably their flexible, linear shape and their susceptibility to enzymatic cleavage in vivo.

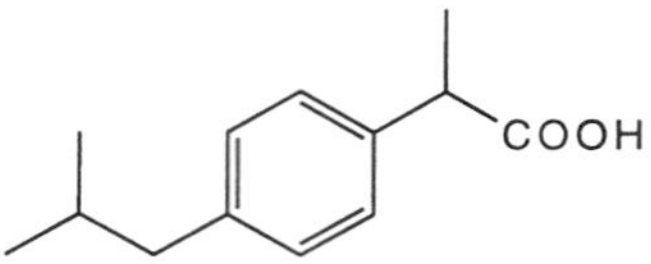

Figure 5.1 The drug ibuprofen.

While the latter may be overcome by incorporating nonnatural building blocks such as D-amino acids, the former characteristic is intrinsic to peptides. By nature, a peptide is a chain that must fold into a specific conformation to achieve a bioactive structure. Most of today's drugs, however, are much more rigid, with the positioning of their functionalities set by a well-defined carbon or heterocyclic skeleton. Ibuprofen (Fig. 5.1) is a very simple example, with two flexible moieties attached to a benzene backbone. Such a skeleton overcomes much of the entropy barrier that looms before any unfolded peptide, instantly conferring an active shape to the drug's functional groups.

A major challenge to researchers in the field of combinatorial chemistry has thus become the application of combinatorial methods to produce small, drug-related molecules. The current list of successes includes benzodiazepines (8), peptoids (9), oligocarbamates (10), and other synthetic compounds recently termed "diversomers" (11,12). The synthesis, characterization, and screening of the polyfunctionalized molecules produced in our group will be the subject of this chapter.

5.2 SYNTHESIS OF LIBRARIES

The ideal combinatorial method for the discovery of pharmaceutically valuable chemicals would produce large libraries of small organic molecules with a drug-related structure, yet would still lend itself to rapid synthesis, screening, and compound structure determination. We recently reported a procedure that approaches this goal of the ideal library (13,14). The idea behind our method of generating libraries of small organic molecules is summarized in Figure 5.2: Combine a rigid core molecule supporting multiple reactive sites with a mixture of building blocks to produce a random mixture of polyfunctionalized structures. To illustrate, a molecule such as cubane tetra acid chloride (Fig. 5.3) could be combined with four molar equivalents of an equimolar mixture of amines A–Z to produce tetra-substituted cubane compounds A,A,A,A through Z,Z,Z,Z.

This method of library generation has several advantages. First, it is a powerful method of generating molecular diversity; in a single combinatorial step, the cubane core **1** and 26 amines A–Z would produce theoretically 38,701 different cubane tetra amides. Second, unlike some methods of generating peptide libraries [the split-bead method, e.g. (4,5)], these compounds are not on a solid support but free in solution. This allows assaying of the compounds without worry of the solid support giving artifactual results. Third, the molecules all have a rigid carbon backbone as

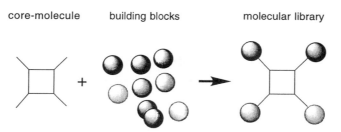

Figure 5.2 Schematic representation of the procedure used to generate libraries of small organic molecules.

defined by the core molecule. This scaffold determines the basic shape of the compounds and can range from a very symmetrical cubane core to a completely asymmetric carbon or heterocyclic skeleton. If a particular bioassay is known to be predisposed to a certain molecular shape or pharmacophore, a suitably configured core molecule may be chosen. Finally, this combinatorial strategy allows for the

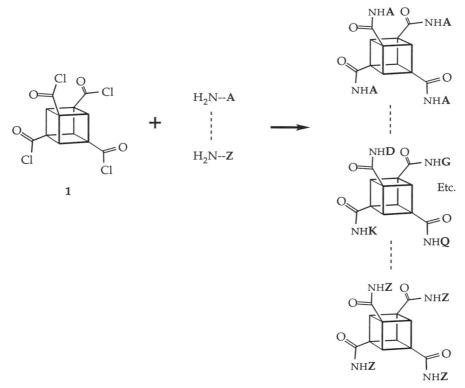

Figure 5.3 Synthesis of a combinatorial library from cubane core **1** and amines A–Z.

display of a nearly limitless variety of functionalities, as determined by the building blocks used. In the example in Figure 5.3, one could make use of hundreds of commercially available amines as building blocks.

This method of generating small-molecule libraries has two drawbacks, both of which are surmountable. First, since compounds are generated in a single solution (not in wells or on beads as in some schemes), a method of screening must be employed that can assay a large mixture of molecules and eventually select one or more individual compounds of highest activity. As described later in detail, we designed an iterative screening procedure modeled after Houghten et al. (15) that was successful in this regard. A second problem is that not all building blocks will be compatible with the reactive sites of a given core molecule; for instance, lysine **2** (Fig. 5.4) might react with cubane tetra acid chloride at the lysine amino terminus, carboxy terminus, or at its amine side chain. This problem was easily circumvented by protecting potentially active sites during the combinatorial step and then deprotecting afterward in a second step. Lysine, for example, could be introduced as **3,** and after reaction with the core, the *t*-butyl and Boc groups could be removed with trifluoroacetic acid.

In our initial studies we investigated three core molecules: the three acid chlorides **1, 4,** and **5** shown in Figures 5.3 and 5.5. The compact, highly symmetric cubane core **1** displays its four acid chloride groups in a tetrahedral array, while the larger xanthene core molecule **4** is planar in overall shape. The less rigid benzene triacetic acid chloride **5** sweeps out a different shape space than either the xanthene or cubane in orientation of its functional groups.

The cubane compound **1** was prepared from cubane monoacid by photolysis in oxalyl chloride (16). The xanthene **4** was prepared from commercial xanthenone via methylation of the 9 position (toluene, trimethylaluminium, 12 h, room temperature, 95% yield), followed by tetrabromination (Br$_2$, cat. Fe powder, CH$_2$Cl$_2$, 2h, 20°C, 4 h reflux, 98% yield). Br/CN exchange (CuCN, N-methyl-2-pyrrolidinone, 2 h, reflux; 20% nitric acid 10 h, reflux, 98% yield) and subsequent hydrolysis of the tetracyano compound (NaOH, water, 14 h, reflux, 98% yield) provided 9,9-dimethyl xanthene-2,4,5,7-tetracarboxylic acid, which was converted to the tetra acid chloride with oxalyl chloride [CH$_2$Cl$_2$, cat. dimethylformamide (DMF), reflux, 4 h]. The benzene compound **5** was prepared from 1,3,5-*tris*-carboxymethylbenzene (17) with oxalyl chloride (CH$_2$Cl$_2$, cat. DMF, reflux, 4 h).

The theoretical number of different molecules created by reaction of an acid chloride core with a mixture of amine nucleophiles under ideal reaction conditions (identical reactivity and equimolarity of all building blocks) can be calculated from

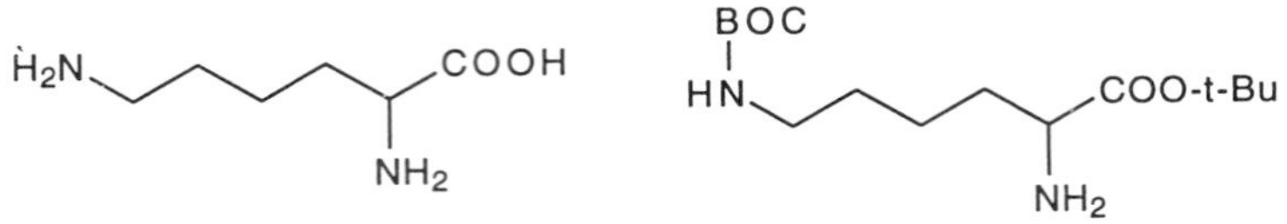

Figure 5.4 Lysine and its protected equivalent.

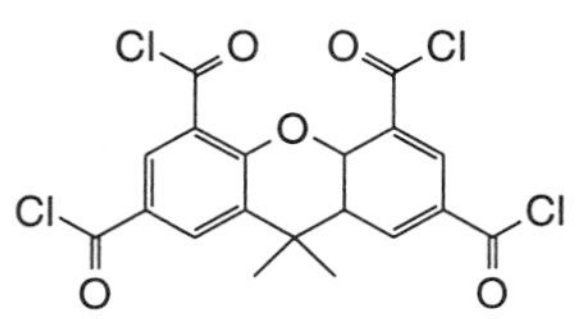

4 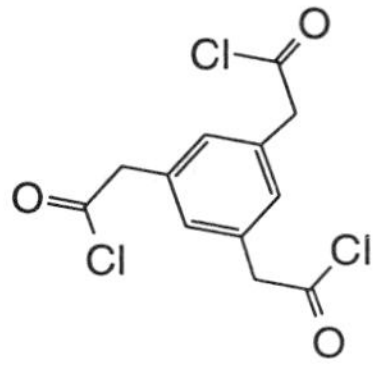   **5**

Figure 5.5 Two aromatic core molecules used for the generation of diverse molecular libraries.

the combinatorial rule* (18) and a set of symmetry factors. These factors depend on the symmetry of the core and are determined individually for each core; the higher the symmetry of the core structure, the fewer compounds are generated with a given set of building blocks. For example, 21 different building blocks combined with the highly symmetric cubane core molecule generate theoretically 16,611 possible compounds, while the same building blocks, when combined with the xanthene core, generate theoretically 97,461 compounds.

For the preparation of the libraries, a two-step procedure of synthesis and deprotection was employed (13,14). First, one equivalent of each acid chloride core molecule was reacted with three or four equivalents (depending on the number of acid chlorides on the core) of an amine mixture. The amine mixtures contained equimolar mixtures of 4–21 of the building blocks listed in Table 5.1 (set 1 and later in set 2). With a few exceptions, these building blocks were L-amino acid derivatives, although clearly a wide variety of nucleophiles could be used in this context. The L-amino acids represent a natural set of biologically relevant functionalities commercially available in their protected forms and were therefore selected to establish a methodology for our scheme.

In order to extend the diversity of functional groups that were introduced into our libraries, we used three non-amino acid derived amines: p-methoxybenzylamine, furfurylamine, and N-methylpyrrol-2-ethylamine. In addition, four amino acids were further functionalized at their carboxyl termini by reaction of the 9-fluorenyl-

---

*Calculation of the theoretical number of tetra-functionalized compounds produced with xanthene core **2** and m building blocks is shown in the table below (libraries **L1–L4**). The total number of compounds equals the sum of the number of compounds with one (AAAA), two (AABB, AAAB), three (AABC), and four (ABCD) different building blocks.

Combination Type	C_{2v} Symmetry Multiplier	Combinatorial Rule (19)	Combinations for $m =$			
			4	7	12	21
AAAA	1	$m!/1!(m-1)!$	4	7	12	21
AAAB/AABB	8	$m!/2!(m-2)!$	48	168	528	1,680
AABC	18	$m!/3!(m-3)!$	72	630	3,960	23,940
ABCD	12	$m!/4!(m-4)!$	12	420	5,940	71,820
		Total combinations	136	1,225	10,440	97,461

TABLE 5.1   List of Amine Building Blocks Used to Create Libraries[a]

Set 1:	L-alanine-methyl ester (Ala), N^g-4-methoxy-2,3,6-trimethylbenzene-sulfonyl-L-arginine-*p*-methoxy-benzylamide (ArgA), O^4-*tert*-butyl-L-aspartic acid methyl ester (Asp), *S*-trityl-L-cysteine-benzylamide (CysA), Furfurylamine (Fur), O^5-*tert*-butyl-L-glutamic acid methyl ester (Glu), N^{im}-trityl-L-histidine-*n*-propylamide (His), L-isoleicine-*tert*-butyl ester (Ile), L-leucine-methyl ester (Leu), N^ϵ-Boc-L-lysine-methyl ester (Lys), L-methionine-methyl ester (Met), 4-methoxybenzyl-amine (Mba), *N*-methylpyrrol-2-ethylamine (Pyr), L-phenylalanine-methyl ester (Phe), L-proline-methyl ester (Pro), *O*-*tert*-butyl-L-serine-methyl ester (Ser), *O*-*tert*-butyl-L-threonine-methyl ester (Thr), L-tryptophane-methyl ester (Trp), *O*-*tert*-butyl-L-tyrosine-methyl ester (Tyr), L-valine-cyclohexylamide (ValA), L-valine-methyl ester (Val).
Set 2:	L-alanine-*tert*-butyl ester (Ala), N^g-4-methoxy-2,3,6-trimethylbenzene-sulfonyl-L-arginine (Arg), L-asparagine-*tert*-butyl ester (Asn), O^4-*tert*-butyl-L-aspartic acid *tert*-butyl ester (Asp), *S*-trityl-L-cysteine (Cys), O^5-*tert*-butyl-L-glutamic acid *tert*-butyl ester (Glu), glycine-methyl ester (Gly), N^{im}-trityl-L-histidine (His), L-isoleucine-*tert*-butyl ester (Ile), L-leucine-*tert*-butyl ester (Leu), N^ϵ-Boc-L-lysine-methyl ester (Lys), L-methionine-methyl ester (Met), L-phenylalanine-*tert*-butyl ester (Phe), L-proline-*tert*-butyl ester (Pro), *O*-*tert*-butyl-L-serine-*tert*-butyl ester (Ser), *O*-*tert*-butyl-L-threonine-methyl ester (Thr), L-tryptophane-methyl ester (Trp), *O*-*tert*-butyl-L-tyrosine-methyl ester (Tyr), L-valine-*tert*-butyl ester (Val).

[a]Set 1: Building blocks used to prepare libraries for HPLC analysis. Set 2: Building blocks used to prepare libraries for mass spectrometric investigations and screening purposes.

methoxycarbonyl (FMOC)-protected amino acids: Fmoc-Arg(Mtr)-OH, Fmoc-Cys(Trt)-OH, Fmoc-His(Trt)-OH, and Fmoc-Val-OH with *p*-methoxybenzylamine, benzylamine, *n*-propylamine, and cyclohexylamine, respectively [DMF, benzo-triazole-1-yl-oxy-tris-(dimethylamino)-phosphonium-hexafluorophosphate (BOP), triethylamine]. Subsequent cleavage of the FMOC protection groups yielded four novel building blocks. This two-step procedure allows the creation of any number of highly functionalized amines that could serve as building blocks for the preparation of libraries.

To ensure that all building blocks reacted with the core molecules in high yields, we reacted the xanthene core molecule **4** separately with the 21 amines in Table 5.1, set 1. Each amine listed gave the expected tetra-functionalized product in excellent yield within 30 min reaction time. Additional functional groups in the building blocks other than the desired amines that might react with acid chlorides (e.g., Ser side chain) were blocked with acid-labile protecting groups (19). The hydrophobic nature of the libraries produced with the protected building blocks allowed their separation from unreacted amines and hydrolyzed core material by extraction with solutions of citric acid and sodium hydrogen carbonate. The resulting protected libraries were obtained as white powders even though they contained large mixtures of molecules.

As a qualitative check on the viability of this synthesis up to the deprotection step, protected libraries with theoretically increasing complexity were synthesized and analyzed by high-pressure liquid chromatography (HPLC). For this purpose, the xanthene tetra acid chloride **4** was condensed with 4, 7, 12, and 21 different amines from Table 5.1, set 1, resulting in the preparation of mixtures **L1–L4** with theoretically 136, 1225, 10,440, and 97,461 different compounds respectively. (See note on p. 99). The HPLC chromatograms obtained from these mixtures are shown in Figure 5.6. They reveal changes in complexity and resolution that one would expect with increasing diversity, indicating that increasing the number of building blocks does in fact increase diversity.

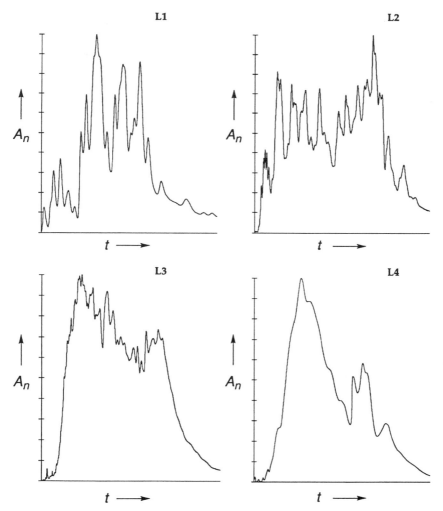

Figure 5.6 Analytical HPLC chromatograms (normalized) obtained from libraries **L1–L4.** Assuming ideal reaction conditions, library **L1** contains theoretically 136 compounds, **L2** contains 1225, **L3** contains 10,440, and **L4** contains 97,461. The libraries were constructed with the xanthene tetra acid chloride **4** and 4, 7, 12, and 21 of the amines in Table 5.1, set 1.

In the second step of library production, the protected libraries were treated with reagent K [trifluoroacetic acid, water, phenol, thioanisol, ethanedithiol (82.5:5:5:5:2.5)] (20), which cleaved the acid-sensitive protecting groups and converted the protected libraries into their more water-soluble forms. The deprotected libraries were then precipitated with an ether/*n*-hexane mixture (1:1). After deprotection, however, the libraries that had been created with the building blocks in Table 5.1, set 1, were not found to be sufficiently water soluble for screening purposes. It was assumed that a preponderance of methyl ester derivatives, which had given the protected libraries excellent organic phase solubility for HPLC analysis, lay at the root of the problem. New libraries were therefore synthesized using the set of 19 building blocks listed in Table 5.1, set 2. The new set of building blocks incorporated more *tert*-butyl esters; unlike methyl esters, these would be cleaved in the deprotection step. After the new libraries were deprotected with reagent K, precipitation with ether gave white powders with solubility in 10:1 water/dimethylsulfoxide sufficient for screening purposes. Thus, in a two-step synthetic procedure, mixtures of small organic molecules with a complexity of 10^4–10^6 different compounds were efficiently generated.

5.3 ANALYZING THE LIBRARIES

To establish that a sizable fraction of the expected compounds are produced in the above synthesis of water-soluble molecular libraries, we analyzed several libraries by electrospray ionization (ESI) mass spectrometry (14). Since direct observation of a library of 97,461 compounds was out of the question, and even a library of 136 compounds appeared daunting in size, smaller yet representative libraries were constructed. Mass spectrometric analysis of these model libraries allowed us to probe the effectiveness of the general synthesis in forming complex mixtures of molecules (21).

Based on three criteria, the diacid chloride **6** (Fig. 5.7) was selected to serve as the core molecule for the model libraries (22). First, condensation of **6** with nine amines from Table 5.1 leads to theoretically only 45 disubstituted compounds, a seemingly manageable number. Second, the two amides formed are at positions 4 and 5 of the xanthene scaffold. As these positions are most susceptible to problems of steric crowding about the xanthene core, **6** provided a realistic test for determin-

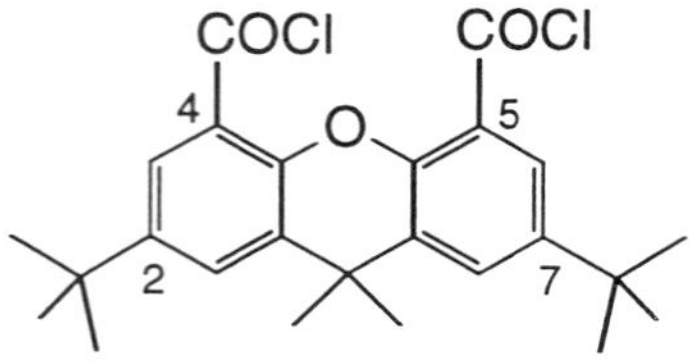

6

Figure 5.7   Truncated core molecule **6** for mass spectrometric determination of model library diversity.

ing any building block combinations that, because of their bulk, would be disfavored in the synthesis. Third, the two *tert*-butyl groups occupying positions 2 and 7 allowed examination of the precipitation behavior of highly hydrophobic library compounds in the final treatment with ether/*n*-hexane.

For the synthesis of the model libraries, five sets of building blocks were selected from the 19 building blocks listed in Table 5.1, set 2: three sets of eight amines and two of nine amines. Condensation of these sets of amines with the core molecule **6** was expected to give libraries of 36 and 45 compounds, respectively. With the help of a simple computer program, the building blocks were grouped in a set such that nearly all of the compounds in the water-soluble library produced would possess a unique molecular weight. This simplified individual detection of each compound present in the libraries. After their formation, the protected model libraries were deprotected with reagent K (20) and then further treated with a solution of trifluoroacetic acid/dichloromethane (4:1) to assure that all protection groups were cleaved. Finally, the water-soluble model libraries were precipitated with ether and *n*-hexane to give white powders.

All model libraries were analyzed in both positive and negative ion modes. The ESI mass spectra showed negligible fragmentation under the ion optics settings used, and thus, taken together, the molecular ion peaks obtained from these measurements are a set of data directly correlated to the diversity of a given molecular library. The molecular ion peaks in the mass spectra were compared with the molecular weights expected for each model library, highlighting which compounds had been formed and which had not.

Results of the mass spectroscopic (MS) analysis of the model libraries are compiled in Figure 5.8. On the x and y axes are the abbreviations of the building blocks used. Each filled square in the charts represents the presence of one of the expected compounds in that model library. Because the truncated core molecule possesses C_{2v} symmetry, only half of the possible building block combinations give rise to new compounds. The pattern of the squares indicates whether the corresponding compound was detected as its positive ion (gray), its negative ion (black), or in both modes (striped).

Out of 198 expected compounds in the model libraries, 173 (87%) were detected. Missing were predominantly those compounds that contained tryptophan residues; less than 50% of the expected Trp compounds were detected. Outside of the compounds containing Trp, only two other combinations, the Gly-Gly and Tyr-Tyr compounds, were not detected in one or more of the model libraries. The absence of Trp compounds may be due to degradation; Trp is an amino acid known to be vulnerable to strongly acidic deprotection conditions. However, as each model library contained some of the expected Trp-substituted xanthenes, this building block was included in the set of building blocks eventually used for large libraries.

Following the success of these experiments, chromatographic techniques coupled on-line to MS were used to add another dimension of resolving power to the system. Omitting tryptophan, a library of diacid **6** plus the 12 amino acids Ala, Arg, Asp, Glu, His, Leu, Phe, Pro, Ser, Thr, Tyr, and Val was synthesized. When the mixture was analyzed by MS coupled to capillary electrophoresis (CE-MS), *all* 78 expected di-amino acid compounds were detected (14). MS-MS was needed to unam-

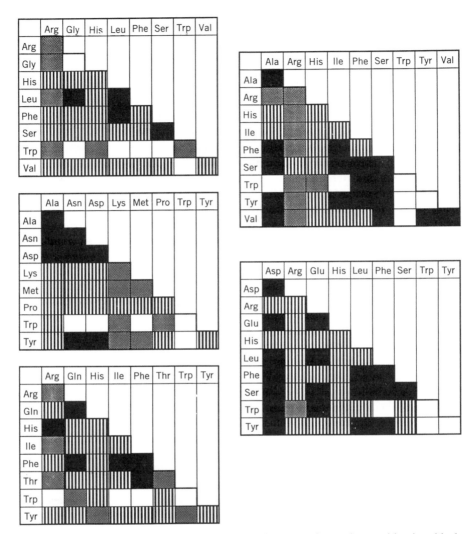

Figure 5.8   Mass spectrometric analysis of libraries: gray, detected as positive ion; black, detected as negative ion; striped, detected as both positive and negative ion.

biguously assign structures in two cases of isobaric molecular ion peaks: the disubstituted xanthene pairs Ser-Pro/Ala-Leu and Val-Glu/Leu-Asp (isobaric molecular weights 594 and 638, respectively). In both cases the resulting MS-MS spectra contained the characteristic fragments of both molecules, confirming the presence of each in the model library.

The mass spectrometric analyses of the model libraries revealed that most of the amines chosen as building blocks generate the expected condensation products with the truncated core molecule **6.** The exceptions were primarily tryptophan-methyl ester derivatives. If one makes the reasonable assumption that reaction at the 2 and 7 positions of **4** is no more difficult than reaction at the 4 and 5 positions of **6,** it follows that most of the compounds expected in a large tetra-acid-chloride-based library will be formed. The compounds that are most probably absent in such libraries contain one or more Trp or multiple Gly building blocks, either because of acidic degradation or failure to precipitate in the final isolation step of ether/ *n*-hexane. However, even if 75% of the expected Trp-containing compounds are absent in a condensation of **4** with 19 building blocks (see screening libraries below), the water-soluble library created still contains over 50,000 different molecules. With the above mass spectrometric data in hand, we were confident that our synthetic methodology produced highly diverse libraries of well-defined composition, and we were able to put faith in the results of subsequent screening assays.

5.4 SCREENING THE LIBRARIES

We chose inhibition of the enzyme trypsin (23) as a test of our system of combinatorial library generation. Trypsin is a digestive enzyme that is a member of the important class of serine proteases (24,25) and is readily available commercially. We sought to isolate a compound able to inhibit the trypsin-catalyzed cleavage of the amide bond in N^α-benzoyl-DL-arginine-*p*-nitroanilide (25,26) by screening compounds from our libraries in an iterative selection process. Our iterative selection procedure was designed through modification and generalization of a screening method first employed by Houghten et al. for the identification of active peptides in a hexapeptide library solution (15).

For screening purposes, we created three libraries **A1, A2,** and **A3** based on core molecules **1, 4,** and **5,** respectively. Each acid chloride core was condensed with the 19 amino acid derivatives listed in Table 5.1, set 2. This procedure gave three libraries of theoretically 11,191 (cubane core) 65,341 (xanthene core), and 1,330 (benzene core) different compounds. To evaluate the potency of each library, 2.5 mg of a given library was added to the trypsin assay and its inhibitory activity was correlated inversely to the rate of *p*-nitroaniline released from trypsin-catalyzed hydrolysis. The results of this experiment are depicted in Chart A of Figure 5.9.

The xanthene-based library **A2** caused significant reduction of the enzyme's activity (approximately 30%). More importantly, even though all three libraries were constructed with the same set of building blocks, only the xanthene library showed significant inhibition. This result hinted that the inhibition was specific to a type of molecule, the functional group orientation of which was best produced by the xanthene core.

To determine which of the 19 building blocks were most responsible for this interaction, six sublibraries were synthesized. First, cysteine (an amino acid known to cause artifactual results in some enzyme assays) was removed summarily from the set of building blocks, leaving 18 amines. These were grouped into the six sets Gr1–Gr6 listed in Table 5.2: smaller hydrophobic side chains, larger hydrophobic side chains, basic side chains, hydroxyl side chains (plus Met), aromatic side

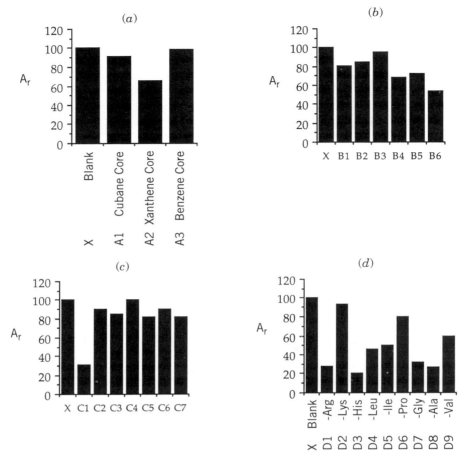

Figure 5.9 A_r: Percent of trypsin activity in the presence of added libraries relative to a blank (**X**) containing no added library material. Each bar represents average trypsin activity for four measurements. Libraries were considered inhibitory if they reduced trypsin activity by > 10%. The activity of the blank was set to 100%. Library solutions added in charts A–D: 2.5 mg in 50 μL DMSO. Chart A: A_r: percent of trypsin activity with the initial libraries **A1, A2,** and **A3** constructed from the core molecules **1, 4,** and **5,** respectively, plus the 19 amino acid building blocks listed in Table 5.1, set 2. Chart B: A_r: percent of trypsin activity with the six sublibraries **B1–B6** constructed from core molecule **2** and 15 of the 19 amino acid building blocks. **B1:** Group G1 omitted. **B2:** Group G2 omitted. **B3:** Group G3 omitted. **B4:** Group G4 omitted. **B5:** Group G5 omitted. **B6:** Group G6 omitted. Groups G1–G6 are listed in Table 5.2. Chart C: A_r: percent of trypsin activity with the seven sublibraries **C1–C7** constructed from the core molecule **2** and 9–12 of the building blocks listed in Table 5.1, set 2. **C1:** Arg, Lys, His, Leu, Ile, Pro, Gly, Ala, Val. **C2:** His, Leu, Ile, Pro, Ala, Val, Phe, Try, Trp, Ser, Thr, Met. **C3:** Arg, Lys, His, Gly, Phe, Tyr, Trp, Glu, Asp, Asn. **C4:** His, Leu, Ile Pro, Ala, Val, Phe, Trp, Glu, Asp, Asn. **C5:** Arg, Lys, His, Gly, Phe, Tyr, Trp, Ser, Thr, Met. **C6:** His, Leu, Ile, Pro, Gly, Ala, Val, Phe, Trp, Glu, Asp, Asn. **C7:** Arg, Lys, His, Pro, Gly, Trp, Glu, Asp, Asn. Chart D: A_r: percent of trypsin activity with the nine sublibraries

TABLE 5.2 List of Amino Acids Present
in the Six Groups of Building Blocks Gr1–Gr6
Used to Generate the Sublibraries B1–B6[a]

Gr1	Gr2	Gr3	Gr4	Gr5	Gr6
Gly	Leu	Arg	Ser	Phe	Glu
Ala	Ile	Lys	Thr	Tyr	Asp
Val	Pro	His	Met	Trp	Asn

[a]For the list of abbreviations see Table 5.1, set 2.

chains, and acidic side chains (plus Asn). Sublibraries **B1–B6** were then prepared with the xanthene core molecule **2** and 15 building blocks from five of the six groups. Sublibrary **B1** was created with all building blocks *except* those in group Gr1, **B2** was created with all building blocks *except* those in group Gr2, and so on. Each sublibrary was calculated to consist of theoretically 25,425 different tetra-substituted xanthenes.

The screening results of the six mixtures are depicted in chart B of Figure 5.9, and show that the sublibrary **B3,** generated without the basic side chain group Gr3, did not inhibit enzyme activity. This result was not entirely unexpected, given the known preference of trypsin for lysine and arginine at the carbonyl side of the cissile amide bond (often referred to as the P_1 position) (27). The next two most important groups were the aliphatic side chain groups Gr1 and Gr2. The nine building blocks present in these three groups were therefore deemed to be most responsible for the presence of inhibitors in the initial library **A2.**

As a control for this result, a library **C1** was constructed with the nine building blocks of groups Gr1–Gr3: Gly, Ala, Val, Leu, Ile, Pro, Arg, Lys, and His. Activity of the control library was measured relative to other libraries **C2–C7** generated with a random set of 9–12 of the 19 amines initially used in library **A2.** Chart C in Figure 5.9 shows clearly that only the control library **C1** possesses significant biological activity. This experiment helped to rule out the possibility that the observed differences in inhibitory activity of the sublibraries resulted from differences in library synthesis and handling rather than the absence of certain important building blocks. Because the control library **C1** contains in theory only 3321 compounds compared to 65,341 present in the initial library **A2,** and building block selection has increased the content of inhibitors (2.5 mg of material now produce 69% inhibition), the process of building block selection and sublibrary synthesis can be viewed as an "amplification" step.

To further narrow the field of possible inhibitors, nine new xanthene sublibraries were prepared using eight of the nine building blocks already selected, with each

---

D1–D9 constructed from the core molecule **2** and eight of the nine building blocks Arg, Lys, His, Leu, Ile, Pro, Gly, Ala, Val. **D1:** Arg omitted. **D2:** Lys omitted. **D3:** His omitted. **D4:** Leu omitted. **D5:** Ile omitted. **D6:** Pro omitted. **D7:** Gly omitted. **D8:** Ala omitted. **D9:** Val omitted.

sublibrary missing one of these nine amino acids. The screening results obtained from this experiment are presented in chart D of Figure 5.9. A sublibrary that showed low inhibitory activity signaled that the building block omitted from that group was crucial for trypsin inhibition. For generation of an active trypsin inhibitor, lysine methyl ester appeared to be the most important building block, followed by proline, valine, isoleucine, and leucine.

In order to establish the most potent combination of the five building blocks, xanthene libraries were constructed with three or four of these five. (It was by no means clear at this stage that the most potent molecule would contain four *different* building blocks.) Trypsin assay results are shown in chart E of Figure 5.10. Even though each compound in a sublibrary constructed with three building blocks was present in *higher* concentration than each compound in a sublibrary constructed with four building blocks, the xanthene library **E1** had the highest inhibitory activity. Library **E1** was synthesized with building blocks lysine, valine, proline, and isoleucine. Omission of any one of these four building blocks gave libraries with a lower potency. Thus, the search for a trypsin inhibitor was narrowed to a sublibrary containing 136 compounds, which included 12 structural isomers of the Lys-Ile-Pro-Val-xanthene derivative. Since Chart E (Fig. 5.10) stipulated that the most potent trypsin inhibitor in our libraries was created with four different building blocks, it was clear that one or more of these 12 isomers was the inhibitor in question.

To narrow the remaining possibilities for the structure of the most potent isomer from 12 to 2, 6 more sublibraries were prepared using the dibenzylester xanthene diacid chloride derivative **7**. The new core molecule **7** was easily prepared from the xanthene tetra acid chloride **4:** by reaction of **4** with benzylalcohol (CH_2Cl_2, pyridine, 12 h, room temperature, 75% yield), the tetrabenzylester compound was obtained, from which the two benzylester groups in positions 4 and 5 were selectively removed by brief treatment with HBr in dichloromethane (3 h, 0°C, 72% yield). The resulting xanthene dibenzylester diacid compound was converted into the diacid chloride with oxalyl chloride in dichloromethane (4 h, reflux).

Using xanthene **7**, six new sublibraries (**F1–F6**, Table 5.3) were synthesized in the two-step procedure outlined schematically in Figure 5.11. Compound **7** was treated in a first "randomization" step with two of the four amines—Lys, Ile, Pro, and Val—followed by deprotection of xanthene positions 2 and 7 by hydrogenolysis (ethyl acetate/ethanol, 10% Pd/C, H_2 atmosphere, 2 h, room temperature). Coupling of the resulting material with the two other building blocks (BOP) and deprotection of the acid-sensitive protection groups with trifluoroacetic acid in CH_2Cl_2 yielded six sublibraries, each with a unique distribution of the four selected building blocks around the xanthene core. Table 5.3 lists the building blocks used in the first and second randomization steps.

The screening results of these six sublibraries are presented in chart F, Figure 5.10. They revealed that only those compounds possessing the combination Lys/Val or Lys/Ile at positions 4 and 5 and the corresponding Pro/Ile or Pro/Val combination at positions 2 and 7 were active as trypsin inhibitors. Other arrangements of the four selected building blocks on the xanthene core were inactive. Furthermore, of the two active libraries **F1** and **F2**, library **F2** (containing the Lys/Ile combination at

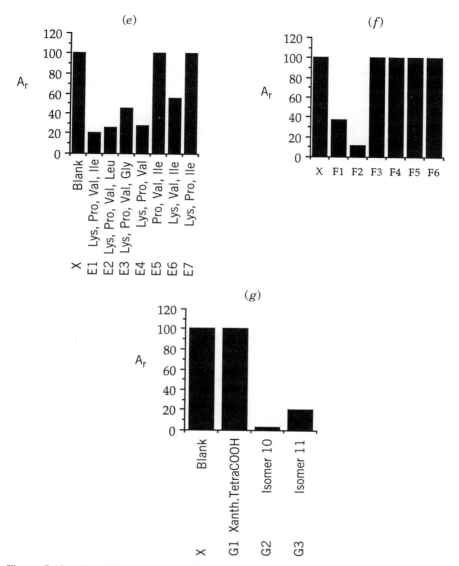

Figure 5.10 Chart E: A_r: percent of trypsin activity with the seven sublibraries **E1–E7** constructed from the core molecule **2** and three or four of the building blocks Lys, Leu, Ile, Pro, Gly, Val. **E1:** Lys, Pro, Val, Ile. **E2:** Lys, Pro, Val, Leu. **E3:** Lys, Pro, Val, Gly **E4:** Lys, Pro, Val. **E5:** Pro, Val, Ile. **E6:** Lys, Val, Ile. **E7:** Lys, Pro, Ile. Chart F: A_r: percent of trypsin activity with the six sublibraries **F1–F6.** For a description of their compositions see text and Table 5.3. Chart G: A_r: percent trypsin activity with the two final inhibitors. **G1:** control run with 9.9-dimethyl-2,4,5,7-xanthene tetracarboxylic acid. **G2:** isomer **10.** **G3:** isomer **11.** Library solutions added: Chart E: 1.5 mg in 50 μL DMSO; chart F: 0.5 mg in 50 μL DMSO; chart G: 0.25 mg in 50 μL DMSO.

**TABLE 5.3   List of Amino Acid Derivatives
Attached to Xanthene Positions 4 and 5
(A_1 and A_2) and Positions 2 and 7 (B_1 and B_2)
in the Generation of Sublibraries F1–F6**

Sublibrary	Positions 4 and 5	Positions 2 and 7
F1	Lys, Val	Ile, Pro
F2	Lys, Ile	Val, Pro
F3	Lys, Pro	Ile, Val
F4	Val, Ile	Lys, Pro
F5	Val, Pro	Lys, Ile
F6	Ile, Pro	Lys, Val

xanthene positions 4 and 5) was the most active. This result narrowed the structure of a final most potent inhibitor to the two isomers **10** and **11** shown in Figure 5.12.

Compounds **10** and **11** were individually prepared via a four-step synthesis from **7**, as outlined in Figure 5.12. The dibenzyl-protected diacid chloride **7** was reacted with a mixture of Lys and Ile (CH_2Cl_2, triethylamine, 1.5 h, room temperature) and the mixed amide xanthene-monolysine-monoisoleucine compound **8a** isolated by flash chromatography (31% yield). Hydrogenolysis (ethyl acetate/ethanol, 10% Pd/C, 2 h, room temperature) of the benzylester protecting groups yielded the monolysine-monoisoleucin xanthene diacid **8b** (98%). Coupling of **8b** with a Pro/Val building block mixture (BOP, dimethylformamide, triethylamine, 1 h, room temperature) yielded a set of four protected compounds from which two

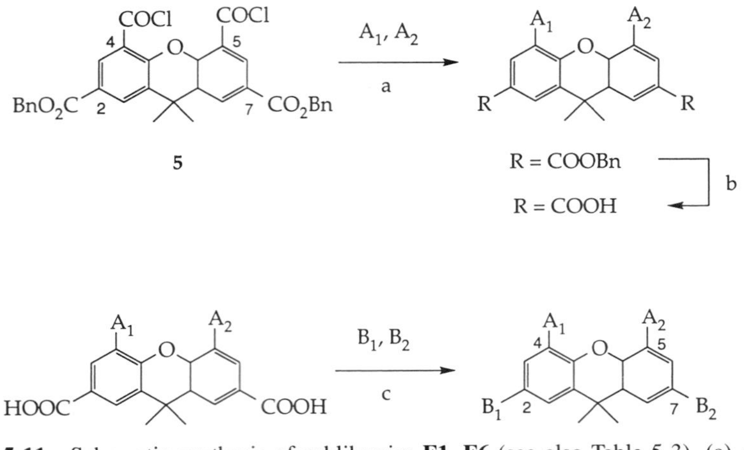

Figure 5.11   Schematic synthesis of sublibraries **F1–F6** (see also Table 5.3). (a) A_1, A_2, triethylamine, 1.5 h, room temperature, 31% yield. (b) ethyl acetate/ethanol, 10% Pd/C, H_2 atmosphere, 2 h, room temperature. (c) B_1, B_2, dimethylformamide, BOP, triethylamine, 1 h, room temperature.

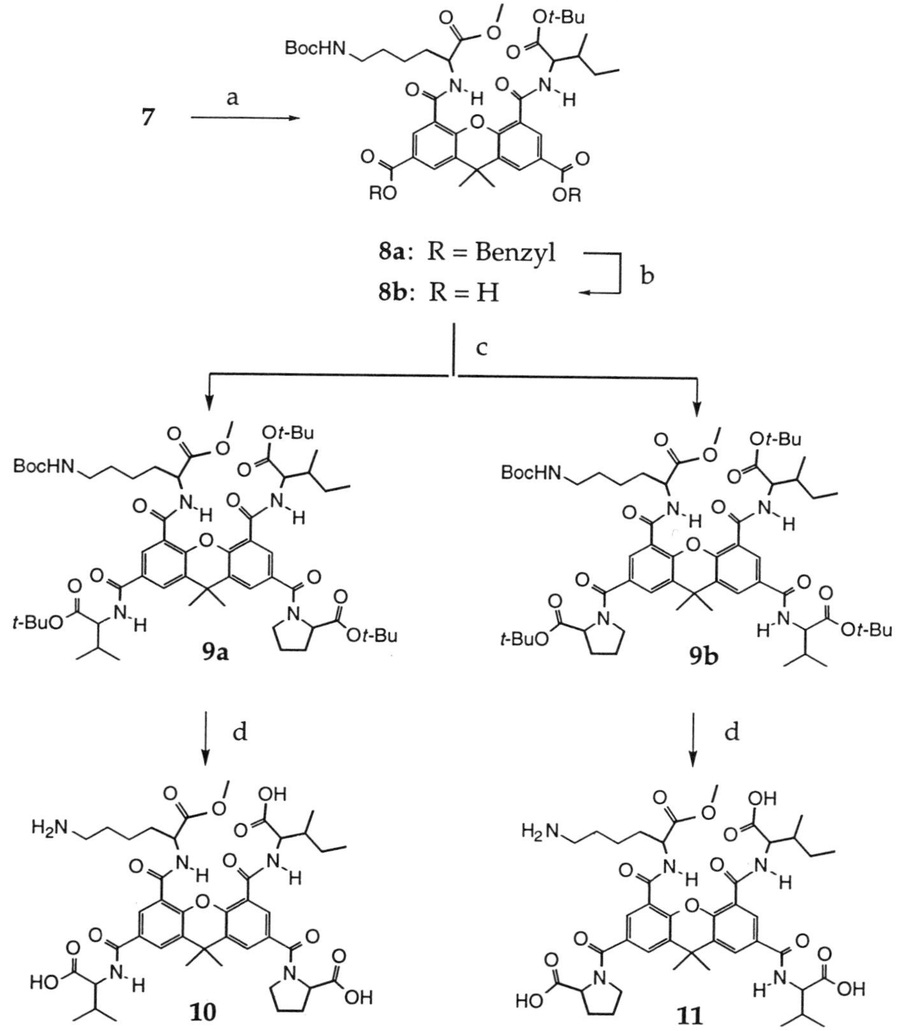

Figure 5.12 Synthesis of the final trypsin inhibitor **10** and its isomer **11**. (a) H-Lys(Boc)-OMe, H-Ile-*O-tert*-butyl, CH$_2$Cl$_2$, triethylamine, 1.5 h, room temperature, 31% yield. (b) ethyl acetate/ethanol, 10% Pd/C, H$_2$ atmosphere, 2 h, room temperature, 98% yield. (c) H-Pro-*O-tert*-butyl, H-Val-*O-tert*-butyl, dimethylformamide, BOP, triethylamine, 1 h, room temperature, 30% yield (**9a**), 28% yield (9b). (d) CH$_2$Cl$_2$, TFA, thioanisol, 4 h, room temperature, 91% yield (**10**), 97% yield (**11**).

isomeric compounds A and B—both containing all four building blocks (A_1 = Lys, A_2 = Ile, B = Pro and Val)—were isolated by flash chromatography and purified by normal phase-preparative HPLC.

The assignment of the isomers to the structures of protected **9a** and **9b** was possible by evaluating two nuclear Overhauser enhancement (NOE) measurements and a correlated spectroscopy (COSY) spectrum of isomer B. Individual irradiation at the absorption frequencies (δ = 8.00 and 7.93) of two aromatic xanthene protons connected to the same six-membered ring gave strong nuclear Overhauser effects with two NH protons. These protons were assigned to the valine and isoleucine substructures through the COSY spectrum of isomer B. Isomer B therefore corresponds to protected compound **9b,** in which isoleucine and valine are connected to the same benzene ring. Comparison of the chemical shifts of the four aromatic xanthene protons of the isomers **9a** and **9b** with other tetra-amino-acid-substituted xanthenes confirmed this assignment.

In the final step of the synthesis, **9a** and **9b** were deprotected with trifluoroacetic acid in dichloromethane (4 h, room temperature, 91% yield for **10;** 97% yield for **11**). The products **10** and **11** were purified by reverse-phase preparative HPLC and characterized by fast atom bombardment mass spectrometry in combination with a detailed study of the fragments by tandem mass spectrometry. The assignment of signals in the nuclear magnetic resonance (NMR) spectra was difficult due to several slow conformational interconversions such as cis/trans isomerization of the proline amide bond. Some of the protons could be assigned to signals in a spectrum measured at 90°C with the help of a COSY spectrum obtained at 90°C. NOE studies of compound **9b** revealed that on an NMR time scale, the amide proton of the lysine side chain is locked into a bifurcated hydrogen bond with the xanthene oxygen and the carbonyl oxygen of the adjacent isoleucine. Similar hydrogen bonding was observed in previous work with xanthene structures in our laboratory (23).

Screening of **10** and **11** in the standard assay (chart G, Fig. 5.10) revealed that both isomers are trypsin inhibitors, with **10** being the most potent. The K_i values of both compounds **10** and **11** were obtained by nonlinear regression of kinetic data according to the equation for competitive inhibition and additionally by evaluation of Lineweaver–Burk plots. The kinetic data were obtained by measurement of the rate of p-nitroaniline released by tryptic cleavage of the substrate benzoyl-L-arginine-p-nitroanilide at increasing concentrations with an increasing presence of either **10** or **11** (28). These measurements clearly show that both isomers **10** and **11** are competitive trypsin inhibitors, with a K_i of 9.4 $\pm$ 0.8 μM for **10** and a K_i of 72 $\pm$ 7 μM for **11**. Thus, structure **10** represents the most potent trypsin inhibitor that was selected from our initial xanthene library **A2.**

5.5 EXPANDING DIVERSITY

Through the above iterative screening procedure, we were able—in 4 weeks of work—to extract from our libraries an inhibitor of trypsin. Although this result is clearly propitious for a method of lead structure discovery, two main concerns must be addressed. Most importantly, one must ask if inhibitor **10** is truly the most active compound that was present in the initial xanthene library of 65,341 compounds. Second, given that amide structures may be poor drug candidates, one must ask how the process can be moved from the realm of amide-based small molecules to libraries of non-amide compounds.

Inhibitors **10** and **11,** although reasonable inhibitors of trypsin, cannot mathematically account for the observed activity in the xanthene-based library **A2.** All compounds were present in very low concentration (on the order of $0.1 \mu M$), and other inhibitory compounds beside **10** and **11** must have been present in the starting library of some 60,000 species. Based on the activities of libraries **E1–E7** and several computer simulations (14), it seems likely that molecule **10** is merely the most active of a family of inhibitors. The family contains other less potent inhibitors (such as **11**), which nevertheless contribute to the activity of library **A2** as a whole; this explains the relatively high activity of the initial xanthene library **A2.** Thus, our method of screening initially operates by selecting groups of molecules rather than individual compounds. The groups selected become more and more focused, until a single highly potent structure is elucidated.

Does this mean that the selection strategy may have skipped over compounds far more potent than isomer **10?** Computer simulations demonstrated that by employing our selection strategy, it was impossible to miss an active compound orders of magnitude more potent than compound **10,** but it was possible to overlook a compound with comparable or even slightly higher activity. While the selection strategy of ever narrowing sublibraries will result in the isolation, if they exist, of one or more of the most active compounds present in a combinatorial library such as **A2,** some active structures could be missed in the process.

The question then becomes, is this drawback a fatal flaw? We would argue that it is not. As long as a procedure is effective in identifying *at least one* of the active lead compounds in a library, and as long as the *potential for generating new libraries is limitless,* it is of little consequence that some other active compounds escape unnoticed. As an analogy, nature could never hope to sort through all 20^{200+} possible peptide structures to find *the best* enzyme for a given task, but it is able to select *useful* enzymes from this pool in a relatively short period of time.

One of the above stipulations, of course, is that a limitless number of libraries can be synthesized. We are therefore expanding our base of core molecules and building blocks. Other acid chloride core molecules that we have explored include the adamantane, biphenyl, and isopthalic acid-based structures shown in Figure 5.13, and there is no shortage of commercially available amines bearing various functional groups. Understanding that all such libraries have the drawback of being amide based, however, we are currently constructing cores with the aim of creating non-amide libraries. Figure 5.14 shows three such possible strategies, creating ureas or carbamates from isocyanates, and finally forming actual carbon–carbon bonds from a polylithiated core. Having proven the concept of our polyfunctionalized molecules through mass spectrometry and solution-phase screening against trypsin,

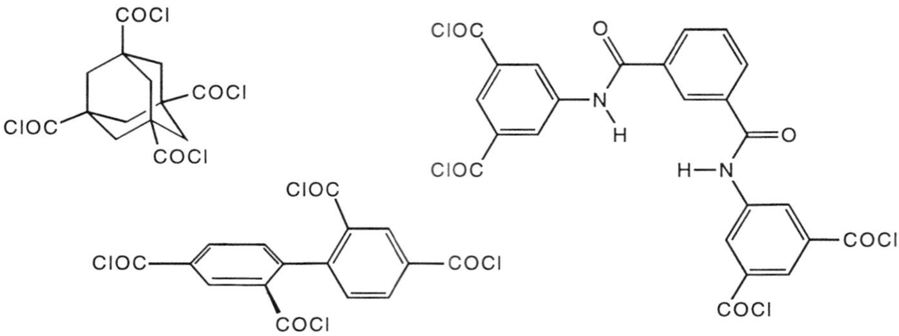

Figure 5.13 Adamantane, biphenyl, and isopthalic acid-based structures.

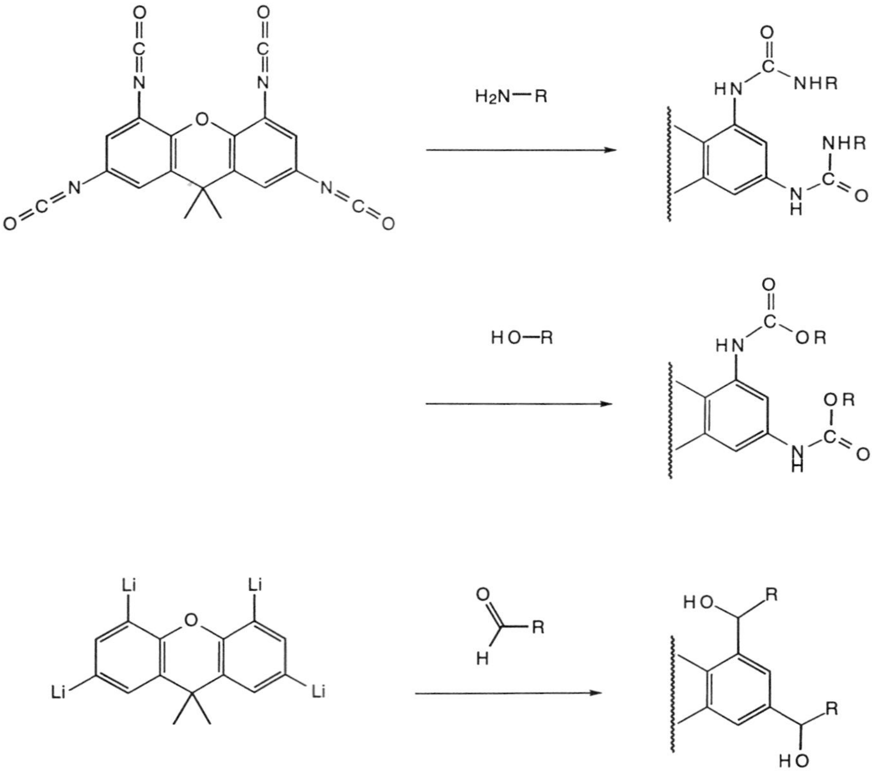

Figure 5.14 Three possible strategies for creating non-amide libraries.

we are hopeful that our combinatorial methods may be a valuable tool in the search for potent therapeutic lead compounds, complementing the existing repertoire of combinatorial procedures to explore the structural landscape of small molecules.

ACKNOWLEDGMENT

The experiments detailed herein are in great part the work of Postdoctoral Fellow Dr. Thomas Carell (see Refs. 15 and 16). We thank Dr. B. Tsao for the measurement of COSY spectra and NOE experiments, J. S. Nowick and Ken Shimizu for the descriptions of the syntheses of **2** and **5,** Dr. Andrew J. Sutherland for confirming trypsin results, Dr. Bashir-Hashemi for providing cubane-1,3,5,7-tetracarboxylic acid chloride **1,** and Prof. J. Stubbe for advice regarding the enzyme assay. The work depicted in Figure 5.14 is being carried out by Dr. Urs P. Spitz, Gerald W. Shipps, Jr., and Kent E. Pryor. This research was supported by the National Institutes of Health, the Alexander-von-Humboldt Foundation (Feodor-Lynen post-doctoral fellowship to Dr. T. Carell), the National Science Foundation, and the American Chemical Society, Organic Division (predoctoral fellowship and graduate fellowship, respectively, to E. A. W.).

REFERENCES

1. Jung, G., and Beck-Sickinger, A. G., *Angew. Chem. Int. Ed. Engl.* **31,** 367–383 (1992).

2. (a) Geysen, H. M., Meloen, R. M., and Barteling, S. J., *Proc. Natl. Acad. Sci. (USA)* **88,** 3998–4002 (1984); (b) Geysen, H. M., Rodda, S. J., Mason, T. J., Tribbick, G., and Schoofs, P. G., *J. Imm. Meth.* **102,** 159–273 (1987).

3. (a) Houghten, R. A., *Proc. Natl. Acad. Sci. (USA)* **82,** 5131–5135 (1985); (b) Hough-ten, R. A., DeBray, S. T., Bray, M. K., Hoffmann, S. R., and Frizzell, N. D., *Bio-Techniques* **4,** 522–528 (1986).

4. (a) Furka, Á., Sebestyén, F., Asgedom, M., and Dibó, G. *Int. J. Pept. Prot. Res.* **37,** 487–493 (1991); (b) Furka, Á., Sebestyén, F., Asgedom, M., and Dibó, G.; *Abstr. 14th Int. Congr. Biochem.,* Vol. 5, Prague, Czechoslovakia, 1988, p. 47.

5. (a) Lam, K. S., Salmon, S. E., Hersh, E. M., Hruby, V. J., Kazmierski, W. M., Knapp, R. J., *Nature (London)* **354,** 82–84 (1991); (b) Salmon, S. E., Lam, K. S., Lebl, M., Kondola, A., Khattri, P. S., Wade, S., Pátek, M., Kocis, P., Krchnak, V., Thorpe, D., and Felder, S., *Proc. Natl. Acad. Sci (USA)* **90,** 11708–11712 (1993).

6. Brummel, C. L., Lee, I. N. W., Zhous, Y., Benkovic, S. J., and Winograd, N. *Science* **264,** 399–402 (1994).

7. (a) Tuerk, C., and Gold, L. *Science* **24,** 505–510 (1990); (b) Beaudry, A. A., and Joyce, G. F., *Science* **257,** 635–641 (1992); (c) Brenner, S., and Lerner, R. A., *Proc. Natl. Acad. Sci (USA)* **89,** 5381–5383 (1992); (d) Bartel, D. P., and Szostak, J. W., *Science* **261,** 1411–1418 (1993); (e) Nielsen, J., Brenner, S., Janda, K. D., *J. Am. Chem. Soc.* **115,** 9812–9813 (1993); (f) Ohlmeyer, M. H. F., Swanson, R. N., Dillard, L. W., Reader, J. C., Asouline, G., Kobayashi, R., Wigler, M., and Still, W. C., *Proc. Natl. Acad. Sci (USA)* **90,** 10922 (1993); (g) Borchardt, A., and Still, W. C., *J. Am. Chem.*

Soc. **116**, 373–374 (1994); (i) Nestler, H. P., Bartlett, P. A., and Still, W. C., *J. Org. Chem.* **59**, 4723–4724 (1994).

8. Bunin, B. A., and Ellman, J. A., *J. Am. Chem. Soc.* **114**, 10997–10998 (1992).

9. (a) Zuckermann, R. N., Martin, E. J., Spellmeyer, D. C., Stauber, G. B., Shoemaker, K. R., Kerr, J. M., Figliozzi, G. M., Goff, D. A., Siani, M. A., Simon, R. J., Banville, S. C., Brown, E. G., Wang, L., Richter, L. S., and Moos, W. H., *J. Med. Chem.* **37**, 2678–2685 (1994); (b) Simon, R. S., Martin, E. S., Miller, S. M., Zuckermann, R. N., Blaney, J. M., and Moos, W. H., *Techniques in Protein Chem. Part V,* Wiley, San Diego, 1994; (c) Kessler, H., *Angew. Chem. Int. Ed. Engl.* **32**, 543–544 (1993).

10. (a) Cho, C. Y., Moran, E. J., Cherry, S. R., Stephaus, J. C., Fodor, S. P. A., Adams, C. L., Sundaram, A., Jacobs, J. W., and Schultz, P. G., *Science* **261**, 1303–1305 (1993); (b) Fodor, S. P. A., Read, J. L., Pirrung, M. C., Stryer, L., Lu, A. T., and Solas, D., *Science* **251**, 767–773 (1991); (c) Rozsnyai, L. F., Benson, D. R., Fodor, S. P. A., and Schultz, P. G., *Angew. Chem. Int. Ed. Engl.* **31**, 759–761 (1992).

11. DeWitt, S. H., Kieley, J. S., Stankovic, C. J., Schroeder, M. C., Reynolds Cody, D. M., and Pavia, M. R., *Proc. Natl. Acad. Sci. (USA)* **90**, 6909–6913 (1993).

12. Liskamp, R. M. J., *Angew. Chem. Int. Ed. Engl.* **33**, 633–636 (1994).

13. (a) Carell, T., Wintner, E. A., Bashir-Hashemi, A., and Rebek, J., Jr., *Angew. Chem. Int. Ed. Engl.* **33**, 2005–2007 (1994); (b) Carell, T., Wintner, E. A., Rebek, J., Jr., *Angew. Chem. Int. Ed. Engl.* **33**, 2007–2110 (1994).

14. (a) Carell, T., Wintner, E. A., Sutherland, A. J., Rebek, J., Jr., Dunayevskiy, Y. M., and Vouros, P., *Chem. Biol.* **2**, 171–183 (1995); (b) Dunayevskiy, Y. M., Vouros, P., Carell, T., Wintner, E. A., and Rebek, J., Jr., *Anal. Chem.* **67**, 2906–2915 (1995).

15. (a) Houghten, R. A., Pinilla, C., Blondelle, S. E., Appel, J. R., Dooley, C. T., and Cuervo, J. H., *Nature (London)* **354**, 84–86 (1991); (b) Pinilla, C., Appel, J. R., Blanc, P., and Houghten, R. A., *BioTechnique* **13**, 901–905 (1992).

16. Bashir-Hashemi, A., *Angew. Chem. Int. Ed. Engl.* **32**, 612–613 (1993).

17. Newman, M. S., and Lowrie, H. S., *J. Am. Chem. Soc.* **76**, 6196–6197 (1954).

18. Weiss, N. A., and Hassett, M. J., *Introductory Statistics,* 3rd ed., Addison-Wesley, New York, 1991, pp. 218–219.

19. (a) Bodanszky, M. *Principles of Peptide Synthesis,* Springer Verlag, Heidelberg, 1984; (b) Bodanszky, M., and Bodanszky, A., *The Practice of Peptide Synthesis,* Springer-Verlag, Heidelberg, 1984.

20. King, D., Fields, C., and Fields, G. *Int. J. Pept. Prot. Res.* **36**, 255–266 (1990).

21. Metzger, J. W., Wiesmüller, K-H., Gnau, V., Grünges, J., and Jung, G. *Angew. Chem. Int. Ed. Engl.* **32**, 894–896 (1993).

22. Nowick, J. S., Ballester, P., Ebmeyer, F., and Rebek, J., Jr. *J. Am. Chem. Soc.* **112**, 8902–8906 (1990). The diacid **4** is commercially available from Aldrich Chemical Company.

23. Eichler, J., and Houghten, R. A. *Biochemistry* **32**, 11035–11041 (1993).

24. (a) Zwaal, R. F. A., and Henker, H. C., *Blood Coagulation,* Elsevier, New York, 1986; (b) Salzman, E. W., *N. Engl. J. Med.* **326**, 1017–1019 (1992); (c) Bock, L. C., Griffin, L. C., Latham, J. A., Vermaas, E. H., and Toole, J. J., *Nature* **355**, 564–566 (1992).

25. (a) Holtz, J., and Goetz, R. M., *Arzneim. Forsch.* **44**(3a), 397–402 (1994); (b) Cody, J. R., *Drugs,* **47**, 586–598 (1954).

26. (a) Erlanger, B. F., Kokowsky, N., and Cohen, W., *Arch. Biochem. Biophys,* **95,** 271–278 (1961); (b) Gaertner, H. F., and Puigserver, A. J., *Enzyme Microb, Technol.* **14,** 150–155 (1992).

27. Laskowski, Jr., M., and Kato, I., *Annu. Rev. Biochem.* **49,** 593–626 (1990).

28. Segel, I. H., *Enzyme Kinetics,* Wiley, New York, 1993.

6

SOLID-PHASE METHODS IN COMBINATORIAL CHEMISTRY

IRVING SUCHOLEIKI

Sphinx Pharmaceuticals, A Division of Eli Lilly & Company, 840 Memorial Drive, Cambridge, Massachusetts 02139

6.1   INTRODUCTION

The application of combinatorial chemistry to pharmaceutical research is an emerging area that will dramatically reduce the time and cost associated with the development of new drugs (1a–g). There are two general combinatorial strategies currently being pursued. One involves making mixtures of compounds and the other involves making single compounds in a spatially addressable format. These strategies can be categorized further as to whether the compounds being produced are peptide or nonpeptide.

We have been interested in developing nonpeptide, single-compound libraries for biological screening. To achieve this goal we feel that a solid-phase approach using room temperature chemistries, followed by cleavage from the solid support is vital. Such an approach substantially reduces the amount of time and effort required for purifying the final product because any unreacted starting material is easily washed off the support. This would also make the simultaneous synthesis and purification of hundreds of compounds easier to automate.

The solid-phase technology used in a combinatorial library can be broken down into three major components (Fig. 6.1). First is the solid support that should be stable to a wide range of organic solvents and reagents. Second is the linker, which connects the support to the scaffold or target molecule. The linker should be cleavable under mild conditions but stable to proposed reaction conditions needed to build the desired product. The cleavage reaction should also be amenable to automa-

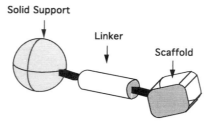

Figure 6.1   Solid support with attached linker connecting the scaffold to the surface of the support.

tion. Third is the scaffold or target molecule, which should be synthesized in high yield and purity.

6.2 CHARACTERISTICS OF VARIOUS SOLID SUPPORTS

The field of peptide synthesis has been one of the engines that has driven the development of new solid-phase supports for broad use in organic chemistry. Early pioneering work by R. B. Merrifield and others in peptide synthesis has made the use of 1–2% crosslinked polystyrene the standard for solid-phase organic chemical reactions (2a,b). In order to understand why this is the case one must first examine the physical nature of the resin-bound substrate. Lightly crosslinked polystyrene (with 1–2% divinyl benzene) can be seen as a sponge with the majority of the active sites located in the cavities (Fig. 6.2). Solvents such as methylene chloride cause the support to expand, while solvents such as methanol cause the support to contract. Higher levels of crosslinking reduce the extent to which the support expands and contracts and also affects the level of reactivity. Work by Regen using electron spin resonance (ESR) spectroscopy of nitroxide radical probes showed that the bound substrate was more restricted than a substrate dissolved in the swollen particle (3a,b). Regen (3a,b) also showed that a higher degree of swelling was associated with a decrease in the rotational correlation time. A decrease in the rotational correlation time can be interpreted to mean that the bound nitroxide probe exhibits a greater mobility in the expanded state of the crosslinked polystyrene. In addition, Regen provided evidence that with greater crosslinking, which translates to less expansion of the support, the internal viscosity of the solvent increased. The use of gel-phase ^{13}C nuclear magnetic resonance (NMR) has also been used to evaluate the extent of mobility of bound substrates (4a–h). Giralt has successfully used gel-phase ^{13}C-NMR to correlate the line widths of amino acids bound to various supports to their peptide coupling yields (4c–e). He found that a broadened ^{13}C line spectrum was related to restricted mobility and that the narrower the line widths the higher the coupling yield was for the bound amino acid. One can dramatically sharpen the line widths by attaching a spacer arm between the bound molecule and the support. Bayer and Rapp have found that attaching a long polyethylene glycol spacer (MW

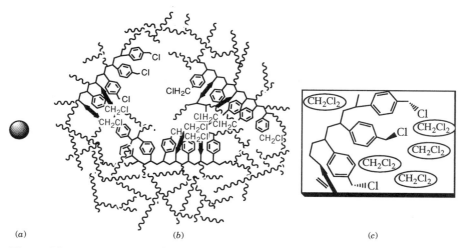

Figure 6.2   Representations of Merrifield resin consisting of 1–2% crosslinked polystyrene under increasing magnification. (a) Low magnification, (b) higher magnification showing spongelike characteristics, and (c) highest magnification showing solvation of support by methylene chloride molecules.

= 2000–3000 daltons) can dramatically sharpen the line widths and increase the relaxation time of the bound component (4g,h). It can be seen then that the extent of mobility of the bound substrate can be affected, not only by the internal viscosity of the area surrounding the bound substrate but also by the length and solubility properties of the spacer arm connecting the substrate to the support.

In solid-phase organic chemistry a dichotomy exists between solvents that expand the crosslinked polystyrene support and solvents that help dissolve and expand the bound substrate. The development of continuous-flow solid-phase peptide synthesis has introduced new supports showing less variability in their expanding and contracting properties when exposed to different polar solvents. The advantage of this for the organic chemist is that more solvents now become available for use in solid-phase organic reactions. The following are some of the new composite materials available for solid-phase organic chemistry.

1. Kieselguhr–Polyacrylamide Composite. This is a composite consisting of polyacrylamide (PAA) gel trapped in the porous structure of kieselguhr. The loading is typically 0.1–0.2 mmol amine/gram resin (5a–c).

2. Polystyrene–Polyacrylamide Composite (also known as Polyhype-based composites). This is a composite of crosslinked polystyrene (PS) containing a very high pore volume (≈90%) containing polyacrylamide inside the cavities. Both covalently attached polystyrene–polyacrylamide and noncovalently attached polystyrene–polyacrylamide composites are available with substitutions ranging from 0.1 to 2.0 mmol amine/gram resin (6a,b).

3. Polystyrene–Polyethylene Glycol Composite. This is a composite of 1% crosslinked polystyrene and covalently attached polyethylene glycol (PEG) (2000–3000 daltons). One form, sold under the name TentaGel, is made by polymerizing ethylene oxide on to a primary alcohol located on the crosslinked polystyrene (7a,b). A second form, sold under the name PEG–PS, is made by attaching, through the formation of an amide bond, an already formed amino terminal polyethylene glycol chain (Jeffamine) to 1% crosslinked polystyrene (7c). The loading capacities for both types of supports are typically in the range of 0.2–0.3 mmol amine/gram resin. Recently, both supports have incorporated lysine branching, raising their available amine substitution to as high as 1 mmol amine/gram resin (7d).

The organic chemist interested in utilizing these and other supports must consider two factors; the level of substitution on the resin and the extent to which the bound component's mobility may be affected by the supports environment. In our laboratory, we found that to produce milligram quantities of hundreds of compounds (MW ≈ 500) in a multiple simultaneous reaction format, a high resin substitution is of prime importance. Supports that typically exhibit substitution levels of less than 0.2 mmol reactive group/gram of resin, such as available silica based supports, were not pursued (8).

We have also found that gel-phase ^{13}C-NMR can successfully be used to quickly evaluate the extent of mobility of components bound to various supports. It was therefore possible to quickly evaluate some of the previously mentioned composite supports to determine which gave the greatest mobility to the bound component and, hence, possibly allow greater reactivity (9a,b). First, we coupled *p*-methoxyl-benzyl-protected cysteine to each of the supports using standard diisopropylcarbo-diimide (DIC) coupling methods. We then acquired a gel-phase ^{13}C-NMR for each of the supports and compared the line widths of the spectra. Those supports incorporating PEG had dramatically narrower line widths (Table 6.1). Of the two PEG-

TABLE 6.1   Line Widths at Half-height of *p*-Methoxy Carbon of Resin-bound Cysteine

Support	Amine Substitution (mmol/g)	Line Width at Half-height of Methoxy Carbon (Hz)
1% crosslinked polystrene	0.7	23
Polyhype P500[a]	0.5	29
Polyhype SU2000[a]	2.0	20
TentaGel[b]	0.3	9
PEG–PS[c]	0.2	9

[a]Polyacrylamide–polystyrene composite, Ref. 6a,b.
[b]PEG-polystyrene composite, Ref. 7a,b.
[c]PEG-polystyrene composite, Ref. 7c.

containing polystyrene supports that were examined, the TentaGel support was found to be more resistant to harsh chemical conditions such as sodium in liquid ammonia (9b).

6.3   CURRENT LINKER TECHNOLOGY

A great number of the commercially available linkers owe their existence to the field of solid-phase peptide synthesis (2a,b). It is therefore understandable that many of the methods employed to attach molecules to a support rely heavily on formation of an ester or an amide bond. Table 6.2 lists some of the solid-phase peptide synthesis linkers that have been applied to the production of nonpeptide combinatorial libraries. As can be seen in Table 6.2, many of the methods used to cleave the bound component require the use of harsh acids such as trifluoroacetic acid. The total removal of trifluoroacetic acid, for example, typically requires incorporation in the cleavage protocol of a series of ether precipitation steps. Such steps make automation of multiple simultaneous synthesis difficult. We have been interested in the development of linkers that not only can be cleaved selectively and under mild conditions but also have chemistries that are easy to automate. Additionally, we

TABLE 6.2   Solid-phase Synthesis Linkers Used in the Production of Combinatorial Libraries

Linking Group Y	Type of Bond Formed	Peptide Cleavage Conditions (Ref)	Combinatorial References
—CH$_2$Cl Merrifield	Ester	Anhydrous HF (2a)	10a,b
Rink Amide	Amide	Trifluoroacetic acid– methylene chloride (11a,b)	12a,b
Wang	Ester	Trifluoroacetic acid (13)	1e–f
2-Chlorotritylchloride	Ester	Acetic acid-trifluoroethanol- methylene chloride (14)	1g

have been interested in creating a linker that upon cleavage does not leave the typical expected carboxylic acid, amide, or alcohol on the product as a result of the cleavage. We have felt that a photocleavable linker could achieve these goals.

Since the early 1960s there has been a great deal of research on photoactive protecting groups that upon irradiation in solution release the active group. One of the first to adapt these studies to a heterogeneous system for the purposes of cleaving product from a support was Wang (15). Wang treated an α-bromo ketone attached to 1% crosslinked polystyrene with the carboxylic acid end of an amino acid to give the resulting resin-bound amino acid ester **1** (Fig. 6.3). Upon irradiation with 350 nm light, the carbon–oxygen bond was observed to cleave, releasing the amino acid or peptide from the support. Later, Tjoeng and Heavner incorporated the α-halo ketone as a separate linker (**2**) (Fig. 6.3) (16a). The advantage of incorporating an α-halo ketone as a separate linker was that it could then be attached to a variety of different types of supports containing a free amine or alcohol (16a,b). Two years later, Pillai synthesized a peptide on a support consisting of 1% crosslinked polystyrene containing a 3-nitro-4-*N*-methylaminomethyl moiety (**3**) (17). Pillai showed that one can successfully cleave the polymer-bound carbon–nitrogen bond upon irradiation with 350 nm light to give C-terminal N-methylated peptide amides (17).

At present, only a handful of research groups have exploited the use of photocleavable linkers in the production of combinatorial libraries (18). The most commonly used photocleavable linker derives from earlier work on photosensitive protecting groups that incorporate an aromatic nitro compound having a C–H bond in the ortho position (19). This idea was subsequently applied as a peptide synthesis linker, **4** (Fig. 6.3) (20a,b). Rich and Gurwara showed that peptides composed of up to seven amino acids could be synthesized and photochemically cleaved in 50%

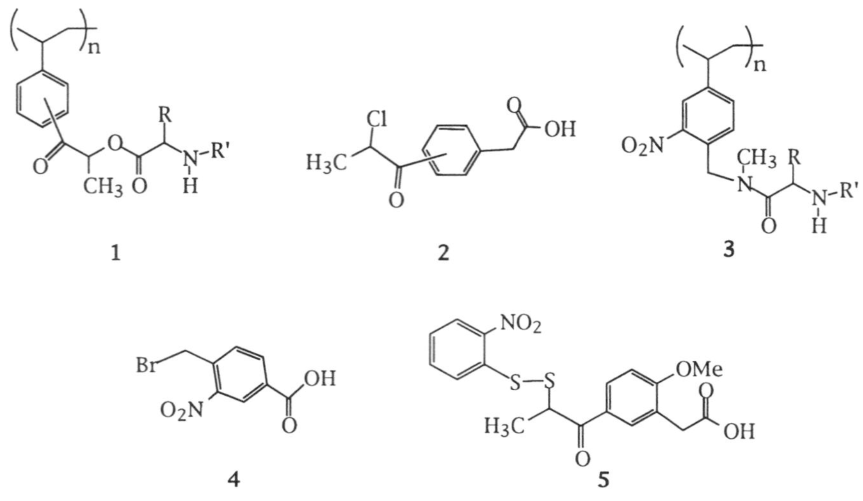

Figure 6.3 Photocleavable linkers used in solid phase organic synthesis.

yield using this linker (**4**) (20b). One drawback is that linker **4** cleaves only pre-formed benzylic carbon–oxygen or carbon–nitrogen bonds releasing the bound component as the free acid, phenol or amide.

We were interested in utilizing photochemistry to cleave molecules from the support, yet we did not want to be restricted to having a hydrogen bond donor such as an acid or a phenol in our compound libraries. Additionally, we were looking at compound libraries with groups such as hydrogen or alkyl positioned at sites formally reserved for carboxylic acids, phenols, and amines. For example, it should be possible to homolytically cleave a benzylic-carbon heteronuclear bond to produce a benzylic radical that subsequently abstracts a hydrogen to form a methyl group. Translating this chemistry to solid support, one cleaves a compound library incorporating a benzylic-heteronuclear bond at the site of attachment. The resulting benzylic radical abstracts a hydrogen to incorporate a methyl group on the cleaved compound.

We have developed a photosensitive linker that upon irradiation with 350 nm

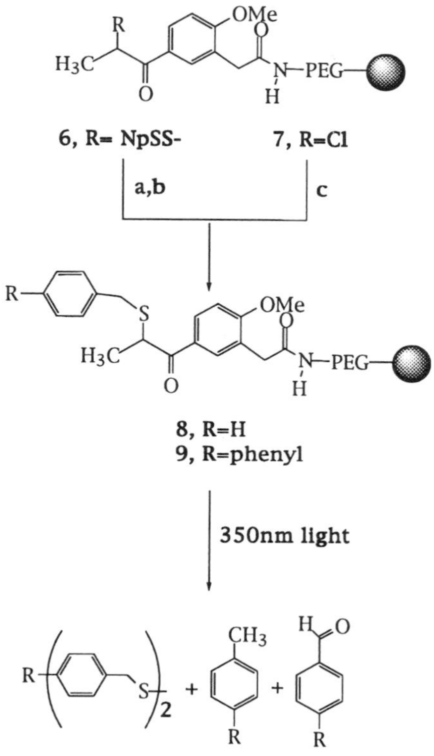

6, R= NpSS-   **7, R=Cl**

8, R=H
9, R=phenyl

350nm light

10   **11**   **12**

Scheme 6.1 Reagents: (a) mercaptoethanol, diisopropylethylamine (DIEA), DMF; (b) 4-phenylbenzylbromide, DIEA, DMF; (c) benzylmercaptan, DIEA, DMF.

light cleaves a thioether carbon–sulfur bond releasing the bound component from the support. This photosensitive linker is an α-mercapto-substituted phenyl ketone that is protected as the disulfide (9,21). The (±)-2-methoxy-5-[2-[(2-nitro-phenyl)dithio]-1-oxopropyl)phenyl acetic acid (NpSSMpact) linker **5** is attached to an amine containing support through an amide bond (Fig. 6.3).

Both the NpSSMpact linker **5** and its precursor (α-chloro derivative) were coupled to a PEG–PS (TentaGel) support using standard diisopropylcarbodiimide coupling methods to give supports **6** and **7** (Scheme 6.1). Support **7** was treated with benzylmercaptan and diisopropylethylamine (DIEA) to give the resulting benzyl-thiolether derivative **8**. Support **6** was first treated with β-mercaptoethanol (BME) and diisopropylethylamine (DIEA) to give the free thiol form of the linker (HSMpact), which was then alkylated with 4-phenylbenzylbromide to give the resulting biphenylthioether adduct **9** (21).

Irradiation of the β-keto-sulfide **8** (R = H) produces, as the sole product, disulfide **10** (Scheme 6.1). Irradiation of resin **9** (R = phenyl) gives biphenyl compounds **11** and **12** in a ratio of 94:6 and with an isolated yield for the major product **11** of 58% (21). The tolyl biphenyl **11** is the first case of a solid-phase photolytic cleavage not to incorporate a hydrogen bond donor or acceptor on the cleavage site of the molecule. The half-life for the release of biphenyl **11** was found to be around 30 min.

6.4   EXAMPLE SOLID-PHASE SYNTHESIS OF A TARGET MOLECULE

Once the support and the linker have been chosen, it is then possible to begin to plan the synthesis of the library. Many research groups have been making a series of amide bonds on a scaffold to produce combinatorial libraries. Because of the extensive early work in solid-phase peptide synthesis, the formation of amide bonds has become routine. In such cases, one could expect a high yield and purity of the final product. More synthetically challenging targets are now being pursued and will require a great deal of research and development to meet similar yield and purity standards. A major point that one must consider is how the synthesis conditions will affect the yield and purity of the final product. There are many problems that one encounters in making nonamide-containing libraries. One such problem is the incompatibility of some reaction solvents with certain supports. For example, reactions that utilize a nonexpanding solvent such as hexane may fail if they are attempted on crosslinked polystyrene. Another problem is the possible incompatibility of the support to high temperature and/or pressure. As discussed in Section 6.2, the restricted mobility of the bound support may negatively affect the rate of the reaction so that one may need to apply energy to the system in order to compensate.

One class of compounds we wished to produce as a library was biphenyls. Biphenyls are commonly found in many important natural products that exhibit both antitumor and antiviral activity (22). For a library approach to have a long-term and cost-effective advantage over classic modes of production certain requirements must be met. The chemistry should be amenable to running hundreds of multiple simultaneous reactions and, most importantly, should be fully automatable. Given present robotic technology, it is easier to meet such requirements by having the chemistries run at room temperature and under atmospheric conditions. Although many synthetic strategies have been used to make biphenyls, the palladium-catalyzed cross-coupling reaction between aryl electrophiles and aryl stannanes (Stille reaction) has been one of the most useful (23a–i). These reactions are reported to go in high yield, although in almost every instance prolonged heating as well as an inert atmosphere are required. We were interested in exploring the application of the Stille reaction to the solid-phase, room temperature synthesis of biaryls (24). Such an application would substantially reduce the amount of time and effort required for purifying the biaryl product, since any unreacted starting material could easily be washed off the support. This would make the simultaneous synthesis and purification of hundreds of biphenyl compounds easier to automate.

In a typical Stille biaryl formation, one combines the aryl electrophile with the aryl stannane in the presence of palladium, a phosphine ligand, and lithium chloride (Scheme 6.2). While the reaction conditions have been optimized for conventional solution coupling, they are just starting to be explored for heterogeneous systems (23j).

Our initial experiments began by attaching an aryl stannane on the Rink amide resin (24). The initial biaryl coupling conditions were adapted from the published work of Stille, Saá, and Farina (23a–h). The conditions were subsequently varied. We were next interested in transferring the best of our biaryl coupling conditions from the Rink amide resin to the NpSSMpact support. The free thiol of the NpSSMpact support (**17**) was treated with 4-iodobenzylbromide (**18**) in the presence of an excess of DIEA in DMF to give the resulting benzylthioether **19** (Scheme 6.3). The support was then treated with various quantities of trifurylphosphine (TFP), LiCl, Pd_2dba_3, and trialkylphenylstannane and subsequently irradiated with 350 nm light to cleave the product from the support.

When our earlier coupling conditions were applied to support **19**, only a very small amount of the corresponding biaryls **11** and **12** were isolated (Table 6.3) (24). Interestingly, beside the expected biaryls **11, 12** and unreacted phenyliodide ring

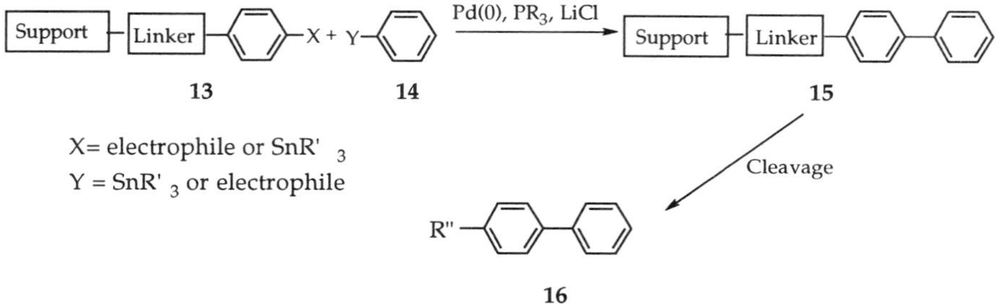

X= electrophile or SnR'$_3$
Y = SnR'$_3$ or electrophile

Scheme 6.2   Solid phase Stille coupling and cleavage to form biphenyls.

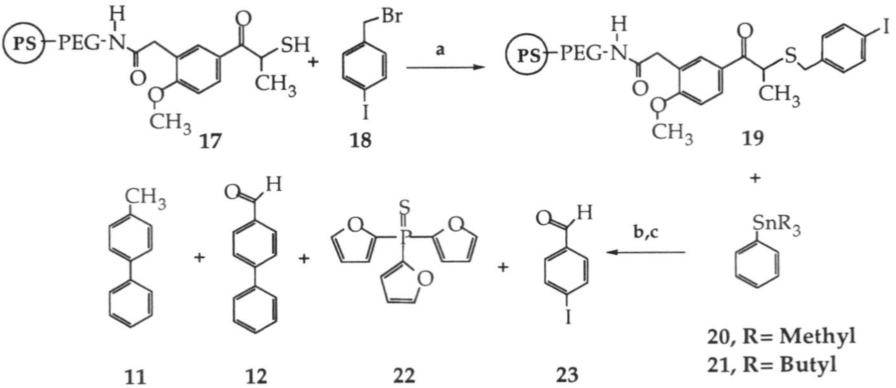

Scheme 6.3   Reagents: (a) DIEA, DMF; (b) Pd$_2$dba$_3$, LiCl, TFP, NMP, 25°C; (c) 350 nm light, acetonitrile.

(**23**), trifurylphosphine sulfide was also produced (entry 1 and 2). It was possible to eliminate this sulfide by-product by simply reducing the number of equivalents of TFP used. The results also showed that the quantities of palladium catalyst and trimethylphenylstannane needed were much higher than in the previous biaryl coupling experiments with the Rink amide resin (**24**). Fortunately, it was possible to adjust the number of equivalents of each of the various reagents to give exclusively biaryl product in modest yield (entry 6).

We were next interested in determining the extent of heterogeneous biaryl coupling with a functionalized trialkylphenyltin. Although ether-functionalized trialkyl-

TABLE 6.3   Product Distribution[a] and Percent Yield[b] of Biphenyl (11) after Biaryl Coupling at 25°C for 24 h in NMP[c] Followed by Photolytic Cleavage[d] of Solid Support

No.	R, Equivalents	TFP[c] (eq.)	Pd$_2$dba$_3$[c] (eq.)	LiCl (eq.)	11	12	22	23	Percent Yield of 11[b]
1	CH$_3$, 1.5	0.21	0.11	1.4	1	0.25	1.67	0.29	3
2	CH$_3$, 2.9	0.43	0.23	1.4	1	0.20	0.57	0	10
3	CH$_3$, 2.9	0.12	0.21	1.4	1	0.7	0	0	4.5
4	CH$_3$, 4.9	0.22	0.29	2.6	1	0.1	0.12	0	10
5	Butyl, 4.3	0.23	0.28	2.8	1	0.7	<0.05	0	3
6	CH$_3$, 12	0.18	0.23	2.0	1	0.1	0	0	27

[a] Product distribution obtained by ^{1}H-NMR.
[b] HPLC yield using an internal standard, Ref. 24.
[c] TFP = trifurylphosphine; Pd2dba3 = *tris*(dibenzylideneacetone)dipalladium; NMP = 1-methyl-2-pyrrolidinone.
[d] 350 nm light in acetonitrile, Ref. 21.

phenyltins have been widely reported to successfully undergo Stille couplings with aryl electrophiles, incorporation of an ester functional group was of interest because they are more easily capable of undergoing further conversion after biaryl coupling. 3-Acetoxytrimethylphenyl tin (**24**) was then coupled to support **19** using Pd$_2$dba$_3$, LiCl, and TFP in NMP to isolate after photolytic cleavage a 21% yield of biphenyl **25** (Scheme 6.4) (24). Recent work suggests the modest yield to be due to both incomplete cleavage of the biaryl compound from the support as well as a relatively low rate of biaryl coupling at room temperature. When biaryl-coupling reactions are run on standard ester-linked, crosslinked polystyrene at elevated temperatures (~80°C), a more than doubling of the biaryl product yield is seen.

Integrating the heating of multiple parallel solid-phase reactions with filtering and washing of the supports can pose significant challenges to automation. One way to circumvent the problem is by planning the library synthesis in such a way that steps requiring the application of heat be conducted as a batch process at the beginning of the synthetic pathway, before dividing up the resin for the multiple reaction well format.

An alternative to heating is the direct application of high-energy ultrasound to the solid-phase coupling reaction. In sonochemistry, enhancement of the rate of a chemical reaction is due not to the transfer of the sound itself but to the phenomenon of cavitation. In cavitation, microbubbles are produced as a result of the application of sound waves to a liquid medium. It is the collapse of these microbubbles that transfers energy to the chemical species. It has been theorized that the collapse of the microbubbles can cause the localized microenvironment surrounding the collapsed bubbles to reach temperatures of 5000 K and pressures of several thousand atmospheres (25).

We have found that one can apply high-energy ultrasound to the solid-phase coupling of a benzoate-protected trialkylphenyl tin **28** and a solid-supported aryl iodide **27** and achieve biaryl-coupling yields similar to that of heating (Scheme 6.5) (26). Applying high-energy ultrasound to solid-phase reactions has several advantages over heating: (1) It degasses the solvent while the reaction is running. (2) It

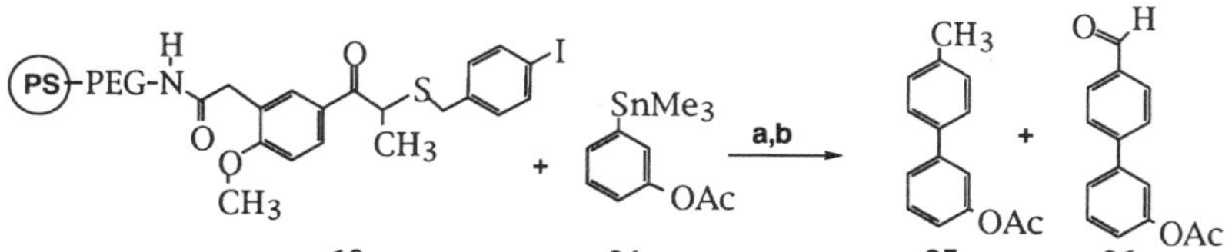

| | | Product Ratios[a] | 1 | : | 0.12 |
| | | % Yield of 25[b] | 21 | | |

[a] Obtained by ^{1}H NMR; [b] Ref. 24.

Scheme 6.4 Reagents: (a) 15 equiv. phenyltin **24**, 0.29 equiv. Pd$_2$dba$_3$, 2.5 equiv. LiCl, 0.35 TFP, NMP, 25°C; (b) 350 nm light, acetonitrile.

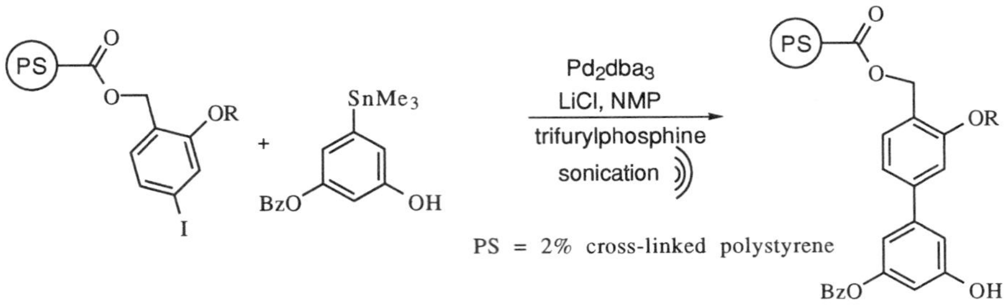

Scheme 6.5   The use of ultrasound in solid phase Stille biaryl couplings.

produces microbubbles that mix the heterogenious reaction, negating the need for stirring. (3) It forces resin that has inadvertently remained above the solvent level to gradually slide into the reaction mixture. Sonication has also been found to aide in resin washing by decreasing the time it takes solute particles located in the inner and outer surface of the support to reach equilibrium (27).

Upon completion of the resin-bound biphenyl scaffold, an array of different functionality can then be attached through the use of the Mitsunobu reaction (28,29). For example, exposing the resin-bound biphenyl **29** (Scheme 6.5) to a primary alcohol under Mitsunobu reaction conditions derivatizes the free phenol (**29**) to the corresponding phenylether. Subsequent deprotection of the phenylbenzo-ate followed by a second Mitsunobu reaction completes the derivatization process (29). By varying the positioning and functionalization of the phenols around the biphenyl scaffold a library composed of a diverse set of compounds can then be produced.

6.5   SUMMARY AND CONCLUSION

The use of a solid support for the synthesis of libraries of organic compounds has the primary advantage of giving one the ability to quickly separate the product from the soluble components of the reaction mixture. With this capability comes a multi-tude of new issues that one must address. Issues such as the support's loading capacity as well as the bound component's mobility must be taken into account. Additionally, the support's stability under the planned reaction conditions must be examined. Once a support has been chosen, one must then look at the type of chemistry that will be used to attach the target molecule to and cleave from the support. One must make certain that the conditions necessary to cleave a linker is compatible with those of the target compound. Once the synthesis of the target compound begins, one must be able to determine the extent to which the reactions have gone to completion and then modify such conditions accordingly. Lastly, if one of the goals is to automate the process, one must look at the entire sequence and determine whether it is more efficient to develop the chemistry to fit the automation or vice versa. At present, a current challenge to the organic chemist is to quickly and efficiently create libraries that are more sophisticated in the types of bonds created without dramatically sacrificing yield or purity. This will require the organic chemist to pursue more carbon–carbon bond forming reactions on solid support. As the field of combinatorial chemistry matures, new challenges will arise that will test the combinatorial research.

REFERENCES

1. (a) Moos, W. H., Green, G. C., and Pavia, M. R., in *Annual Reports in Medicinal Chemistry,* Vol. 28, J. A. Bristol (Ed.), 1993, p. 315; (b) Pavia, M. R., Sawyer, T. K., and Moos, W. H., *Bioorg. Med. Chem. Lett.* **3,** 387 (1993); (c) Terrett, N. K., Gardner, M., Gordon, D. W., Kobylecki, R. J., and Steele, J. *Tetrahedron* **51,** 8135 (1995); (d) Früchtel J. S., and Jung, G., *Angew. Chem. Int. Ed. Engl.* **35,** 17 (1996); (e) Dewitt, S. H., Kiely, J. S., Stankovic, C. J., Schroeder, M. C., Cody, D. M. R., and Pavia, M. R. *Proc. Natl. Acad. Sci. U.S.A.* **90,** 6909 (1993); (f) Bunin, B. A., and Ellman, J. A., *J. Am. Chem. Soc.* **114,** 10997 (1992); (g) Chen, C., Ahlberg Randall, L. A., Miller, R. B., Jones, A. D., and Kurth, M. J., *J. Am. Chem. Soc.* **116,** 2661 (1994).

2. (a) Barany, G., and Merrifield, R. B., in *The Peptides,* Vol. 2; E. Gross, and J. Meienhofer (Eds.), Academic, New York, 1980, pp. 1–284; (b) Fréchet, J. M. J., in *Polymer-supported Reactions in Organic Synthesis,* P. Hodge, and D. C. Sherrington (Eds.), Wiley, 1980, p. 294.

3. Regen, S. L., *J. Am. Chem. Soc.* **96,** 5275 (1974); (b) Regen, S. L., *Macromolecules* **8,** 689 (1975).

4. (a) Epton, R., Goddard, P., and Irvin, K., *J. Polymer* **21,** 1367 (1980); (b) Fréchet, J. M. J., *Tetrahedron* **37,** 663 (1981); (c) Giralt, E., Albericio, F., Bardella, F., Eritja, R., Feliz, M., Pedroso, E., Pons, M., and Rizo, J., in *Innovations and Perspectives in Solid Phase Synthesis,* R. Epton (Ed.), Hartnolls, Bodmin, Cornwall, U.K., 1990, pp. 111–120; (d) Albericio, F., Pons, M., Pedroso, E., and Giralt, E., *J. Org. Chem.* **54,** 360 (1989); (e) Giralt, E., Rizo, J., and Pedroso, E., *Tetrahedron,* **40,** 4141 (1984); (f) Look, G. C., Holmes, C. P., Chin, J. P., and Gallop, M. A. *J. Org. Chem.* **59,** 7588 (1994); (g) Bayer, E., and Rapp, W., in *Poly(ethylene Glycol) Chemistry: Biotechnology and Biomedical Applications,* J. M. Harris (Ed.), Plenum Press, New York, 1992, p. 325; (h) Bayer, E., Albert, K., Willisch, H., Rapp, W., and Hemmasi, B., *Macromolecules* **23,** 1937 (1990).

5. (a) Atherton, E., Brown, E., Sheppard, R. C., Rosevear, A., *J. Chem. Soc. Chem. Commun.* 1151 (1981); (b) Gait, M. J., Matthes, H. W., Singh, M., Sproat, B. S., and Titmas, R. C., *Nucleic Acid Res.* **10,** 6243 (1982); (c) Minganti, C., Ganesh, K. N., Sproat, B. S., and Gait, M. J., *Analytical Biochem.* **147,** 63 (1985).

6. (a) Small, P. W., and Sherrington, D. C., *J. Chem. Soc. Chem. Comm.* 1589 (1989); (b) Bhaskar, N. K., King, B. W., Meyers, P., and Westlake, J. P., in *Innovation and Perspectives in Solid Phase Synthesis, Peptides, Proteins and Nucleic Acids,* R. Epton (Ed.), Mayflower Worldwide, Birmingham, U.K., 1994, p. 451.

7. (a) Bayer, E., and Rapp, W., in *Chemistry of Peptides and Proteins,* Vol. 2, 1986, p. 3; (b) Bayer, E., U.S. patent 4,908,405, 1990; (c) Zalipsky, S., Albericio, F., and Barany, G., *Peptides: Structure and Function. Proceedings of the Ninth American Peptide Sympo-*

sium, V. J. Hruby, C. N. Deber, and K. D. Kopple (Eds.), Pierce Chemical, Rockford, IL, 1986, p. 257; (d) Butz, S., Rawer, S., Rapp, W., and Birsner, U., *Peptide Res.* **7**, 20 (1994).

8. Keana, J. F. W., Shimizu, M., and Jernstedt, K. K., *J. Org. Chem.* **51**, 1641 (1986).

9. (a) Sucholeiki, I., *Med. Chem. Res.* **5**, 618 (1995); (b) Sucholeiki, I., in *Fourth International Symposium—Solid Phase Synthesis & Complementary Technologies*, R. Epton, (Ed.), Mayflower Worldwide, Birmingham, U.K., 1996.

10. (a) Frenette, R., and Friesen, R. W., *Tetrahedron Lett.* **35**, 9177 (1994); (b) Kurth, M. J., Ahlberg Randal, L. A., Chen, C., Melander, C., Miller, R. B., McAlister, K., Reitz, G., Kang, R., Nakatsu, T., and Green, C., *J. Org. Chem.* **59**, 5862 (1994).

11. (a) Rink, H., *Tetrahedron Lett.* **28**, 3787 (1987); (b) Bernatowica, M. S., Daniels, S. B., and Köster, H., *Tetrahedron Lett.* **30**, 4645 (1989).

12. (a) Zuckermann, R. N., Kerr, J. M., Kent, S. B. H., and Moos, W. H., *J. Am. Chem. Soc.* **114**, 10646 (1992); (b) Zuckerman, R. N., Martin, E. J., Spellmeyer, D. C., Stauber, G. B., Shoemaker, K. R., Kerr, J. M., Figliozzi, G. M., Goff, D. A., Siani, M. A., Simon, R. J., Banville, s. C., Brown, E. G., Wang, L., Richter, L. S., and Moos, W. H., *J. Med. Chem.* **37**, 2678 (1994).

13. Wang, S. S., *J. Am. Chem. Soc.* **95**, 1328 (1973).

14. Barlos, K., Gatos, D., Papaphotiu, G., Schäfer, W., and Wenqing, Y., *Tetrahedron Lett.* **30**, 3947 (1989).

15. Wang, S. S., *J. Org. Chem.* **41**, 3258 (1976).

16. (a) Tjoeng, F. S., and Heavner, G. A., *Tetrahedron Lett.* **23**, 4439 (1982); (b) Uggeri, F., Giordano, C., and Brambilla, A., *J. Org. Chem.* **51**, 97 (1986).

17. Pillai, V. N. R., and Ajayaghosh, A., *Indian J. Chem.* **27B**, 1004 (1988).

18. Nestler, H. P., Bartlett, P. A., and Still, W. C., *J. Org. Chem.* **59**, 4723 (1994).

19. Barltrop, J. A., Plant, P. J., and Schofield, P., *Chem. Commun.* **22**, 823 (1966).

20. (a) Rich, D. H., and Gurwara, S. K., *Chem. Commun.* 610 (1973); (b) Rich, D. H., and Gurwara, S. K., *J. Am. Chem. Soc.* **97**, 1575 (1975).

21. Sucholeiki, I., *Tetrahedron Lett.* **35**, 7307 (1994).

22. Okuda, T., Yoshida, T., and Hatano, T., in *Phenolic Compounds in Food and Their Effects on Health*, Vol. II, M. Huang, C. Ho, C. Lee (Eds.), ACS Symposium Series 507, American Chemical Society, Washington, DC, 1992, p. 160.

23. (a) Stille, J. K., *Angew. Chem. Int. Ed. Engl.* **25**, 508 (1986); (b) Echavarren, A. M., and Stille, J. K., *J. Am. Chem. Soc.* **110**, 1557 (1988); (c) Thompson, W. J., Jones, J. H., Lyle, P. A., and Thies, J. E., *J. Org. Chem.*, **53**, 2052 (1988); (d) Miyaura, N., Ishiyama, T., Sasaki, H., Ishikawa, M., Satoh, M., and Sazuki, A., *J. Am. Chem. Soc.* **111**, 314 (1989); (e) Martorell, G., García-Raso, A., and Saá, J. M., *Tett. Lett.* **31**, 2357 (1990); (f) Farina, V., and Krishnan, B., *J. Am. Chem. Soc.* **113**, 9585 (1991); (g) Saá, J. M., Martorell, G., and García-Raso, A., *J. Org. Chem.* **57**, 678 (1992); (h) Farina, V., Krishnan, B., Marshall, D. R., and Roth, G. P., *J. Org. Chem.* **58**, 5434 (1993); (i) Ritter, K., *Synthesis*, 735 (1993); (j) Deshpande, M. S., *Tetrahedron Lett.* **35**, 5613 (1994).

24. Forman, F. W., and Sucholeiki, I., *J. Org. Chem.* **60**, 523 (1995).

25. Suslick, K. S., *Science* **247**, 1373 (1990).

26. Forman, F. W., and Sucholeiki, I., unpublished results.

27. Takahashi, S., and Shimonishi, Y., *Chem. Lett.***XL,** 51 (1974).

28. Krchnák, V., Flegelová, Z., Weichsel, A. S., and Lebl, M., *Tetrahedron Lett.*, **36,** 6193 (1995).

29. Pavia, M. R., Cohen, M. P., Dilley, G. J., Dubuc, G. R., Durgin, T. L., Forman, F. W., Hediger, M. E., Milot, G., Powers, T. S., Sucholeiki, I., Zhou, S., and Hangauer, D. G., *Biorg. Med. Chem.* **4**(5), 659–666 (1996).

7

RADIOFREQUENCY ENCODING AND ADDITIONAL TECHNIQUES FOR THE STRUCTURE ELUCIDATION OF SYNTHETIC COMBINATORIAL LIBRARIES

Xiao-yi Xiao and Michael P. Nova

IRORI Quantum Microchemistry, 11025 N. Torrey Pines Road, Suite 100, La Jolla, California 92037

As one of the most promising approaches to generate large molecular diversity, combinatorial chemistry (1–4) attracts ever increasing scrutiny from the drug discovery community. Synthetic chemical libraries with 10^2 to $>10^6$ compounds have been constructed and screened during the past few years utilizing modern solution and solid-phase synthetic chemistry methodology and advanced robotic instrumentation. Split synthesis (or pool and split synthesis, Fig. 7.1) (5–7) is by far the most efficient method for the construction of large combinatorial chemical libraries. Although library design, synthetic methodology development, library construction, and screening are important issues in the application of combinatorial chemistry, the biggest challenge (or the bottleneck) of the combinatorial process is the structural elucidation of the interested member(s) within a particular library. Strategies addressing this identification issue can be grouped into three major categories: (1) microanalysis, (2) iterative deconvolution, and (3) encoding by chemical or the newly demonstrated remote radiofrequency methods. Parallel synthesis of spatially addressable compound arrays (8,9) is more suitable for small-size libraries and will not be discussed in this chapter. Microanalysis and chemical encoding methods use complex chemical and microanalytical procedures to solve the structures of library members. Deconvolution addresses the issue by tedious, iterative resynthesis and assay of smaller and smaller sublibraries. Radiofrequency encoding is a concep-

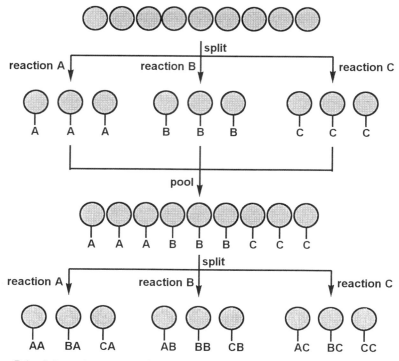

Figure 7.1   Schematic representation of a 3 × 3 split combinatorial synthesis. A, B, and C are building blocks.

tually new, noninvasive method employing chemically benign microelectronic memory to encode combinatorial synthesis.

7.1   MICROANALYSIS

Direct microanalysis is the very first technique used to characterize synthetic chemical libraries. In general two types of microanalysis are utilized: microsequencing and mass spectrometry. Members in peptide libraries can be sequenced by Edman degradation, and oligonucleotides libraries can be analyzed by Sanger dideoxy sequencing (10,11). For libraries other than peptides and oligonucleotides, mass spectrometry can be used to elucidate structures of library members.

7.1.1   Off-bead Mass Spectrometry

Individual compounds can be cleaved from individual resin beads, worked up, and analyzed conventionally (12,13). Mixtures of a small number of compounds cleaved from pools of beads can also be analyzed by electrospray mass spectrometry (ES-MS) coupled with chromatographic methods such as gas chromatography (GC) and high-pressure liquid chromatography (HPLC) (GC-MS and HPLC-MS) (14–17). Metzger et al. (17) employed electrospray mass spectrometry coupled with tandem mass spectrometry (MS-MS) in the determination of the composition and purity of 100 synthetic 48-component peptide mixtures. Very little mass discrimination effects were observed among the structurally similar peptides in the mixtures. Therefore the relative concentrations of the individual components with different molecular weights can be estimated using the peak heights of the ES-MS spectra. The identification of isobaric peptides and by-products was achieved by the application of tandem mass spectrometry analysis.

Affinity capillary electrophoresis (ACE) has been coupled with mass spectrometry (ACE-MS) to select and identify ligands for receptors. A mixture of compounds (i.e., a peptide library) is passed through an affinity capillary. The tighter a ligand binds to the target receptor, the longer it takes to pass through the capillary (retention time). Thus ligands with different binding properties are separated and are identified by on-line MS. Chu et al. (18) demonstrated this technique using vancomycin (19) as the model receptor and a 100-member all-D tetrapeptide library as the ligand mixture. Three tight-binding ligands (Fmoc-DDYA, Fmoc-DDFA, and Fmoc-DDHA) as well as the natural ligand (Fmoc-DDAA) were unambiguously identified. Only nanograms of ligands are required for this procedure.

7.1.2 On-bead Mass Spectrometry

More direct procedures, in which the cleaved compounds are analyzed while still resting on the resin beads, have been discussed recently. Brummel et al. (20) used imaging time-of-flight secondary ion mass spectrometry (TOF-SIMS) (21,22) to identify the molecular weights of peptides attached through an acid-labile linker to polystyrene beads. The beads were placed on a Cu grid and briefly exposed to trifluoroacetic acid/methylene chloride vapor to cleave the covalent bonds between the peptides and the polystyrene while leaving the detached peptides resting in place on the beads. A TOF-SIMS image was then recorded directly from the beads residing on the Cu grid. Since the beads are spatially defined on the Cu grid, mixtures of beads with different peptides (or other molecules) can be analyzed in parallel.

Fitzgerald et al. (23) have demonstrated the application of photolytic cleavage and matrix-assisted laser desorption/ionization (MALDI) mass spectrometry in the direct analysis of molecules bound on solid supports. Peptides were synthesized on polystyrene beads through a photolabile linker. Resin beads were deposited on a MALDI sample plate, added with an ethanol solution of the matrix, and dried at room temperature. The matrix was photolyzed *and* ionized at the same time with an ultraviolet (UV) laser, and the mass spectrum was then recorded. Because only a very small amount of material is cleaved from the resin by the laser irradiation used in the MALDI analysis (24), the resin can be easily recovered from the sample for further reactions/manipulations. A similar procedure employing an acid-labile linker and trifluoroacetic acid vapor as the cleavage reagent was reported by Egner et al. (25).

Microanalysis of synthetic chemical libraries is advantageous in the sense that the compounds are analyzed directly; therefore the structural information obtained has a high degree of reliability. However, there are several limitations associated with this strategy. At present, microsequencing can only be applied to peptide and oligonucleotide libraries. Although mass spectrometry can be used to analyze a far greater variety of compounds, it can only identify compounds with a unique mass. When compounds with the same molecular weights are to be distinguished, complex, time-consuming fragmentation analysis or other delicate techniques are required.

7.2   DECONVOLUTION

7.2.1   Iterative Deconvolution

The iterative deconvolution strategy has been extensively investigated in the last decade. In essence, this method consists of the screening of compound pools, identifying the active pool(s), resynthesizing and rescreening sublibraries (smaller pools). The number of compounds in the sublibraries gets smaller and smaller, until only a single compound is present in each pool, therefore leading to the identification of the active library member(s).

Geysen et al. (26) first used the iterative process to identify peptide ligands for monoclonal antibodies in epitope analyses. In the synthesis of an octapeptide library using the multipin method (27), the fourth and fifth positions were defined, and 400 sublibraries were made using the 20 natural L-amino acids (represented as $XXXA_4A_5XXX$ where A_4 and A_5 are the defined positions with a single amino acid, and X is the random positions through coupling of mixtures of activated amino acids). The sublibraries were assayed with an ELISA (enzyme-linked immunosorbant assay), and the most active library was identified, therefore defining the best A_4 and A_5. A third position was then fixed and 20 new, smaller sublibraries were resynthesized and assayed to define the third best residue. This iterative process was repeated until all the residues were defined. The above method is called the "mimotope strategy."

In the study of a library of more than 34 million hexapeptides in a general formula of Ac-XXXXXX-NH_2, Houghten et al. (28) synthesized 324 sublibraries by fixing the first two positions and varying the other four positions ("dual-defined iterative method") with 18 natural L-amino acids (represented by Ac-A_1A_2XXXX-NH_2). In a similar fashion to the mimotope strategy, the sequence Ac-DVPDYA-NH_2 was identified as the most effective inhibitor (IC_{50} = 0.03 μM) against a specific antibody binding event.

The same process has also been employed in the deconvolution of oligonucleotide libraries (29) and small molecule organic libraries (30). In an example of a small molecule library, Patel et al. (30) prepared a 100-member dihydropyridine library with two degrees of variations (10 building blocks for each). After the addition of the second sets of building blocks, the 10 pools were kept separate (each containing 10 dihydropyridines) and assayed using a cortex membrane binding assay (31). Members in the most active pool(s) were resynthesized and assayed using the crude cleavage products and the most active compounds were then purified by HPLC, fully characterized, and used to determine precise IC_{50} values. Dihydropyridines with IC_{50} values in the 10 nM range were successfully identified.

A variation of the above described iterative process termed "recursive deconvolution" is presented by Erb et al. (32) in their pentapeptide library study. During the split synthesis of the library, a portion of the resin in each pool was saved after each coupling. These saved pools were then used in the resynthesis of the sublibraries during the iterative deconvolution process. This method saves sublibrary synthesis work by providing partially built pools for resynthesis use.

7.2.2 Positional Scanning

Positional scanning is a term for the deconvolution process in which all sublibraries, each having one position defined, are synthesized up front. Taking a hexapeptide library as an example, the six positional scanning sublibrary series can be represented as A_1XXXXX, XA_2XXXX, XXA_3XXX, $XXXA_4XX$, $XXXXA_5X$ and $XXXXXA_6$. Each series consists of 20 sublibraries if all 20 L-amino acids are to be used, giving a total of 120 sublibraries to be screened. The most active sublibrary or sublibraries in each series define the best residue(s) at that particular position. These preferred amino acids for each position are then used to synthesize the sequence(s) with the best activities. Positional scanning eliminates the need to resynthesize and assay sublibraries but does not have the advantage of activity enrichment along the process as observed in the mimotope strategy. Pinna et al. (23) and Dooley and Houghten (34) successfully identified opioid receptor ligands from synthetic peptide libraries employing the positional scanning strategy. A 54-member carbamate library was constructed and deconvoluted by Pirrung et al. (35) employing an almost identical strategy called "indexed library."

Iterative deconvolution eliminates the need for direct microanalysis. It also can be applied in the synthesis of "un-encodable" libraries where the different building blocks are connected together in one single step [i.e., a library formed by a Ugi reaction (36)] rather than sequentially. However, it creates the need to synthesize and assay sublibraries, which is obviously very time consuming. Any inconsistency during the synthesis and assay process will very likely give erroneous results. The total concentration limit of all the components, and possible combinational biological effects of multiple components in a pool, only further diminish the effectiveness of this technique.

7.3 ENCODING

To overcome some of the problems associated with microanalysis and deconvolution, various encoding (or tagging) strategies have been applied in synthesizing combinatorial libraries. The basic principle of synthetic combinatorial library encoding is that a unique tag (chemical or nonchemical, T_a, T_b, or T_c; Fig. 7.2) is

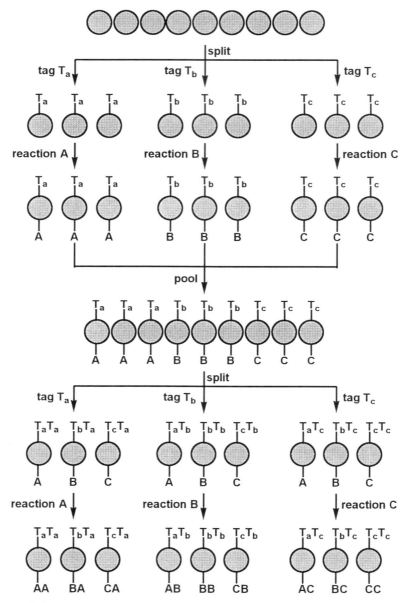

Figure 7.2 Schematic representation of a 3 × 3 encoded combinatorial library. A, B, and C are building blocks. T_a, T_b, and T_c are tags.

associated sequentially with each bead when each building block (A, B, C) is appended, therefore recording a histogram of building block additions, which each bead has been subjected to, during the entire synthesis. The complete structure of the compound synthesized on any bead can then be reconstructed by reading this histogram recorded by the associated tags. The scheme for binary encoding is somewhat different from this and will be discussed separately. If chemical tags are to be used, dual chemical compatibility between the chemistry for both the tags and ligands is clearly essential for the entire tagging strategy to be effective. A noninvasive encoding scheme can only be realized when nonchemical tags, such as radiofrequency memory units, are utilized.

7.3.1 Chemical Encoding

Oligonucleotides, peptides, halocarbons, and secondary amines have been used to chemically encode synthetic libraries.

7.3.1.1 Oligonucleotide Tags The concept of oligonucleotide encoding was proposed and tested by two independent groups. Brenner and Lerner (37) and Nielsen et al. (38) demonstrated this procedure by encoding an eight-member tripeptide library with two sequences of hexanucleotides: CACATG for Gly, ACGGTA for Met. The first polymerase chain reaction (PCR) primer (GGGCCCTATTCTTAG) was synthesized on one end of an orthogonally protected bifunctional linker attached to the peptide synthesis resin. The split synthesis of the tripeptides using the two amino acids was then carried out from the other end of the linker, with the addition of the corresponding oligonucleotide code following each amino acid coupling. The second PCR primer (AGCTACTTCCCAAGG) was finally added. The identities of the peptides in the library were decoded by PCR amplification and sequencing of the DNA tags.

Needles et al. (39) independently proposed and investigated the same concept of DNA encoding of synthetic libraries by the construction on 10-μm polystyrene beads of a much larger pentapeptide library (7^7 = 823,543) encoded with seven dinucleotides (TA, TC, CT, AT, TT, CA, and AC) for the seven amino acids (Arg, Gln, Phe, Lys, Val, D-Val, and Thr). The beads were then subjected to a fluorescence activated cell sorting (FACS) analysis of antibody (mAb D32.39) binding. Individual beads with the most binding were sorted out and the bead-bound DNA tags were amplified by PCR and sequenced to identify the peptides synthesized on the beads.

7.3.1.2 Peptide Tags A 200-peptide library (Ac-RAX$_3$HTTGX$_2$IX$_1$-NH$_2$) was encoded with tripeptide tags containing Leu, Phe, Gly, and Ala. An orthogonally protected lysine (N^α-Fmoc-N^ϵ-Moz-lysine) was used as the bifunctional linker (40). Thus, the ligand peptides reside on the "binding strand" and the tagging tripeptides on the "coding strand." The four pools of 50 peptides corresponding to the four building blocks for X$_3$ were kept separate and cleaved into solution. The pools were subjected to a competition assay and three highest affinity peptides were isolated from the most active pool by affinity selection (41,42) with the antibody anti-gp120 and HPLC chromatography. Edman sequencing of the coding strands on the high-affinity components identified the structures of the three decapeptides with IC_{50} values between 10^{-6} and 10^{-7} M, which were confirmed by subsequent independent synthesis and assay. Separate control study indicated that the coding strand did not interfere with the binding strand at least in this case.

A rather different approach of using peptides as tags was reported recently by Youngquist et al. (43). Peptide libraries are synthesized using a process termed "termination synthesis." During the synthesis of peptide libraries, a small percentage of the growing chains are terminated at each coupling step by a mixture of a capping reagent (i.e., N-acetyl-D,L-alanine) and the individual amino acid in a ratio of 1:9. Therefore, the composition of the final product on any individual bead in the synthesis of, say, a hexapeptide library will be $X_6X_5X_4X_3X_2X_1$-bead (full length, major product), $CAP-X_5X_4X_3X_2X_1$-bead, $CAP-X_4X_3X_2X_1$-bead, $CAP-X_3X_2X_1$-bead, $CAP-X_2X_1$-bead, $CAP-X_1$-bead, and CAP-bead, where CAP represent the capping reagent and X_n for amino acid residues. The sequence-specific termination products so generated are then cleaved, together with the full length peptide, from a single positive bead after in vitro screening. This mixture of full length and termination peptides are then analyzed with MALDI-MS and the sequence of the full length peptide is deduced from the mass differences between the termination products. Different capping reagents can be used to differentiate building blocks with the same molecular weights. Using this tagging strategy, the above authors (43) synthesized peptide libraries of up to 10^6 members and identified peptide ligands to streptavidin and an anti-HIV-1 gp120 monoclonal antibody. The same procedure was also applied in the study of a methyl phosphonate oligodeoxyribonucleotides (44).

7.3.1.3 Molecular Tags
A different tagging strategy called "binary encoding" has been developed (45–47). Unlike the above-described approaches, the sequence and building block information is recorded by a set of binary codes assigned to a set of molecular tags (and their mixtures) rather than by the sequence in which the tags are linked. The way the molecular tags link together is not important. A set of n-bit binary codes can sufficiently represent a set of (2^n-1) building blocks used in a synthetic step. An m-step synthesis can then be described with a string of $(n \times m)$ binary digits (assuming each step uses the same number of building blocks). To chemically represent these binary digits, a set of $(n \times m)$ distinguishable, easily detectable molecular tags (i.e., fluoro- or chlorocarbons) are used where the presence and absence of a particular tag corresponds to a binary digit 1 or 0.

As an example, a set of three building blocks (A, B, C) can be represented by the following 2-bit binary codes: $01 = A$, $10 = B$, and $11 = C$ (Fig. 7.3). For simplicity, let us assume the complete synthesis is two steps with the same set of building blocks for each step. The synthesis on any individual bead can then be described by a string of four binary digits, which in turn requires a total of four molecular tags (T_4, T_3, T_2, T_1) to represent the 1's and 0's starting from right to left of the binary string. For the first step of the addition of the building blocks A, B, and C, the tags (or tag mixtures) T_1, T_2 and $(T_1 + T_2)$ are added, respectively, and

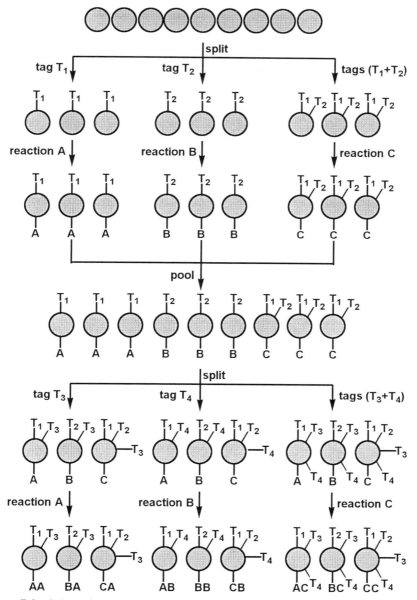

Figure 7.3 Schematic representation of a 3 × 3 binary encoded combinatorial library. A, B, and C are building blocks. T_1, T_2, T_3, and T_4 are tags.

T_3, T_4, and ($T_3 + T_4$) for the second step. The amount of tags is controlled so that only a small percentage (0.5%) of the growing ligands (i.e., peptides) is terminated or modified by the tags. After synthesis and screening, tag mixtures from positive beads are cleaved and analyzed by the highly sensitive electron capture gas chromatography (ECCO) method (48). If the tag mixture cleaved from a particular bead after the complete synthesis contains only T_4, T_2, T_1, the corresponding binary string would be 10/11, which in turn represents a structure of B-C-bead.

In practice, two tag attaching and detaching mechanisms have been developed (Fig. 7.4). The nitrobenzoic acid linker was first used to attach the tags to amines on solid supports through an amide bond (45,49). The tag detachment was conveniently achieved by UV irradiation. A second linker was developed using a diazoketone functionality as the attaching group and an oxidatively cleavable catechol diether moiety as the detaching mechanism (46,50). Using the above binary encoding strategy, a peptide library containing 7^6 members was encoded and screened with an anti-c-MYC mAb to identify binding sequences (45). A synthetic receptor substrate library (49) as well as a smaller molecule, amide bond formation-based library (50) were also encoded with this technique.

Ni et al. at Affymax (51) recently reported a variation of the above binary encoding procedure. Instead of using halocarbons, the Affymax group used sets of secondary amines whose dansyl derivatives can be readily analyzed by reverse-phase HPLC. The tags were easily prepared by opening the anhydride of a protected iminodiacetic acid with the selected secondary amines. The tag addition was accomplished by amidation of the orthogonally differentiated amino groups on the resin (or the secondary amine on the tag strand after the first step) by the carboxylic acid moiety of the tags. Tag detachment was achieved by acidic hydrolysis (Fig. 7.5).

Molecular tagging or binary encoding partially solves the tag stability problems

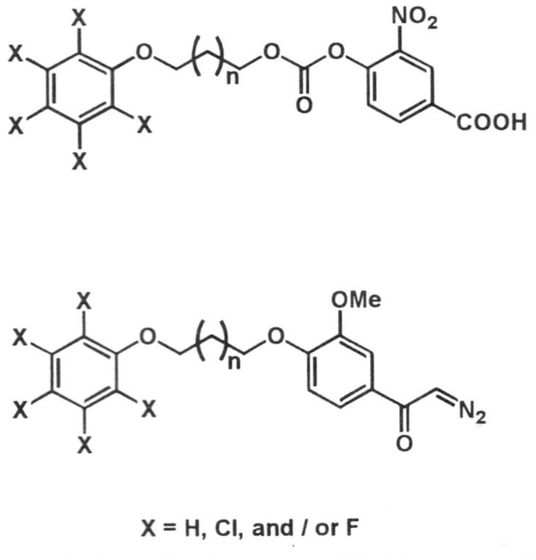

X = H, Cl, and / or F

Figure 7.4   Molecular tags used in binary encoding.

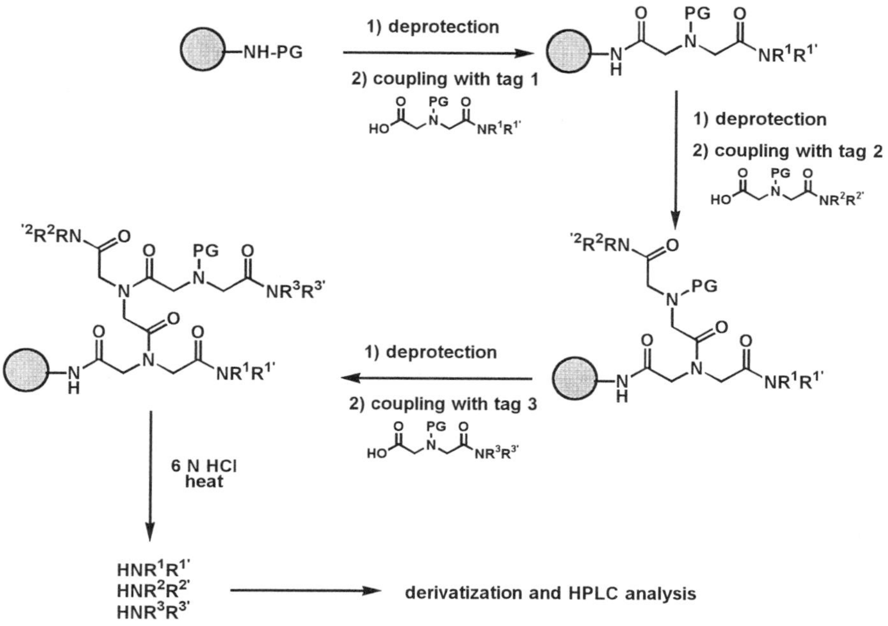

Figure 7.5   Attaching and detaching of secondary amine binary tags.

associated with oligonucleotide and peptide tagging by introducing chemically more stable tags such as halocarbons and secondary amines (in a form of poly secondary amides). It avoids, to a partial degree, the possible interference from the oligonucleotide or peptide tags during biological assays. However, the application of a binary coding system requires a set of specially crafted molecular tags since both the identities and the sequences of the building blocks have to be represented unambiguously by the tag mixtures. Due to its chemical or invasive nature, any molecular tagging system not only more than doubles the synthetic work during library construction but also requires tedious tag analysis for subsequent decoding, which further limits the potential applications.

7.3.1.4   Isotope Encoding   Recently, Geysen et al. (56) reported a method for isotopically tagging resin beads during combinatorial synthesis. The tags are encoded via a controlled ratio of a number of stable isotopes as the tagging molecules, and range from a single to a complex isotopic distribution. The isotopes are cleaved after assay and analyzed by mass spectrometry in an automated fashion.

7.3.2   Radiofrequency Encoding

Microanalysis, deconvolution, and chemical encoding may solve some of the problems in the structure elucidation of synthetic combinatorial libraries; however, these techniques create additional analytical problems. Their limitations are obvious, and the ultimate solution is clear: a straightforward, completely nonchemical, noninvasive encoding strategy.

Nicolaou et al. (52) introduced a conceptually new strategy termed "Radiofrequency Encoded Combinatorial (REC) chemistry." Using small microelectronic memory semiconductors, rather than chemical labels, relevant information along a synthetic pathway within a combinatorial synthesis (i.e., a histogram of the synthesis) is recorded on each Microreactor (or a macro "bead") through remote radiofrequency transmission. The information can be retrieved anytime from a distance (75–150 mm) during or after the synthesis to decode the structure of the compound synthesized in each microreactor. Apparently, this strategy successfully meets the requirement for a completely noninvasive encoding/decoding procedure due to its nonchemical nature.

The microreactor consists of three components (panel a, Fig. 7.6): (1) a chemically inert porous enclosure made of polypropylene or fluoropolymer, which encapsulates the other two components; (2) regular solid-phase synthesis resin (20–50 mg); and (3) a glass-encased Single or Multiple Addressable Radiofrequency Tag (SMART) semiconductor unit capable of receiving, storing, and emitting radiofrequency signals from a distance (53) (an RF tag). This small tag contains standard EEPROM (electrically erasable, programmable, read-only memory) coupled to an antenna core. The antenna not only captures the relevant information to be stored or read but also provides the power source for the chip. No battery is then ever required. Solid-phase reactions take place on the regular resin inside the porous enclosure and the encoding information is recorded on the RF tag. Since each microreactor contains up to 50 mg of resin (and can be increased if desired by using a bigger porous enclosure), multimilligrams of pure (assuming the chemistry works), discrete compounds can be obtained from each microreactor.

A representative 3×3 split synthesis using the microreactors are depicted in Figure 7.7. A pool of microreactors are split into three equal groups. Each group is encoded, through radiofrequency transmission from the encoding/decoding station, with a unique radiofrequency signal (i.e., *a*, *b*, or *c*). Building block additions (i.e., **A, B,** or **C**) are then performed with the corresponding group. The three groups are then combined and resplit equally into three new groups, with which encoding (with *a, b,* or *c*) and building block additions (with **A, B,** or **C**) are performed accordingly. After the completion of the synthesis, the structure of the compound synthesized in any individual microreactor is readily and reliably decoded by simply reading the RF codes recorded on the memory of the RF tag inside the microreactor. The authors successfully demonstrated this new concept by the split synthesis of a 24-member tetrapeptide library using 96 microreactors. The structures of all the library members were decoded from the radiofrequency codes and confirmed by electrospray mass spectrometry and ¹H-NMR. Complete correlation between the RF codes and compound structures were evident. Utilities with large organic libraries have also been demonstrated by us recently (54).

A second form of the microreactor is a RF tag directly coated with a layer of solid-phase synthesis polymer such as polystyrene and properly functionalized (55),

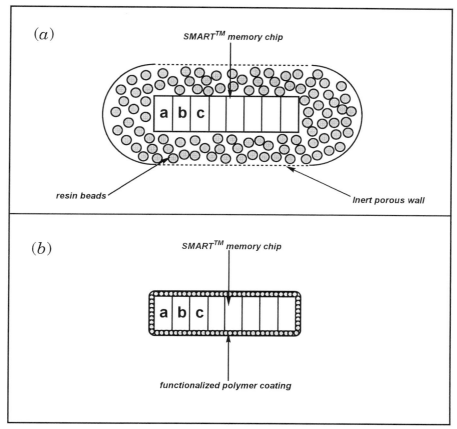

Figure 7.6 Schematic representation of the Microreactors used in Radiofrequency Encoded Combinatorial (REC) chemistry.

shown in panel b, Figure 7.6. While microreactor a (Fig. 7.6) has the advantage of greater versatility in terms of solid support selection (one can use essentially any type of resin desired), the directly coated microreactor (b, Fig. 7.6) is more compact, easier to manipulate, and potentially provides greater purity of compounds.

Radiofrequency Encoded Combinatorial (REC) chemistry overcomes all the limitations associated with any previously existing structure elucidation methods for combinatorial synthesis by relying entirely on chemically benign radiofrequency signals and micro memory electronics. Its obvious advantages include (but are not limited to): (a) reliable and straightforward encoding/decoding; (b) large encoding capacity [current RF memory chips can hold a 16-bit alphanumeric (26 letters and 10 numbers) string]. That translates to a 16-split-step synthesis with up to 36 building blocks for each step if a one-letter code is used to encode one building block, producing a library of $36^{16} = 8 \times 10^{24}$ members! Two-letter codes can be used if a

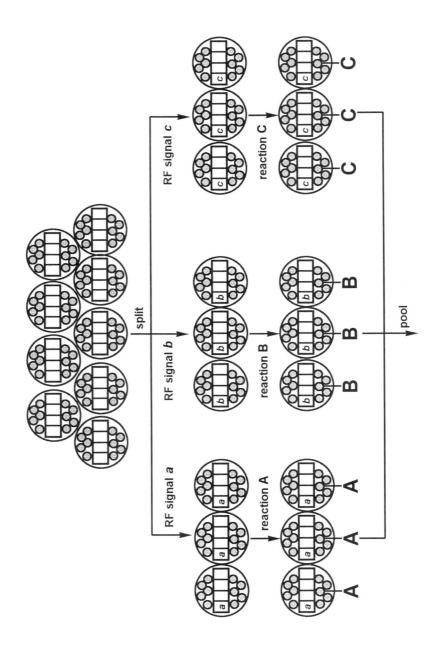

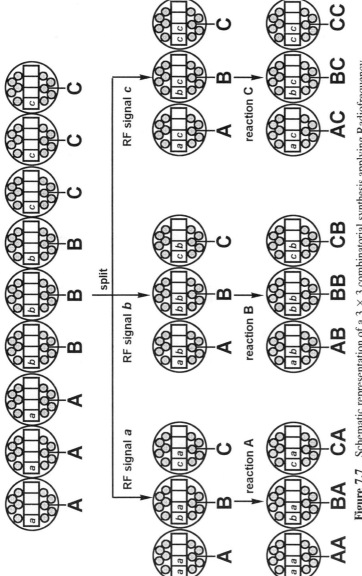

Figure 7.7 Schematic representation of a 3 × 3 combinatorial synthesis applying Radiofrequency Encoded Combinatorial (REC) chemistry. A, B, and C are building blocks; *a*, *b*, and *c* are radio-frequency signals used for encoding.

split step uses more than 36 building blocks.]; (c) storage of other relevant information along the synthetic pathway; (d) capability of producing multimilligram quantities of pure, discrete compounds; and (e) ready automation. REC chemistry clearly combines the advantages of split synthesis to achieve high synthesis efficiency, and the advantages of parallel synthesis to produce pure, discrete library compounds in good quantities. The huge potential of the REC technology will make it the method of choice for future combinatorial and other chemistry and biology applications.

REFERENCES

1. Gallop, M. A., Barret, R. W., Dower, W. J., Fodor, S. P. A., and Gordon, E. M., *J. Med. Chem.* **37,** 1233 (1994).

2. Gordon, E. M., Barret, R. W., Dower, W. J., Fodor, S. P. A., and Gallop, M. A., *J. Med. Chem.* **37,** 1385 (1994).

3. Jung, G., and Deck-Sickinger, A. G., *Angew. Chem. Int. Ed. Engl.* **31,** 367 (1992).

4. Pavia, M. R., Sawyer, T. K., and Moos, W. H., *Bioorg. Med. Chem. Lett.* **3,** 387 (1993).

5. Lam, K. S., Salmon, S. E., Hersh, E. M., Hruby, V. J., Kazmierski, W. M., and Knapp, R. J., *Nature* **354,** 82 (1991).

6. Lam, K. S., Hruby, V. J., Lebl, M., Knapp, R. J., Kazmierski, W. M., Hersh, E. M., and Salmon, S. E., *Bioorg. Med. Chem. Lett.* **3,** 419 (1993).

7. Furka, Á., Sevestyén, F., Asgedom, M., and Dibó, G. *Int. J. Peptide Res.* **37,** 487 (1991).

8. Fodor, S. P. A., Read, J. L., Pirrung, M. C., Stryer, L., Lu, A. T., and Solas, D., *Science* **251,** 767 (1991).

9. Meyers, H. V., Dilley, G. J., Durgin, T. L., Powers, T. S., Winssinger, N. A., Zhu, H., and Pavia, M. R., *Mol. Diversity* **1,** 13 (1995).

10. Stevanocic, S., and Jung, G., *Anal. Biochem.* **212,** 212 (1993).

11. Ellington, A. D., and Szostak, J. W., *Nature* **346,** 818 (1990).

12. Brown, B. B., Wagner, D. S., and Geysen, H. M., *Mol. Diversity* **1,** 4 (1995).

13. Lebl, M., Pátek, M., Kociš, P., Krchňák, V., Hruby, V. J., Salmon, S. E., and Lam, K. S., *Int. J. Peptide Protein Res.* **41,** 201 (1993).

14. Stevanovic, S., Wiesmüller, K.-H., Metzger, J. W., Beck-Sickinger, A. G., and Jung, G., *Bioorg. Med. Chem. Lett.* **3,** 436 (1993).

15. Metzger, J. W., Wiesmüller, K.-H., Stevanovic, S., and Jung, G., in *Peptides: 1992 Proceedings of the 22nd European Peptide Symposium,* C. H. Schngder and A. N. Eberle (Eds.), Escom, Leiden, 1993, p. 481.

16. Metzger, J. W., Wiesmüller, K.-H., Gnau, V., Brünjes, J., and Jung, G., *Angew. Chem. Int. Ed. Engl.* **32,** 894 (1993).

17. Metzger, J. W., Kempter, C., Wiesmüller, K.-H., and Jung, G., *Anal. Biochem.* **219,** 261 (1994).

18. Chu, Y.-H., Kirby, D. P., and Karger, B. L., *J. Am. Chem. Soc.* **117,** 5419 (1995).

19. Williams, D. H., and Waltho, J. P., *Biochem. Pharmacol.* **37,** 133 (1988).

20. Brummel, C. L., Lee, I. N. W., Zhou, Y., Benkovic, S. J., and Winograd, N., *Science* **264,** 399 (1994).

21. Winograd, N., *Anal. Chem.* **65,** 622A (1993).

22. Benninghoven, A., Hagenhoff, B., and Niehuis, E., *Anal. Chem.* **65,** 630A (1993).

23. Fitzgerald, M. C., Harris, K., Shevlin, C. G., and Siuzdak, G., *Bioorg. Med. Chem. Lett.* **6,** 979 (1996).

24. Cerpapoljak, A., Jenkins, A., and Duncan, M. W., *Rapid Commun. Mass Spectrom.* **9,** 233 (1995).

25. Egner, B. J., Langley, G. J., and Bradley, M., *J. Org. Chem.* **60,** 2652 (1995).

26. Geysen, H. M., Rodda, S. J., Mason, T. J., Tribbick, G., and Schoofs, P. G., *J. Immunol. Methods* **102,** 259 (1987).

27. Geysen, H. M., Meloen, R. H., and Barteling, S. J., *Proc. Natl. Acad. Sci. U.S.A.* **81,** 3998 (1984).

28. Houghten, R. A., Pinilla, C., Blondelle, S. E., Appel, J. R., Dooley, C. T., and Cuervo, J. H., *Nature* **354,** 84 (1991).

29. Ecker, D. J., Vickers, T. A., Hanecak, R., Driver, V., and Anderson, K., *Nucleic Acids Res.* **21,** 1853 (1993).

30. Patel, D. V., Gordeev, M. F., England, B. P., and Gordon, E. M., *J. Org. Chem.* **61,** 924 (1996).

31. Boecker, R. H., and Guengerich, F. P., *J. Med. Chem.* **29,** 1596 (1986).

32. Erb, E., Janda, K. D., and Brenner, S., *Proc. Natl. Acad. Sci. U.S.A.* **91,** 11422 (1994).

33. Pinna, C., Appel, J. R., Blanc, P., and Houghten, R. A., *Biotechniques* **13,** 901 (1992).

34. Dooley, C. T., and Houghten, R. A., *Life Sci.* **52,** 1509 (1993).

35. Pirrung, M. C., and Chen, J., *J. Am. Chem. Soc.* **117,** 1240 (1995).

36. Ugi, I., in *Isonitrile Chemistry,* A. T. Blomquist (Ed.), Academic, New York, 1971, p. 133.

37. Brenner, S., and Lerner, R. A., *Proc. Natl. Acad. Sci.* **89,** 5381 (1992).

38. Nielsen, J., Brenner, S., and Janda, K. D., *J. Am. Chem. Soc.* **115,** 9812 (1993).

39. Needles, M. C., Jones, D. G., Tate, E. H., Heinkel, G. L. Kochersperger, L. M., Dower, W. J., Barrett, R. W., and Gallop, M. A., *Proc. Natl. Acad. Sci. U.S.A.* **90,** 10700 (1993).

40. Kerr, J. M., Banville, S. C., and Zuckermann, R. N., *J. Am. Chem. Soc.* **115,** 2529 (1993).

41. Zuckermann, R. N., Kerr, J. M., Siani, M. A., Banville, S. C., and Santi, D. V., *Proc. Natl. Acad. Sci.* **89,** 4505 (1992).

42. Kerr, J. M., Banville, S. C., and Zuckermann, R. N., *Biol. Med. Chem. Lett.* **3,** 463 (1993).

43. Youngquist, R. S., Fuentes, G. R., Lacey, M. P., and Keough, T. *J. Am. Chem. Soc.* **117,** 3900 (1995).

44. Keough, T., Baker, T. R., Dobson, R. L., Lacey, M. P., Riley, T. A., Hasselfield, J. A., and Hesselberth, P. E., *Rapid Commun. Mass Spectrom.* **7,** 195 (1993).

45. Ohlmeyer, M. H. J., Swanson, R. N., Dillard, L. W., Reader, J. C., Asouline, G., Kobayashi, R., Wigler, M., and Still, W. C., *Proc. Natl. Acad. Sci. U.S.A.* **90,** 10922 (1993).

46. Nestler, H. P., Bartlett, P. A., and Still, W. C., *J. Org. Chem.* **59,** 4723 (1994).

47. Eckes, P., *Angew. Chem. Int. Ed. Engl.* **33,** 1573 (1994).

48. Grimsrud, E. P., in *Detectors for Capillary Chromatography,* H. H. Hill and D. G. McMinn (Eds.), Wiley, New York, 1992, p. 83.

49. Borchardt, A., and Still, W. C., *J. Am. Chem. Soc.* **116,** 373 (1994).

50. Baldwin, J. J., Burbaum, J. J., Henderson, I. H., and Ohlmeyer, M. H. J., *J. Am. Chem. Soc.* **117,** 5588 (1995).

51. Ni, Z.-J., Maclean, D., Holmes, C. P., Murphy, M. M., Ruhland, B., Jacobs, J. W., Grovdon, E. M., and Gallop, M. A., *J. Med. Chem.* **39,** 1601 (1996).

52. Nicolaou, K. C., Xiao, X.-Y., Parandoosh, Z., Senyei, A., and Nova, M. P., *Angew. Chem. Int. Ed. Engl.* **34,** 2289 (1995).

53. Beigel, M. L., US-A 5266926; 5257011 and 5214409. A read-only radiofrequency tag was used in a study published after the IRORI publication: Moran, E. J., Sarshat, S., Cargil, J. F., Shabbaz, M. M., Lio, A., Mjali, A. M. M., and Armstrong, R. W. *J. Am. Chem. Soc.* **117,** 10787 (1995).

54. Xiao, X.-Y., Shi, S., and Nova, M. P., manuscript submitted

55. Xiao, X.-Y., Zhao, C., and Nova, M. P., unpublished results.

56. Geysen, H. M., *Chem. Biol.* **3**(8), 679 (1996).

8

COMBINATORIAL SYNTHESIS EXPLOITING MULTIPLE-COMPONENT CONDENSATIONS, MICROCHIP ENCODING, AND RESIN CAPTURE

ROBERT W. ARMSTRONG, S. DAVID BROWN, THOMAS A. KEATING, AND PAUL A. TEMPEST

Department of Chemistry and Biochemistry, University of California, Los Angeles, California 90095

8.1 INTRODUCTION

8.1.1 Background

The relatively new discipline of combinatorial chemistry has been driven in part by advances in high-throughput biological screening of potential drug leads. With the increased demand for compounds, the traditional cycle of screening and synthesis of individual structures has proved inadequate. Chemists have responded to this challenge by developing techniques to increase the speed and efficiency of synthesis. Initial efforts in compound libraries of peptides (1–4) and oligonucleotides (5,6) have succeeded in yielding high-affinity ligands to a range of targets. However, the synthetic methodology for these linear biopolymers is well established, and it is only recently that attention has been turned to the larger challenge of generating libraries of small-molecule lead compounds.

A large part of the task of combinatorial chemistry today is the development of new methods to synthesize these small-molecule libraries. These methods will be dictated by (*1*) the particular core structure desired and (*2*) the availability, commercial or synthetic, of inputs that functionalize the core structure. There are many potential routes to a given core structure, and a particular approach may be a linear process, a multiple-component condensation (MCC), or a hybrid of the two. When referring to a linear synthesis in the chapter, we mean a multistep procedure that requires the isolation of intermediates or washing of the solid support resin and reexposure to new reagents for each step of the synthesis. Although the more familiar distinction is made among synthetic organic chemists between "linear" and "convergent" when referring to synthetic strategies, here we define as "linear" any combinatorial library method that builds up a target molecule one step at a time. Thus, we consider not only the well-known peptide and oligonucleotide libraries to be linear but also the majority of the combinatorial libraries in the literature today.

Our group has focused on multiple component condensation reactions (MCCs) as one of the strategies available for library synthesis. While most libraries have been generated using a linear, multistep process, MCCs provide a complementary approach to a number of different core structures. MCCs are reactions in which three or more reactants come together in a single reaction vessel to form a new product that displays aspects of all the components. These reactions may be carried out in solution or on solid support. It is not necessary that all components condense in a single, mechanistically concerted event; however, the MCC reactions detailed here do not require extensive manipulations: They are one-pot reactions. Employing MCCs in library synthesis rather than linear methods often entails differences in techniques, potential library size, and output format. For example, a four-component condensation (4CC) provides, in a single step, a core structure displaying functionality from all components, in a spatially addressable library format. In contrast, a linear strategy targeting the same core may require multiple synthesis and workup cycles to achieve the same library, but could allow for split-and-mix pooling strategies (7). We discuss this further in the sections on Passerini and Ugi reaction-based libraries.

8.1.2   Linear versus MCC Syntheses

Linear strategies for combinatorial synthesis have evolved from the solid-phase synthesis of biopolymers such as peptides and oligonucleotides. We characterize the initial inputs for linear combinatorial synthesis as having one of three features: They must be (a) monofunctional and bireactive, (b) bifunctional (or polyfunctional) and orthogonally reactive, or (c) monofunctional. Only the "capping" inputs (c), those that truncate the extension of a functional group, can be monoreactive or monofunctional (Fig. 8.1). Thus, each step in a linear synthesis, except the last, must provide a point of attachment, or handle, for the successive coupling. For example, a peptide synthesis employs bifunctional, orthogonally reactive inputs (amino acids) exclusively, whereas a synthesis of 1,4-benzodiazepines (accomplished by several groups recently) might involve all three types of inputs.

In a linear synthesis, the library inputs, and thus the "diversity" of the end products, is limited by requirements (a), (b), and (c). While there are many more monofunctional commercially available reagents, the diversity of available structures will be limited compared to chemistry available to bifunctional inputs. That is, monofunctional inputs can be used only to cap a functional group and not to extend

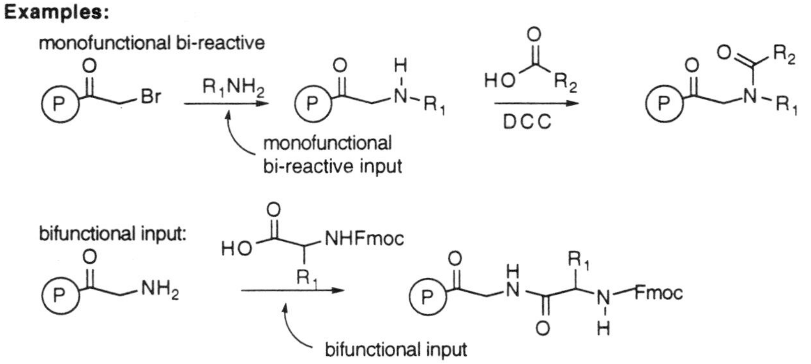

Examples:

monofunctional bi-reactive

monofunctional
bi-reactive input

bifunctional input:

bifunctional input

Figure 8.1 Inputs for a linear combinatorial synthesis.

the skeleton of the molecule. Overall, the main weakness of linear library strategies is that when the inputs are limited in synthetic or commercial availability, the libraries will themselves be limited in size and/or scope.

The alternate approach we focus on is the use of MCCs for the generation of libraries. This is a historically rich area of chemistry, beginning with Strecker's synthesis of amino cyanides (precursors to amino acids) in 1850 (8,9) and continuing up to the present day (Fig. 8.2) (10–18). Most of these reactions have not been adapted to solid-support synthesis nor exploited in a library format (19).

As stated above, an MCC is a reaction in which three or more reactants combine in a single event to yield a product that features aspects of all the inputs. Because each condensation is a single process, each product in a library of compounds can be synthesized in a separate reaction vessel. Standard 96-well microtiter plates are thus well suited for MCC synthesis in a spatially addressable format. We define library synthesis in this manner as *array* synthesis, an array simply being a group of discrete compounds whose structures are unequivocally known by the inputs used at each location in the array. The dimensionality of the array is equal to the number of components in the MCC; thus, a 3CC reaction gives a three-dimensional array of products if all three inputs are varied.

The MCC is a powerful tool for combinatorial chemistry targeting compounds with a common core structure, because the product is formed in a single step, thus saving synthetic time and effort, and because any of the inputs can be varied independently of all others, thus producing a library whose diversity and size is proportional to the number and availability of the inputs. MCC libraries represent a significant departure from linear approaches by not being limited to bifunctional or bireactive inputs. An MCC strategy is the most efficient for generation of discrete (single compound/reaction vessel) libraries because it involves (but is not limited to) a single reaction event. However, additional linear steps can be added either before or after the key MCC reaction. With MCCs, time- and labor-intensive processes such as resin washing and reagent addition are minimized. We have named this approach to combinatorial synthesis the multiple-component condensation array

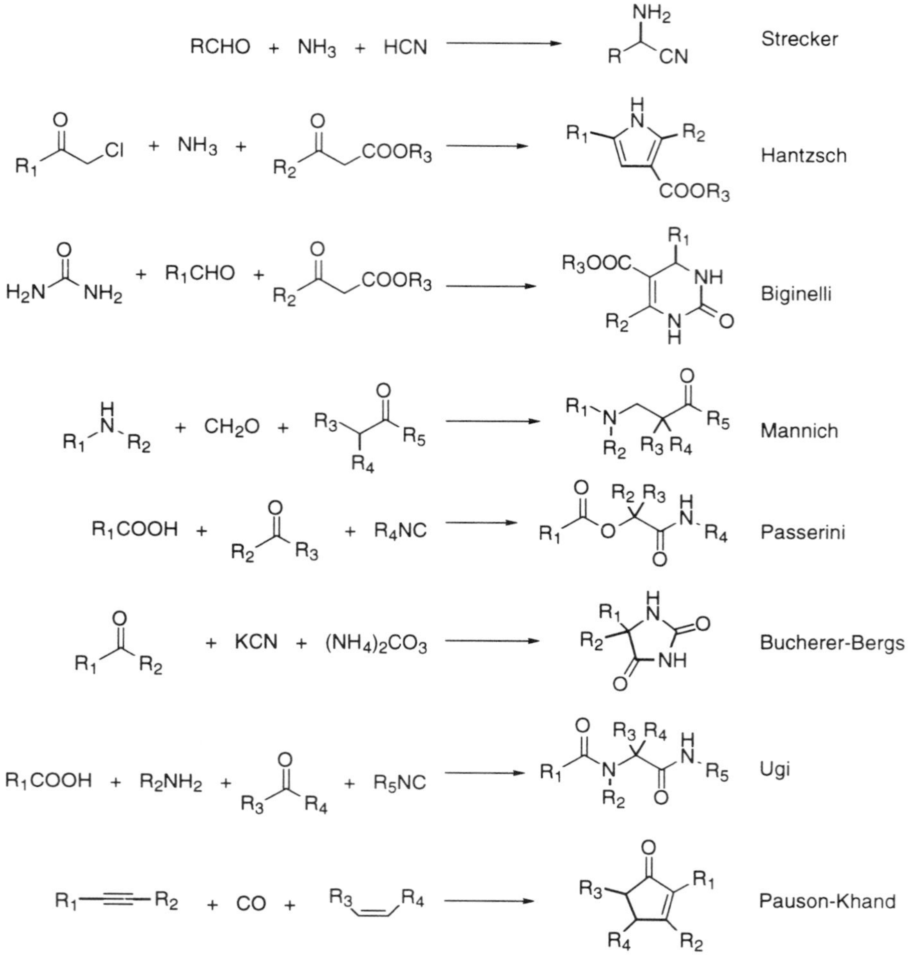

Figure 8.2 Some examples of multiple-component condensations, in chronological order of discovery.

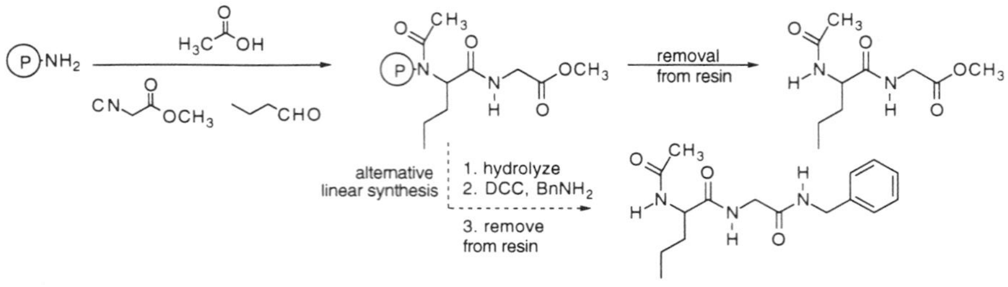

Figure 8.3 Strategy for library synthesis using the Ugi 4CC.

TABLE 8.1 Comparison of Synthetic Steps Required for Libraries Using Either MCC or Linear Strategies

Number of Components	Structural Variants per Input	Compounds Generated	MCC Synthetic Steps	Linear Steps (with deblock)[a]
2	20	400	1	1 (2)
3	20	8,000	1	2 (4)
4	20	160,000	1	3 (6)
5	20	3,200,000	1	4 (8)
6	20	64,000,000	1	5 (10)

[a]Parentheses indicate number of steps if deprotection is required prior to each coupling.

synthesis (MCCAS) (20). It is simply the application of MCC reactions to the synthesis of large arrays of related compounds. One example of this approach is shown in Figure 8.3, and depicts the Ugi four-component condensation, of which more will be said later.

The potential size of a library generated via a linear synthesis is a function of the number of steps and the number of individual inputs in each step. For instance, a four-step synthesis in which each step has 20 different inputs results in a library of 20^4 compounds. In contrast, a 4CC reaction with 20 inputs of each functional group provides the same number of compounds overall. However, in terms of number of steps, the MCC achieves the same library size by a single reaction event. Table 8.1 details this comparison. With a fixed number of 20 variants per input (as an analogy to the number of natural amino acids), the advantage of an MCC over a linear process increases with the number of components. This advantage is even greater if one includes the deprotection steps often necessary in a linear synthesis (peptide synthesis, e.g.), which doubles the number of steps in an iterative, linear synthesis. The box in Table 8.1 highlights the number of components of the MCCs, which will be discussed below, the Passerini 3CC and the Ugi 4CC.

8.2 PASSERINI REACTION AND APPLICATION TO AZINOMYCIN ANALOGS (14,21,22)

Our efforts in the parallel synthesis of compound libraries began as a result of our work toward the total synthesis of the azinomycin (Fig. 8.4) antitumor antibiotics (23,24). Binding studies had established that this cytotoxic natural product cross-linked duplex DNA in the major groove (25). Partial degradation of the crosslinked adduct suggested that the aziridine and epoxide moieties were involved in the alkylation event, perhaps aided by the intercalation of the naphthyl ester. Concurrent with these studies, we had developed a highly convergent synthesis of the left portion of the molecule involving the Passerini three-component condensation (21) in which each of the components contained one of the postulated functionalities

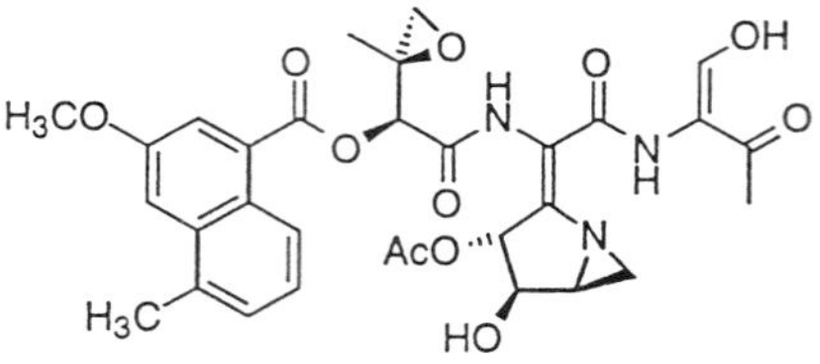

Figure 8.4 Azinomycin B.

involved in binding (see Fig. 8.5). A structure–activity relationship (SAR) study of the natural product, specifically the interrelation of the key functionalities, would therefore be accessible via the Passerini reaction using the appropriate starting materials. A polymer-supported strategy using the Passerini three-component condensation (3CC) was employed to rapidly synthesize azinomycin analogs; however, a photocleavable polymer linker was needed to ensure survival of azinomycin analogs not stable to acid or base polymer cleaving conditions.

Before conducting the Passerini reaction in a combinatorial array, we optimized the Passerini reaction conditions and the photolytic cleavage from the resin for a representative system (Scheme 8.1). The glycine carbamate linker **2.3** was constructed by reacting isocyanate **2.1** with the free hydroxyl of the known photolabile linker **2.2** (26–29). Coupling of linker **2.3** to methylbenzhydrylamine (MBHA)-Gly-resin **2.4** yielded the polymer-supported photocleavable carbamates **2.5**. Hydrolysis of the ester **2.5** afforded the requisite polymer-supported acid **2.6**. A solution of methyl isocyanoacetate and butyraldehyde was then added to polymer **2.6** and the reaction allowed to stand for 2 days affording resin-bound Passerini adduct **2.7**. Photolytic cleavage of the solid-supported Passerini adduct **2.7** and in situ acylation by acetic anhydride afforded the *N*-acyl Passerini adduct **2.10** as the only observable compound.

These methods were then applied to the first solid-phase MCCAS. A solid support 3-(6×5×1)-MCCAS (6 isocyanides, 5 aldehydes, 1 carboxylic acid) array was generated using the MBHA-gly resin **6** in each reaction well, followed by photolysis in the presence of acetic anhydride (Fig. 8.6). The isocyanides (**2.11**–

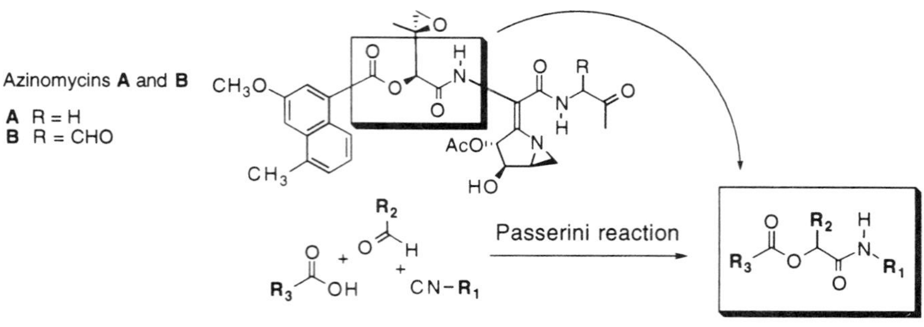

Figure 8.5 Synthesis of azinomycin analogs via Passerini 3CC.

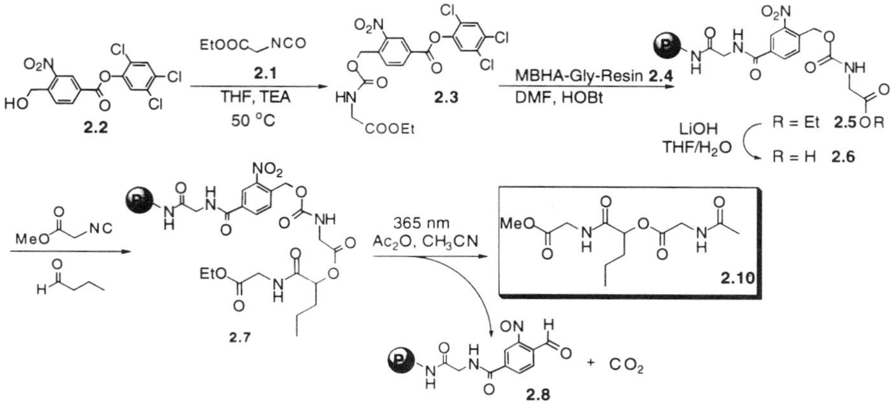

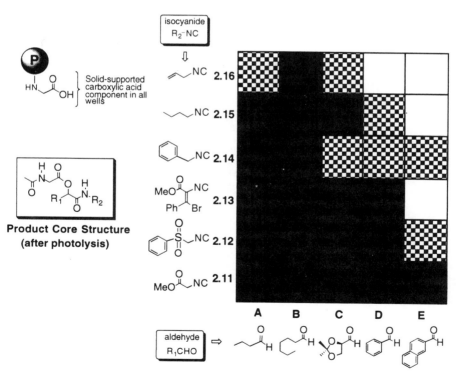

Scheme 8.1 Conditions for Passerini MCCAS of azinomycin analogs.

Figure 8.6 MCCAS of a Passerini library. Dark squares: >70% isolated yield; checkered squares: 30–70% isolated yield; white squares: no product detected.

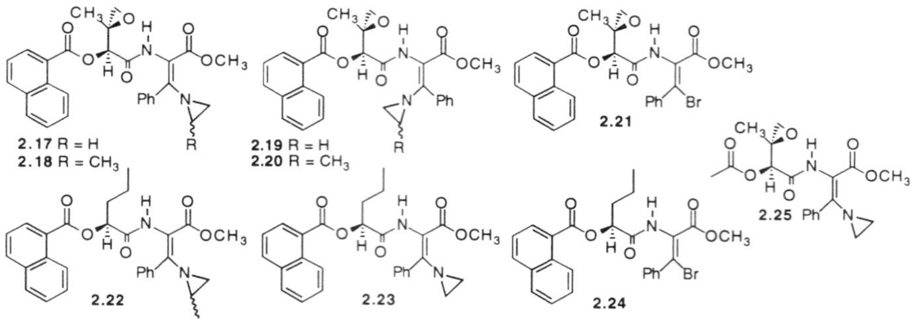

Figure 8.7 Selected members of MCCAS of azinomycin analogs.

2.16) and aldehydes (**A–E**) were chosen in such a manner as to test the generality of the solid-supported Passerini reaction and maximize the structural diversity of products formed. The isolated products were each analyzed by thin-layer chromatography (TLC) and low-resolution mass spectra (LRMS). LRMS of compounds in all wells provided proof of the existence of desired products, while TLC and ^{1}H nuclear magnetic resonance (NMR) demonstrated excellent product purity (only a single product was observed in each). TLC was also particularly diagnostic for determining reaction success, since the relative polarities (R_f's) of the desired products was consistent between rows. Analysis of the reactivity profile of individual reagents revealed the same general trend observed in the MCCAS solution studies. The alkyl aldehydes (**A, B, C**) afforded the desired Passerini products in nearly all wells, whereas the aromatic aldehydes (**D, E**) displayed significantly lower reactivity toward selected isocyanides.

TABLE 8.2 In Vitro Cytotoxicities of Azinomycin Analogs in HCT Human Colon Carcinoma Cell Lines[a]

Compound No.	HCT116	HCT116/VM46	HCT116/VP35
2.17	4.39	5.56	5.27
2.18	5.4	1.6	2.6
2.19	12.4	13.2	11.0
2.20	6.76	7.7	6.4
2.21	>30	>30	>30
2.22E	>30	>30	>30
2.22Z	25.3	27.2	25.5
2.24E/Z	>30	>30	>30
2.23E	>30	>30	>30
2.23Z	28.6	38.4	27.3
2.25Z	>30	>30	>30
2.25E	>30	>30	>30
Azinomycin B	0.838	—	—

[a]IC_{50} (μm), cytotoxicity assessed XTT assay after 72 h continuous drug exposure.

A second, analogous array synthesis was performed in solution, resulting in compounds shown in Figure 8.7. These analogs were then assayed for cytotoxicity toward the HCT116 human colon carcinoma cell line as well as two drug-resistant sublines: HCT116/VM46 expressing the MDR phenotype and HCT116/VP35 resistant to verapamyl and topoisomerase-II-active drugs; data is tabulated in Table 8.2. As can be seen, compounds **2.17, 2.18,** and **2.20** exhibit potencies only fivefold less than that of the natural azinomycin B.

8.3 UGI REACTION AND APPLICATIONS (49)

8.3.1 Solid-Supported Ugi Reaction Libraries (30)

Having completed a 3CCAS, we wished to expand the scope of MCC (31) reactions on solid support and next moved forward to the Ugi reaction. The Ugi (32) reaction is a four-component condensation (4CC) in which an amine, aldehyde, carboxylic acid, and an isocyanide combine in a single transformation to yield an α-acylamino amide (Scheme 8.2).

Proceeding as shown in Scheme 8.3, a Schiff's base is formed with the condensation of the amine and aldehyde, followed by attack at the imine carbon by the isocyanide. The carboxylate then attacks the carbon of the isocyanide. Up to this point the reactions are reversible, but the final step, an intramolecular acylation, drives the reaction forward to the α-acylamino amide. The Ugi reaction gives good yields over a variety of solvents and conditions, with methanol generally giving the best overall performance.

As mentioned in the introduction, MCCs such as the Ugi reaction represent ideal candidates for solid-phase combinatorial synthesis. Solid-phase synthesis holds two key advantages in constructing libraries with respect to solution libraries. The first is that excess reagents can be used to drive reactions to completion. The second is that upon completion of the reaction purification proceeds by simply filtering the resin to wash away products not bound to the solid phase. With these advantages in mind, we developed methodology for running Ugi reactions on solid phase.

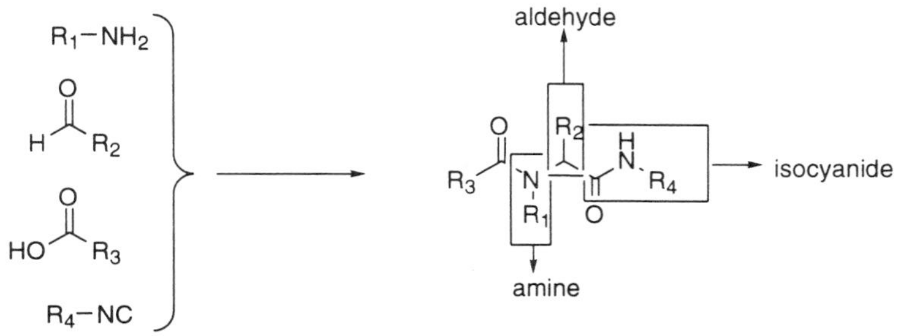

Scheme 8.2 Ugi four-component condensation (4CC) reaction. The unboxed portion of the product derives from the carboxylate.

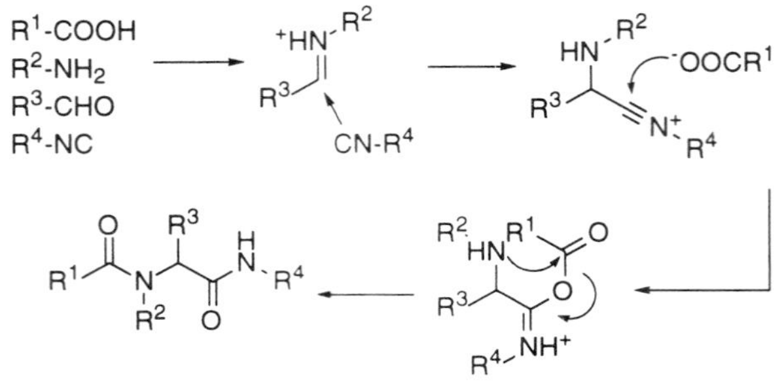

Scheme 8.3 Ugi 4CC mechanism. An intramolecular acylation event drives the reaction forward.

While any of the four components can be covalently tethered to the solid support, we chose the amino functionality as it is available in wide range of resins. Rink amide resin (33), a polystyrene-based resin, was chosen as our solid support due to a number of considerations. The products linked to the amine are readily cleaved from the resin under relatively mild conditions, thus limiting concerns of product compatability to the cleavage procedure. Any unreacted amine would cleave from the resin as ammonia, thus not posing a purity problem. Finally, the products that result from the reactions with the Rink amine input yield secondary amides. Forming secondary amines in solution phase requires ammonia to be used as the amine equivalent, which is known to produce poor yields. Thus, we can generate products on solid support that would otherwise pose difficulties for the same reaction in solution (Scheme 8.4).

Traditionally, linearly assembled libraries need multiple synthetic steps to generate diversity. Multiple steps on solid support necessitate resin manipulation such as washing, transferring, and in addition, often time-consuming compound tracking strategies. Since only one synthetic transformation is necessary to generate compound libraries with the Ugi 4CC, we utilized a one-compound per well, spatially encoded format that obviates the need for extensive resin manipulation. In this manner, we have generated α-acylamino amides on solid support using the Ugi reaction in an MCCAS format.

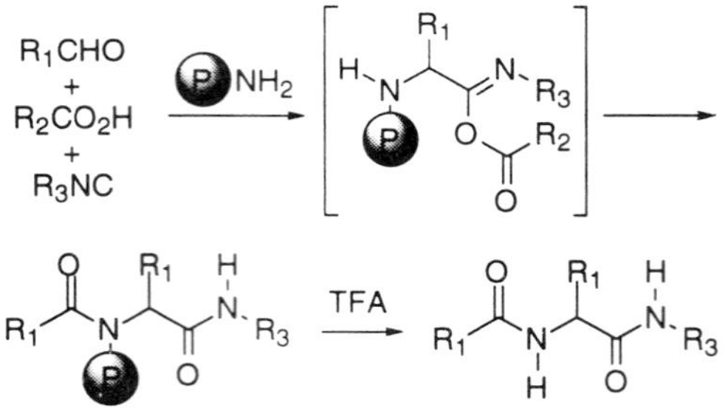

Scheme 8.4 Ugi 4CC on Rink resin to yield secondary amides.

Rink amide resin was evenly dispersed into the 96 wells (0.014 mM of amine per well) of a standard microtiter plate. The wells of the plate have a 2-mL volume capacity and are formed from polypropylene, yielding excellent compatibility with a wide range of solvents. To facilitate addition to the wells, the solution inputs (aldehyde, carboxylic acid, and isocyanide) were first diluted to 1M solutions. Using an eight-channel, variable volume multichannel pipettor, the 1M solutions were added rapidly to the 96 wells. The 8 aldehyde inputs (10 equiv.) in methylene chloride and the 12 carboxylic acid inputs (10 equiv.) in methanol were added first and agitated for 30 min. The single isocyanide (10 equiv.), also in methylene chloride, was then added, and the plate was capped. After 24 h, the excess reagents were washed from the resin with methanol and methylene chloride and the products cleaved from the resin with 30% (v/v) trifluoroacetic acid in methylene chloride. The solvents from the cleavage reaction were stripped in a reduced pressure oven to yield 1–3 mg of compound per well (Table 8.3). By ^{1}H-NMR, the products were recovered in good purity.

A range of inputs was selected in order to produce a substituent effect analysis on the solid support reaction in a single plate (Scheme 8.5). As in solution reactions, the product yields were most sensitive to the structure of the aldehyde inputs. Aliphatic aldehydes and those containing electron-donating groups exhibit good overall yields, compared to those with electron-withdrawing groups even in the presence of large excess of reagents or repeated exposure to fresh reagents. For acid inputs, the yields involving phenolic derivatives were generally low, in part related to their precipitation from solution over the 24-h reaction period. Four larger scale reactions were performed (0.12 mmol of amine). The purity of the recovered compounds was >90% by ^{1}H-NMR and ^{13}C-NMR in yields from 70 to 80%.

8.3.2 Isocyanide Sublibraries (20,30)

One of the limitations of the Ugi reaction as a tool for library generation is lack of available isocyanides: although there are literally thousands of acids, amines, and aldehydes/ketones, there are perhaps fewer than two dozen commercially available isocyanides—a severe impediment. We sought to address this problem via the pregeneration of a library of isocyanides as inputs to an Ugi-based library. In general, this strategy involves the solution condensation of two subunits—an isocyanide anion and an electrophile—prior to solid support synthesis, and then use of this sublibrary of isocyanides as an input into a larger array.

Figure 8.8 details our efforts toward such a library. Isocyanides **c, d,** and **e** were synthesized from benzylisocyanide **b** via α-lithiation with butyllithium followed by an alkyl halide quench. All new isocyanides were carried on as crude reaction mixtures after aqueous wash into the array with aldehydes **N, O,** and **P,** acids **3.2.1, 3.2.2,** and **3.2.3,** and Rink amine polymer. A representative product of this five-component condensation, **3.2.3Pe,** is shown in Figure 8.8. Yields after trifluoroacetic acid (TFA) cleavage from the solid support were variable (11–61%) but all expected products were observed by mass spectrometry, and ^{1}H-NMR indicated >90% purity. The pre-4CC solution condensation of the isocyanide input effec-

TABLE 8.3 Yields for the 96-Well Plate

	3.1.1	3.1.2	3.1.3	3.1.4	3.1.5	3.1.6	3.1.7	3.1.8	3.1.9	3.1.10	3.1.11	3.1.12
A	59	95	95	79	95	45	95	95	85	17	8	51
B	67	14	70	59	52	41	64	71	42	2	9	37
C	81	65	77	57	93	23	71	68	21	2	4	36
D	58	65	95	79	95	98	96	90	93	91	64	50
E	42	86	37	64	61	70	80	76	25	4	78	54
F	46	30	14	11	30	0	48	31	0	35	28	26
G	55	94	46	52	64	33	66	70	0	5	47	33
H	5	0	0	24	45	0	0	30	5	0	21	18

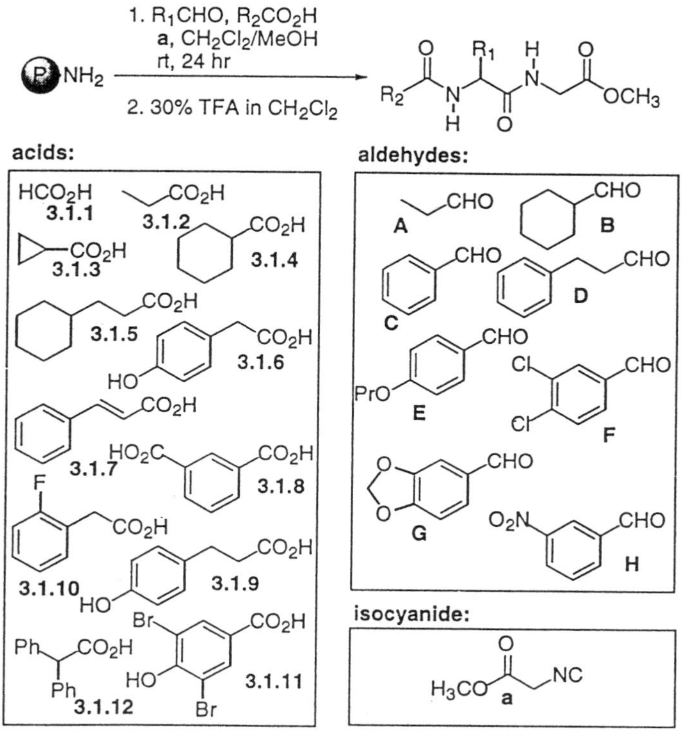

Scheme 8.5 Inputs for the 96-well plate.

tively produces a 5CC library on the solid support. This strategy has been extended to an overall 6CC reaction, by quenching the isocyanide anion with an aldehyde, which is followed by an acylation of the resultant alkoxide. In such a scheme, 10 structural variants of each chemical input in a 6CC reaction generate a 10^6 compound library.

8.3.3 Convertible Isocyanides (34,35)

We have also performed extensive investigations into another solution for the lack of available isocyanides. We envisioned the concept of a "universal isocyanide," an input for the Ugi 4CC that can be converted, postcondensation, into different functionalities, thereby circumventing the lack of commercial isocyanide inputs as well as avoiding the need to synthesize and store a large number of isocyanides should commercial sources prove insufficient. The isocyanide detailed here, 1-isocyanocyclohexene (**3.3.1**), is a remarkably versatile substrate (see Fig. 8.9) whose 4CC product **3.3.2** can be converted in a single step to a variety of products under acidic conditions, including many products that are otherwise inaccessible from the Ugi reaction.

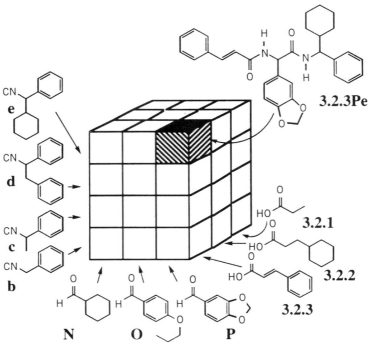

Figure 8.8 Chemical inputs and positional decoding of product structures for a three-dimensional four-component array.

8.3.3.1 Cyclohexenamide Conversions Our initial work in this area demonstrated transformation of Ugi products of type **3.3.3** to new products **3.3.4** [Eq. (3.3.1)]:

$$\text{(3.3.1)}$$

3.3.3   **3.3.4**

Ugi (36) and Geller and Ugi (37) have published work on cleavable carbonamide moieties R^4, but the methods to date require conversion of the amide group into another, more labile functionality, and involve at least three steps from the 4CC product **3.3.3**. In addition, these methods yield only the carboxylic acid derivative of **3.3.4** ($-XR^5 = -OH$).

However, Ugi had earlier demonstrated the use of 1-isocyanocyclohexene (**3.3.1**) in a 4CC and had converted the enamide product **3.3.2** to the primary amide **3.3.5** [Eq. (3.3.2)] through acidic hydrolysis (38):

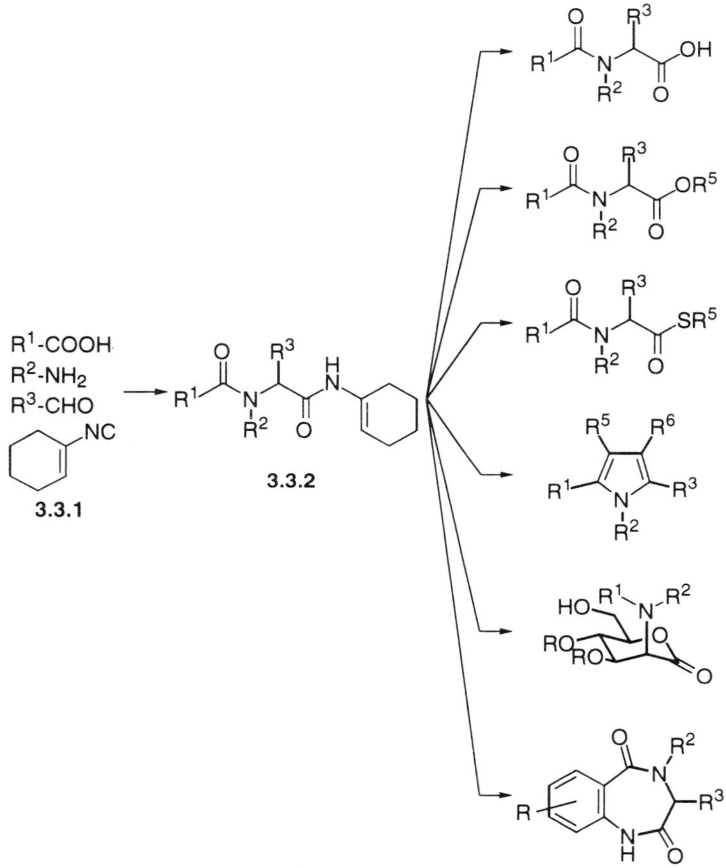

Figure 8.9 Single-step conversions of cyclohexenamide Ugi product **3.3.2**.

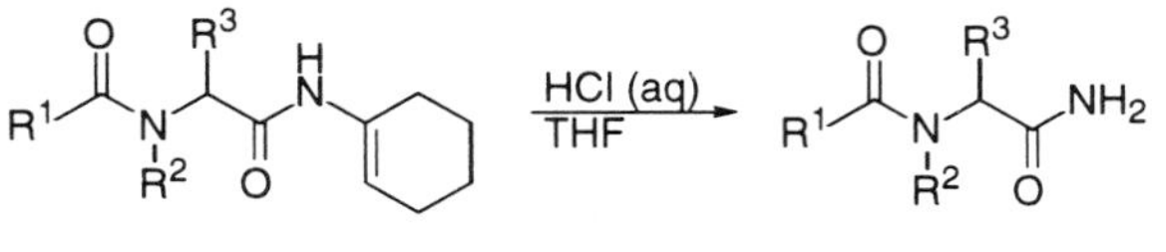

(3.3.2)

We decided to reinvestigate this transformation, prompted by a report that an enamide could be selectively cleaved to the corresponding methyl ester under acidic methanol conditions (39).

Synthesis of 1-isocyanocyclohexene (**3.3.1**) was straightforward and proceeded as shown in Scheme 8.6.

Ugi's original procedure for synthesis of **3.3.1** was modified only in that better yields were obtained when **3.3.6** was purified prior to dehydration and triphosgene

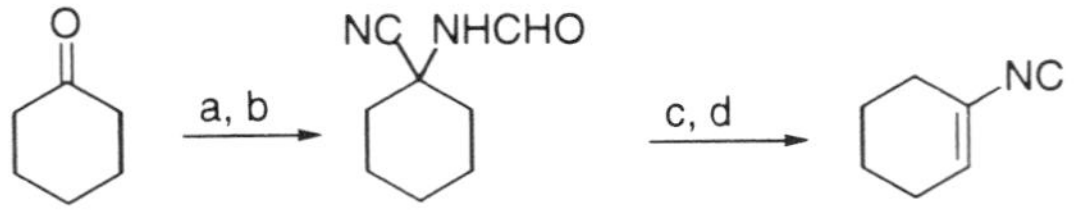

Scheme 8.6 Reagents and conditions: (a) NaCN(aq), NH$_4$Cl(aq), Et$_2$O, 61%; (b) HCOOH, Ac$_2$O, 44%; (c) ^{t}BuOK, THF; (d) triphosgene, DABCO, CH$_2$Cl$_2$, 50% (two steps).

was used as the dehydrating agent in place of phosphorus oxychloride. Other syntheses of **3.3.1** have appeared in the literature (40,41). 1-Isocyanocyclohexene can be stored indefinitely at $-30°C$ under an inert atmosphere but darkens in a short time upon exposure to air. We have succeeded in easily preparing multigram quantities.

Ugi four-component condensations with **3.3.1** proceeded smoothly and in good yield (ca. 50–85%) for a variety of examples illustrated herein. Conversions of the cyclohexenamide moiety were then attempted with various conditions and nucleophiles. When the isolated 4CC products were treated with the acidic conditions detailed in the footnotes to Table 8.4, the products listed were obtained in high isolated yield.

As can be seen, the cyclohexenamide moiety has been converted under mild conditions to a variety of carboxylic esters, thioesters, and carboxylic acids. Not only are products that are not accessible via the Ugi reaction (i.e., esters) obtained, but amides can be synthesized from the carboxylic acids via standard carbodiimide coupling techniques to afford new Ugi products without requiring the appropriate isocyanide. This result greatly expands the scope of the 4CC and reduces the impact of its weakest component, the isocyanide input.

We next turned to in situ conversions of the cyclohexenamide. The goal was to perform some of the conversions of Table 8.4 without isolation of initial cyclohexenamide 4CC product. It was expected that simple acidification of a crude reaction mixture that contained the appropriate nucleophile would result in the cyclohexenamide being converted regardless of other species present. Results are shown in Table 8.5.

After monitoring the Ugi reaction in methanol solution and judging it complete, the introduction of acetyl chloride (to generate HCl) and subsequent heating resulted in the product methyl esters listed in Table 8.5. Hydrolysis products (i.e., carboxylic acids), which might have arisen from the single equivalent of water produced in the 4CC, were not observed. By performing the cyclohexenamide conversion in a one-pot process, an overall five-component condensation is achieved, with the isocyanide input contributing only a single carbonyl carbon atom to the final structure.

We next focused on the mechanism for this transformation. It is unusual that a carboxylic acid would result from acidic hydrolysis of an enamide, as shown in Table 8.4. One would expect instead the primary amide, because under aqueous acidic conditions, protonation of the cyclohexenamide would typically be followed

TABLE 8.4 Results of Cleavage of Cyclohexenamide 4CC Products

Condensation Product[a]

R[1]	R[2]	R[3]	Nu:	Cond.[b]/ Yield[c]	Product
Me-	PMB-	iPr-	H_2O	A/56%	3.3.7
Me-	PMB-	Ph-	H_2O	A/83%	3.3.8
Ph-	Bu-	Ph-	H_2O	A/25%	3.3.9
Ph-	Bu-	Ph-	MeOH	B/98%	3.3.10
Me-	PMB-	Ph-	MeOH	B/100%	3.3.11
Me-	PMB-	Ph-	EtOH	B/57%	3.3.12
Me-	PMB-	Ph-	BnOH	C/75%	3.3.13
Me-	PMB-	iPr-	EtSH	D/68%	3.3.14
Me-	PMB-	-(CH$_2$)$_5$-	tBuOH	E/64%	3.3.15

[a]PMB = p-MeO-benzyl.
[b]Reaction conditions: (A) 1.7% HCl in THF, 23°C, overnight. (B) Indicated alcohol as solvent, 5 eq. AcCl, 55°C, 3 h. (C) 5 eq. AcCl, 10 eq. ROH in THF, 55°C, 3 h. (D) EtSH as solvent, 10 eq. AcCl, 23°C, overnight. (E) 5 eq. AcCl, 10 eq. tBuOH in THF, 55°C, 48 h.
[c]All yields are of isolated, purified product.

**TABLE 8.5   Results of In Situ Acidic Methanolyses
of Four-Component Condensation Products**

R¹COOH	R²NH₂	R³CHO	Product	Isolated Yield
1-Undecyl-	PMB-	Ph-	**3.3.16**	65%
CH₃-	PMB-	Ph-	**3.3.11**	79%
CH₃-	1-Decyl	Ph-	**3.3.17**	99%
PhCH₂-	C₆H₁₁-	ⁱPr-	**3.3.18**	67%
CH₃-	PMB-		**3.3.19**	55%

by hydrolysis of the resulting *N*-acyliminium species to the amide and cyclohex-anone (42). Although cyclohexanone is indeed observed as a product of these reactions, the primary amide is not.

A clue to the mechanism of transformation is given in Scheme 8.7. In attempts to convert **3.3.20** to the methyl ester under the acidic methanol conditions of both Tables 8.4 and 8.5, only the deformylated primary amide was isolated. This is the expected product based on a mechanism of hydrolysis of an *N*-acyliminium species but does not fit with the results in Tables 8.4 and 8.5. In additional experiments on **3.3.22** and **3.3.23,** it was not only established that deformylation under these acidic conditions (43) was very rapid (<30 min) but also that the absence of an acylated amine altogether (**3.3.24**) precludes formation of carboxylic acid as per Table 8.4. Thus, it appears that an *N*-acyl group is essential for the conversions shown in Tables 8.4 and 8.5, and its loss before the crucial step prevents the formation of the Table 8.4 products. This led us to propose (34) the mechanism detailed in Scheme 8.8, which involves an oxazolinium-5-one (münchnone) intermediate.

Protonation of the enamide gives the activated species **3.3.26,** which then cycl-

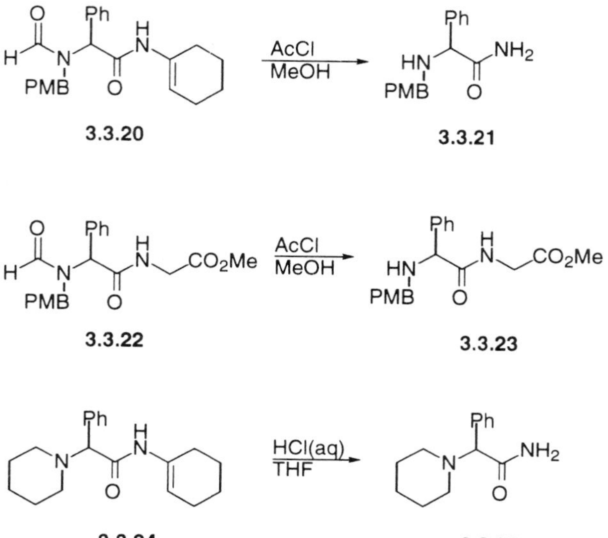

3.3.20 3.3.21 3.3.22 3.3.23 3.3.24 3.3.25

Scheme 8.7

izes to the münchnone (44–47) **3.3.27** and eliminates cyclohexanimine. The reactive münchnone then is opened by a nucleophile to yield the product **3.3.28.** Lack of an acylated amine (**3.3.24**) or its rapid loss (**3.3.20**) prevents the formation of **3.3.27.**

8.3.3.2 ***Pyrroles*** Although these experiments offered some evidence for the intermediacy of a münchnone in the cyclohexenamide conversion, more compelling proof would result from a 1,3-dipolar cycloaddition of a dipolarophile to the proposed intermediate. It is well known that the anhydro-5-hydroxyoxazolium hydroxide species **3.3.29** (Fig. 8.10), which are members of a larger class of azomethine

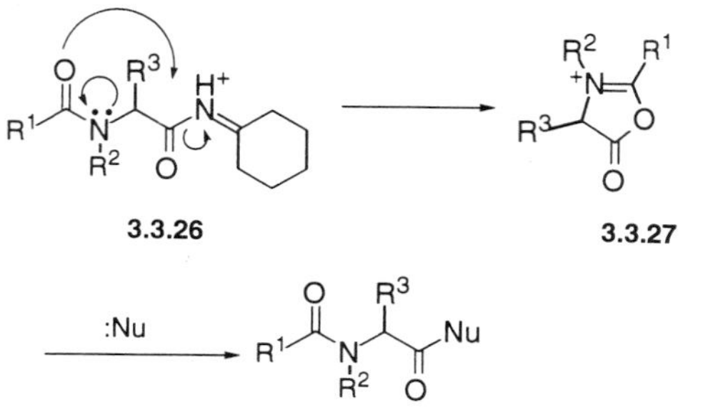

3.3.26 3.3.27 3.3.28

Scheme 8.8 Proposed mechanism of cyclohexenamide conversions.

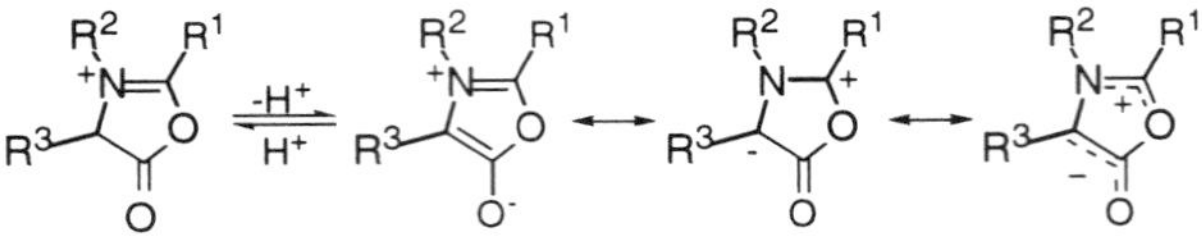

Figure 8.10 Resonance structures of active 1,3-dipoles derived from Ugi products.

ylides, undergo cycloadditions with a wide variety of dipolarophiles (48). Perhaps the most common method of generating such species is the cyclodehydration of *N*-acyl-*N*-alkylamino acids using acetic anhydride and a nitrogenous base at elevated temperatures (50).

Therefore, we attempted cycloaddition of cyclohexenamide Ugi products under various acidic conditions with a selection of acetylenic dipolarophiles, with the expectation that the reaction would proceed as depicted in Scheme 8.9. Protonation of **3.3.2** is followed by cyclization and loss of cyclohexanimine to **3.3.27,** which loses a proton to form 1,3-dipole **3.3.30**. This 1,3-dipole undergoes a [3 + 2] cycloaddition reaction with the acetylene to **3.3.32,** which rapidly aromatizes with loss of CO_2 to the pyrrole **3.3.33**. Results of these reactions are shown in Table 8.6.

Several general trends can be observed. First, unlike cyclodehydration procedures, which are typically run at 50–60°C, higher temperatures and toluene as a solvent were necessary for improved or even observable yields. Second, the more electron withdrawing the acetylenic dipolarophile, the better the yields. Steric hinderance plays a role, as seen in the product ratios of **3.3.36** to **3.3.37** (44), the failure of diphenylacetylene to react to form the tetraphenylpyrrole (50) and the failure to form the bicyclic pyrrole expected from the γ-lactam 4CC product. Optimization of yields by further variation of conditions has not been attempted. Although cycloaddition of münchnones with electron-deficient nitriles such as ethyl cyanoacetate has also been reported (51), we were unable to observe any predicted imidazole products with a variety of conditions and substrates.

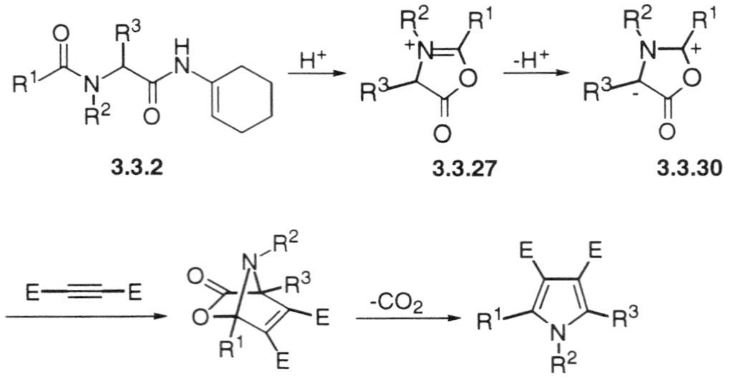

Scheme 8.9

Table 8.6 1,3-Dipolar Cycloadditions of Acetylenic Dipolarphiles with Ugi Products

Condensation Product

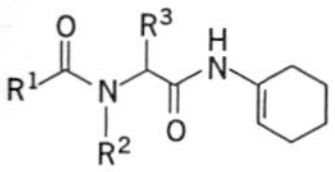

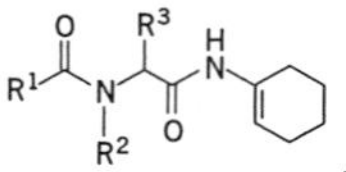

R¹	R²	R³	Dipolar-ophile	Cond.[a]/Yield[b]	Product
Me-	PMB-	Ph-	COOMe / COOMe	A/63%	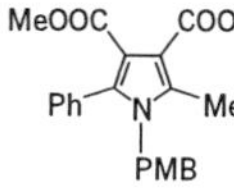 MeOOC, COOMe; Ph–N(PMB)–Me pyrrole 3.3.34
Ph-	Bu-	Ph-	COOMe / COOMe	A/35%	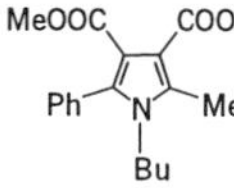 MeOOC, COOMe; Ph–N(Bu)–Me pyrrole 3.3.35
Me-	PMB-	Ph-	COOMe / COOMe	A/63%	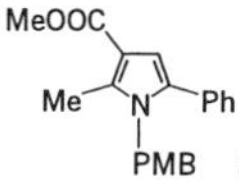 MeOOC; Me–N(PMB)–Ph pyrrole 3.3.36 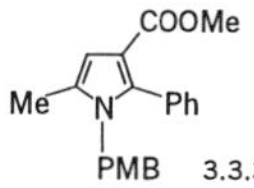 and COOMe; Me–N(PMB)–Ph pyrrole 3.3.37 (1)
Ph-	Bu-	Ph-	H / COOMe	A/24%	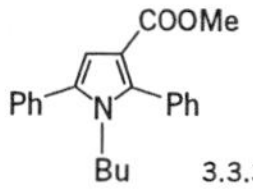 COOMe; Ph–N(Bu)–Ph pyrrole 3.3.38
Me-	PMB-	¹Pr-	COOMe / COOMe	A/13%	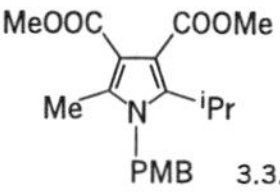 MeOOC, COOMe; Me–N(PMB)–¹Pr pyrrole 3.3.39

Condensation Product

R¹	R²	R³	Dipolar-ophile	Cond.[a]/Yield[b]	Product
Me-	PMB-	Ph-	COOEt / COOEt	A/19%	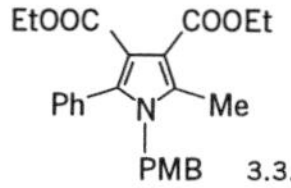 EtOOC, COOEt; Ph–N(PMB)–Me pyrrole 3.3.40
Me-	PMB-	¹Pr-	COOEt / COOEt	A/9%	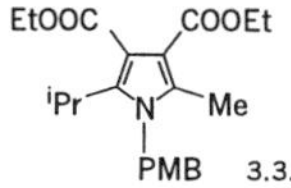 EtOOC, COOEt; ¹Pr–N(PMB)–Me pyrrole 3.3.41
Me-	PMB-	¹Pr-	COOMe / COOMe	A/5%	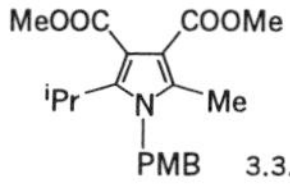 MeOOC, COOMe; ¹Pr–N(PMB)–Me pyrrole 3.3.39
Me-	PMB-	Ph-	H / COOEt	A/0%	N.R.
Ph-	Bu-	Ph-	Ph / Ph	A/0%	N.R.
Ph-	Bu-	Ph-	CN / COOEt	A/0%	N.R.
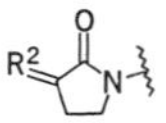 R¹, R² (lactam)		Ph-	COOMe / COOMe	A/0%	N.R.

[a] Reagents and conditions: (A) 5 eq. dipolarophile, 3 eq. HCl, toluene, 100°C; (B) 5 eq. dipolarophile, 3 eq. HCl, THF, 55°C.
[b] Purified, isolated yield.

This 1,3-dipolar cycloaddition reaction represents a novel synthesis of pyrroles, which are important pharmacophores in their own right (52). There are several notable advantages to this method. Instead of reliance upon acylated amino acids as precursors for münchnones **3.3.27,** the larger and more diverse pool of carboxylic acids, amines, and aldehydes can be called upon to furnish the 1, 2, and 5 substituents of pyrrole **3.3.33** resulting from cycloaddition. Thus, even though the cyclohexenamide class of Ugi 4CC products can be seen as precursors of acylated amino acids (as per **3.3.7, 3.3.8,** and **3.3.9** in Table 8.4), it is not necessary to convert them to the free carboxylic acid to access the standard acetic anhydride methods of generating active 1,3-dipoles for cycloaddition; the cyclohexenamide itself is a substrate for münchnone formation. Once again, the cyclohexenamide functionality has been erased in the product pyrrole, with even the single carbon atom present in products **3.3.7–19** lost as CO_2. Finally, the stereocenter created at the α-carbon in the Ugi 4CC (resulting in an enantiomeric mixture of products) is removed by aromatization after cycloaddition, resulting in a single product.

8.3.3.3 *Internal Nucleophile*

As an extension of the work on nucleophilic open-ing of münchnone intermediates to yield products **3.3.7–19,** we investigated teth-ered nucleophiles as a means of forming rings (Fig. 8.11).

The concept in Figure 8.11a is illustrated by using D-arabinose as an aldehyde input in an Ugi reaction followed by cyclization to form the corresponding 2-acetamido-2-deoxy hexose (Scheme 8.10).

Protected D-arabinose **3.3.46** was prepared using standard procedures (53–55). This aldehyde reacted smoothly under standard Ugi conditions to furnish **3.3.47** in high yield as a 3.4-to-1 mixture of inseparable diastereomers at the α-carbon (as determined by ^{1}H-NMR). We expected that acidic treatment of **3.3.47** would cleave the isopropylidene protecting group, protonate the enamide, promote münchnone formation, and either open the münchnone with methanol or the newly deprotected secondary hydroxyl, with the exact sequence of events dependent upon the relative rates. Lactonization should occur under these conditions whether or not the methyl ester is initially formed, and cyclization should occur via the secondary hydroxyl to form a six-membered ring rather than via the primary hydroxyl (seven-membered ring). Treatment of **3.3.47** with acidic methanol conditions (0.1M HCl, 23°C) yielded the protected 2-acetamido-2-deoxy-D-mannonic-δ-lactone **3.3.48** in 29% yield. Attempts to improve the yield either through elevated temperatures or in-creased acidity resulted in β-elimination and formation of the α, β-unsaturated 2-acetamidolactone. The *p*-methoxybenzyl amide protecting group could be oxi-

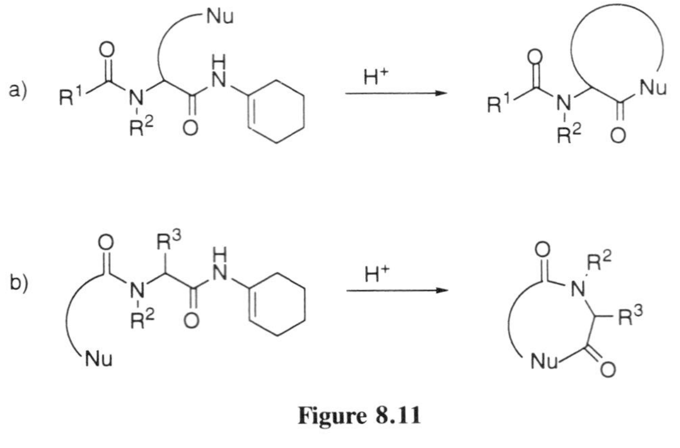

Figure 8.11

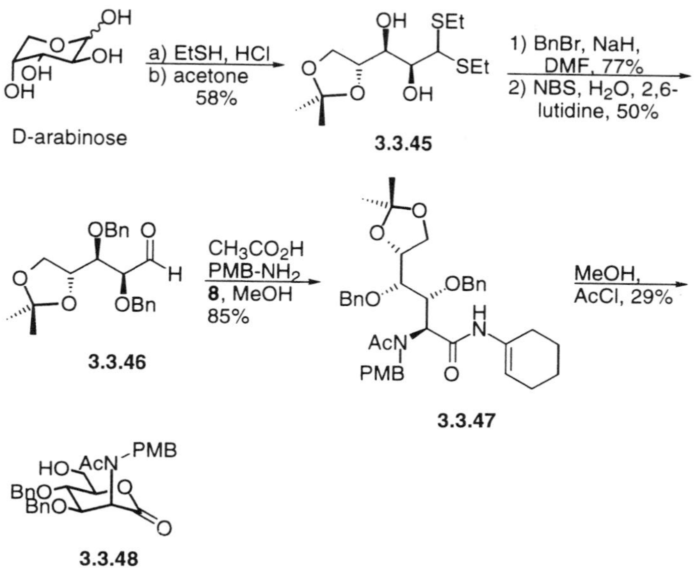

Scheme 8.10

datively removed using ceric ammonium nitrate, and the benzyl ethers by catalytic hydrogenation over Pearlman's catalyst.

8.3.3.4 *1,4-Benzodiazepine-2,5-diones* 1,4-Benzodiazepines (56) **3.3.49** have been the target of several solid-phase combinatorial strategies (57–60). The structurally similar 1,4-benzodiazepine-2,5-diones **3.3.50,** however, have been reported as important pharmacophores in their own right, as anticonvulsants (61), as antitumor agents (62), and as glycoprotein antagonists (63). 1,4-Benzodiazepine-2,5-diones have appeared very recently in several solid- and solution-phase synthesis (64–67).

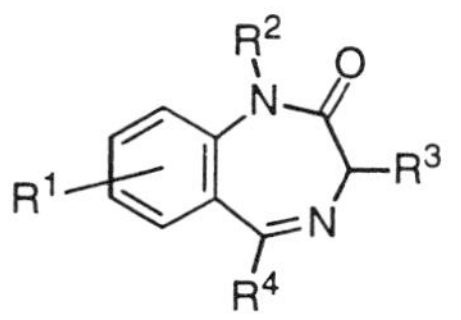

3.3.49 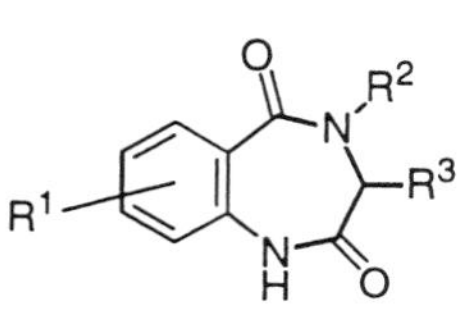   **3.3.50**

Synthesis of this class of compounds would represent an intramolecular cyclization of the type shown in Figure 8.11b. If a Ugi product of type **3.3.51** could be synthesized, cleavage of the cyclohexenamide to an ester or acid and subsequent lactamization with the anthranilic nitrogen would yield the corresponding 1,4-

benzodiazepine-2,5-dione **3.3.50,** in either one or two steps from the Ugi product [Eq. (3.3.3)]:

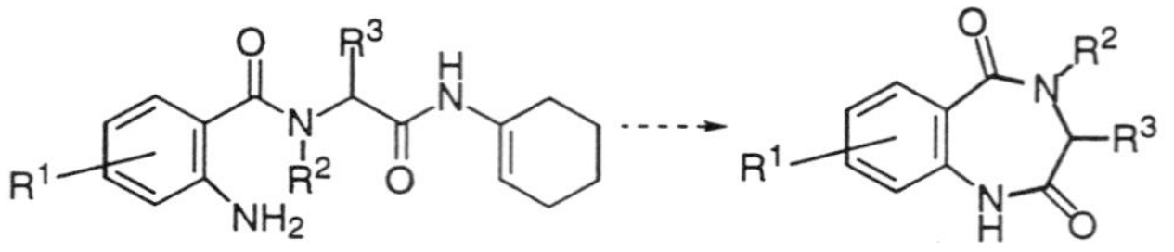

$$\tag{3.3.3}$$

3.3.51   **3.3.50**

The commercially available inputs for a library of such compounds would then consist of over 40 substituted anthranilic acids, and the legion of amines and aldehydes. As before, the isocyanide input would be erased except for a single carbon atom.

In the interests of ease of synthesis, we wished to avoid employing a protecting group for the anthranilic acid nitrogen in the Ugi 4CC. This would allow the use of anthranilic acids "off-the-shelf" and obviate the need for protecting group removal later. We expected that the precondensation of the amine and aldehyde components, along with the reduced nucleophilicity of the anthranilic nitrogen, would avoid this problem. The results are shown in Scheme 8.11.

By combining isobutyraldehyde and *p*-methoxybenzylamine in methanol with 4 Å molecular sieves and stirring for an hour, followed by isocyanide and finally anthranilic acid addition, a 73% isolated yield of 4CC product **3.3.52** was obtained, with some recoverable starting materials, but no observable side products. Treatment of this product with acetyl chloride in methanol resulted in 1,4-benzo-diazepine-2,5-dione **3.3.53** as a single isolable product in 82% yield. A second example with different inputs is shown in Scheme 8.11. Aside from sluggishness of

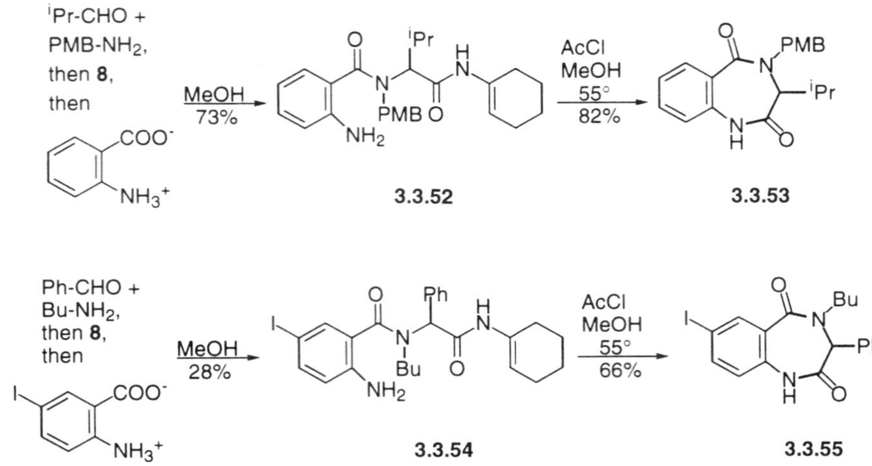

3.3.52   **3.3.53**

3.3.54   **3.3.55**

Scheme 8.11

the 4CC, the reactions proceeded similarly. This accomplishes the synthesis of 1,4-benzodiazepine-2,5-diones extremely rapidly, in good yield, and with remarkable possibilities for diverse functionality.

8.4 MICROCHIP-ENCODED LIBRARIES (68)

MCC reactions, such as the Ugi 4CC, are able to form selective core structures efficiently since compounds can be constructed in a single transformation. In contrast, traditional linear library synthesis allows access to a greater number of core structures, but at the expense of multiple resin manipulations and postsynthesis compound identification. The library described below represents a hybrid of the two strategies, incorporating an MCC reaction as the key step within a linear synthesis, and utilizing an alternative method for compound identification.

Typically, a linear synthesis is performed with a "split-mix" approach (7,69,70), which requires a deconvolution process (71). In this process the component of interest must be identified from the compound mixture and its structure elucidated. Chemical tagging techniques have been used to encode the structure of each of the components of a pool in order to facilitate the identification of selected members of the library (72–74). However, introduction, removal, and decoding of chemical tags can comprise a large portion of the effort to generate and screen the library.

In conceptual terms, introduction of encoded chemical tags at each cycle of a "split synthesis" represents a WRITE function in which information relating to chemical structure is written to the resin. Encoding can also be achieved by a READ function if there is a unique identifier associated with each resin bead in the library that may be read. This latter strategy removes the write steps needed to encode a library. In the strategy described herein, commercially available radiofrequency (rf) transponders (75) commonly used for laboratory animal tagging were chosen to tag each compound in the library (76,77). These transponders are pre-encoded with a unique 10-digit alphanumeric ID and are glass encased and stable to most solvents and reagents. The transponders can be scanned directly through standard laboratory glassware, even while immersed in a solvent. The rf signal emitted is multidirectional, requiring no specific alignment of the transponder to a detector. In order to associate resin with unique IDs, polypropylene mesh "tea bags" containing Wang (78,79) p-benzyloxybenzylhydroxyl polystyrene resin and a single transponder per bag were used. The individual mesh bags used effectively sequestered the resin within while allowing the free exchange of solvent and reagents.

The basic procedure for carrying out the synthesis was similar to the split synthesis method (Fig. 8.12). A library containing 64 members was generated from a linear three-step synthesis (steps a, b, and c) with four inputs (1–4) per step. The tea bags containing the functionalized resin and a single transponder per bag were partitioned into four individual reaction vessels and subjected to reaction with inputs A. The mixture of bags (16/flask) were then removed, washed of excess reagents, scanned, and sorted for the second step of the synthesis (inputs B). Scanning involved passing the transponder near an rf detector, where its unique ID was

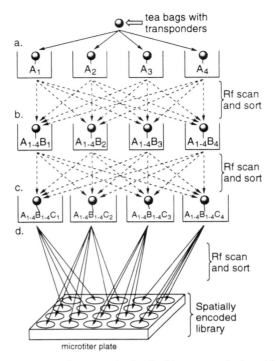

Figure 8.12 (a–c) Three-step linear synthesis of a 64-compound microchip-encoded library plus (d) the deconvolution step.

recorded on a computer. This process was repeated for the B inputs. After the parallel C input cycle was completed, the bags were sorted to 64 individual wells of a 96-well microtiter plate format, and the products were cleaved from the resin. Following removal of the tea bags, a single compound per well format of the discrete library of 64 unique products was obtained. A histogram of the reaction sequence for each unique ID provides the unequivocal structure of the expected single product in each well. Unlike the split synthesis, the use of tea bags means that the scale of synthesis is not limited to the load of individual resin beads, and the bags greatly ease handling and transfer of the resin between steps.

Having previously generated secondary amides with the Ugi reaction on solid support, we also looked to generate tertiary amides. Rather than using Rink amide resin, for this synthesis we incorporated amino acids onto Wang *p*-benzyloxy-benzylhydroxyl polystyrene as our first step (Scheme 8.12). The amine from the amino acid then became the amine input for the Ugi reaction. After a READ function and apportionment to the appropriate reaction vessels, a Ugi four-component condensation with four different aldehydes resulted in **4.2,** keeping constant the phenol and benzyl isocyanide. Subsequent recording of IDs and sorting provided the four sets of tea bag mixtures necessary for the acylation (**4.3**) reactions. The mixtures of bags were then sorted individually to the microtiter plate format and

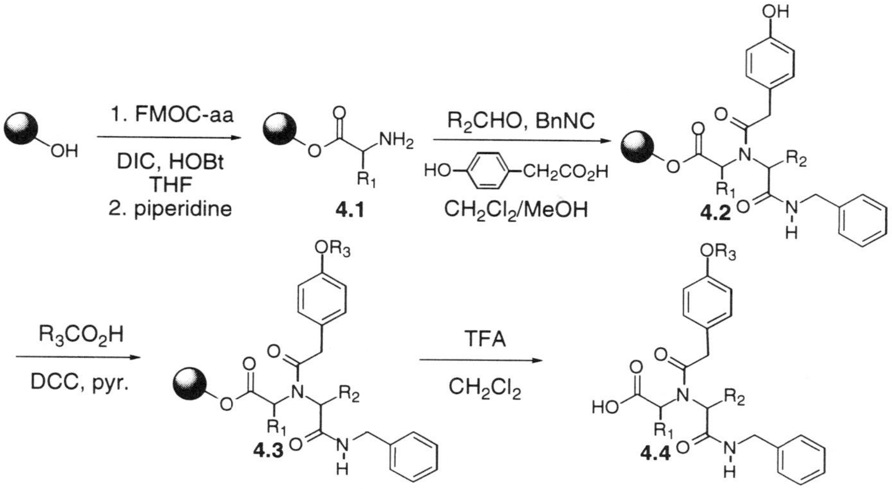

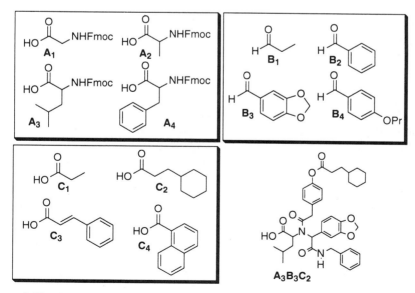

Scheme 8.12 Synthetic procedure for the 64-compound library.

compounds were removed from the resin with TFA. Evacuation of excess solvent in a vacuum oven provided the products **4.4.** The structure of the inputs for the three-step sequence are shown in Figure 8.13. Analysis of the products in the library indicated that all expected products were generated with most yields between 45 and 55% (8–14 mg).

Figure 8.13 Structure of the chemical inputs for the three-step library and the structure of one of the products.

The end products of a microchip-encoded library are single compounds (per well) whose structure is effortlessly decoded from the histogram of each transponder ID. This "decoding" is a facile process that can be software driven. The "read and sort" strategy does not require separate reactions to introduce tags and avoids potential incompatibility issues associated with the library synthesis. It eliminates the need for a biological screen-directed deconvolution of a mixture of compounds and the necessity for the chemical or biochemical analysis of the code. A mixing process to achieve a statistical distribution of beads is unnecessary because the scanning step provides the sorting information for the synthesis of all structures. Thus, the total number of tea bags required is equal to the total theoretical number of compounds that are to be made in the particular library. Because the final product of this library is a discrete array, biological screening of individual compounds of known structure can provide an SAR profile of the complete library.

8.5   RESIN CAPTURE

8.5.1   Introduction

The generation of small-molecule libraries has traditionally followed either a solution phase (80) or a solid supported synthesis. The majority of libraries described to date have used a solid support matrix (20,30,58,81,82) because of the ease in isolation and purification of products. In addition, high yields can often be obtained in a solid-phase synthesis by using multiple equivalents of reagents to drive the reaction toward completion. However, the solution phase has advantages as well: Few reactions have been adapted to the solid phase in comparison to solution phase, solid-phase reactions are more difficult to monitor, and low-yielding reactions are often incompatible with synthesis on solid support. In order to address these issues, we have developed a strategy that combines the strengths of both solution and solid-phase synthesis. In this method, the synthesis of a library is initiated in solution and the material is subsequently transferred to solid support for further transformation. This strategy, which we refer to as resin capture, offers some advantages over a single-phase synthesis.

In resin capture, only the desired product in a crude reaction mixture is trapped on solid support. This is possible when the starting materials and side products lack the functionality that enables the desired product to react with the resin. Resin captures serves a dual purpose: purification of the solution reaction and synthesis of a resin-bound intermediate. In a resin capture strategy, difficult to monitor or low-yielding reactions can be performed in solution, and the following reactions are performed on solid support. This method combines the flexibility of solution synthesis with the purity of solid-phase products.

8.5.2   Resin Capture in Cyclohexenamide Conversion (35)

Our initial resin capture studies employed the Wang (78) p-benzyloxybenzyl alcohol resin as the nucleophile in cyclohexenamide conversion (Scheme 8.13), which was expected to perform similarly to benzyl alcohol in product **3.3.13**.

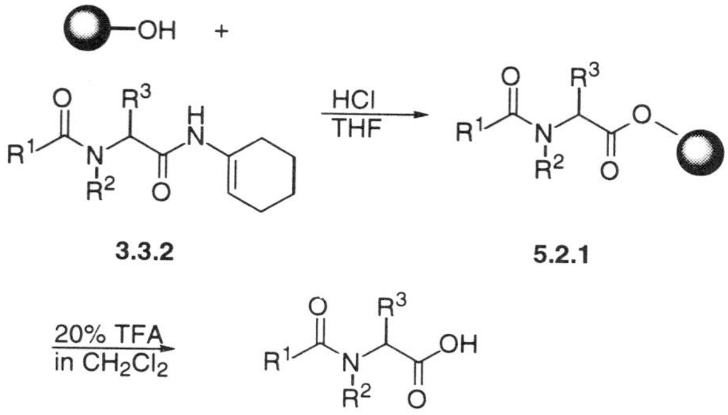

Scheme 8.13

In order to validate the concept of resin capture, these studies utilized purified products rather than crude reaction mixtures. An excess of Ugi 4CC products **3.3.2** were incubated with Wang resin under anhydrous acidic THF conditions, then the resin was washed repeatedly with methanol and CH_2Cl_2. Cleavage from the resin was with a 20% (v/v) trifluoroacetic acid in methylene chloride solution. The products were characterized without purification and were >95% pure by TLC and ^{1}H-NMR. Perhaps most remarkable, as displayed in Table 8.7, are the yields of products recovered from the resin. The yields were calculated based on the manufacturer's stated loading level of the Wang resin. We initially employed a fourfold excess of 4CC products, but discovered that high yields of recovered carboxylic acid were maintained even when the excess of Ugi products was reduced to 1.5 equivalents! Inspection of the solution washes of the resin prior to cleavage revealed a mixture of carboxylic acid and methyl ester derivatives arising from hydrolysis/methanolysis of the excess 4CC starting material during these washes.

Interestingly, when we attempted to capture 1,4-benzodiazepine-2,5-dione precursors **3.3.52** and **3.3.54** on Wang resin, subsequent cleavage yielded no product.

TABLE 8.7   Yields of Products Recovered from Resin Capture

Condensation Product

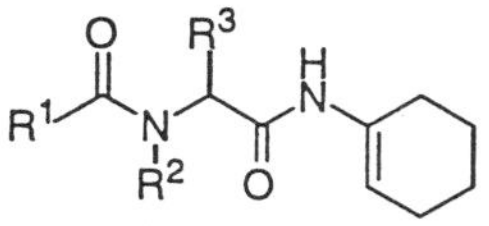

R^1	R^2	R^3	eq of 4CC Prod.	Conditions	Prod./ Yield
Me-	PMB-	Ph-	4	HCl, toluene, 100°	3.3.8/100%
Ph-	Bu-	Ph-	4	HCl, toluene, 100°	3.3.9/62%
Me-	PMB-	Ph-	4	HCl, THF, 55°	3.3.8/100%
Me-	PMB-	^{i}Pr	4	HCl, THF, 55°	3.3.7/100%
Me-	PMB-	^{i}Pr	1.5	HCl, THF, 55°	3.3.7/96%

Characterization of the wash solutions revealed high yields of the 1,4-benzo-diazepine-2,5-diones. Apparently, the cyclization to produce the 1,4-benzo-diazepine-2,5-diones from their 4CC precursors is facile enough that the initially formed Wang benzyl ester is very rapidly displaced by the anthranilic nitrogen, thus the product cleaves itself off the resin (59). This was observed even under milder temperatures and acidity.

8.5.3   Resin Capture of Vinyl Boronates (83)

Using resin capture, we have synthesized a number of tetrasubstituted ethylenes in which all four substituents can be modified. In this example, the crude product of a two-step solution synthesis is selectively captured on solid support. This synthesis provides a route to antiestrogenic triphenylethylene derivatives (84) like tamoxifen (85), which is used to treat breast cancer (86–88).

Recently, Ishiyama et al. (89,90) described the platinum-catalyzed diboration of alkynes to give bis(boryl)alkenes, **5.3.2** with very high cis selectivity (Scheme 8.14). We felt that **5.3.2** was an attractive starting material because the bis-boronate esters could be differentiated to introduce two additional substituents. **5.3.2** could be monoalkylated in a solution Suzuki reaction with alkyl or aryl halides. A second Suzuki reaction with a resin-bound aryl halide would result in the synthesis of substituted ethylenes involving three distinct components in a single-pot transforma-tion. Several groups have reported success in coupling aryl boronic acids to poly-mer-bound aryl halides (65,66,91,92). However, resin capture allows us to exploit the full range of Suzuki substrates in solution: methyl, benzyl, allyl, vinyl, as well as aryl halides (93). The large number of commercially available alkynes also provides access to a variety of bis(boryl)alkenes through diboration.

Following Ishiyama and co-worker's (89,90) procedure, we have diborated a variety of alkynes to give **5.3.2** in good to excellent yield. Isolation of **5.3.2** is unnecessary because the starting alkyne is unreactive in the following Suzuki reac-tion as required by our resin capture strategy. Crude **5.3.2** is reacted with 1.5 equivalent of organohalide to give the mono-addition product **5.3.3** (regioisomers are produced when $R_1 \neq R_2$) along with the di-addition product **5.3.4** (Scheme 8.15). The first coupling is fast in comparison to the second coupling, which produces **5.3.4,** thus most of **5.3.2** is consumed in the reaction. The mixture of **5.3.3** and **5.3.4** is combined with Rink-resin-bound aryl iodide **5.3.5** to initiate a

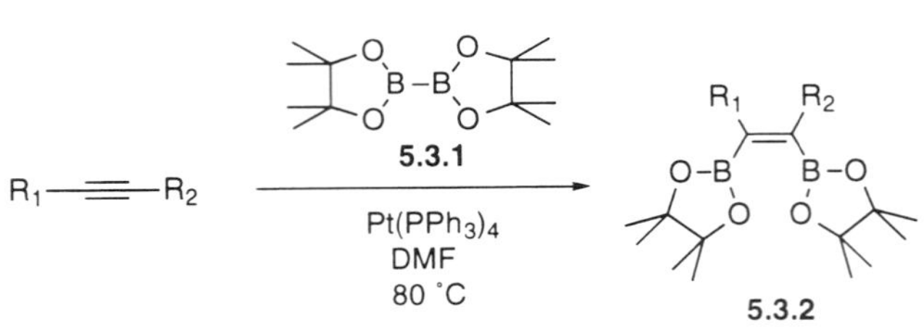

Scheme 8.14

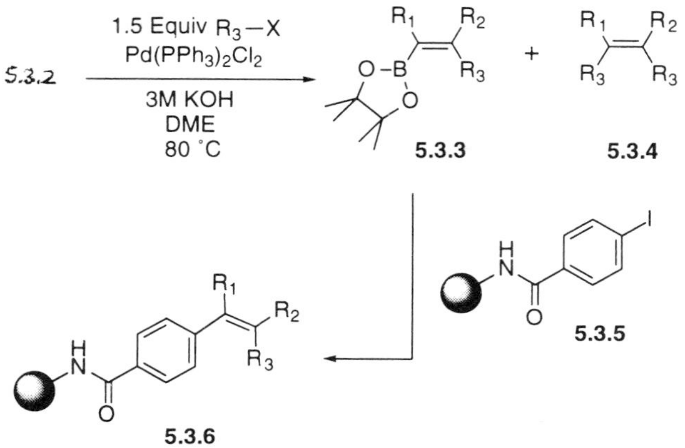

Scheme 8.15

second Suzuki reaction *without* any further addition of palladium catalyst. Only **5.3.3** is captured on solid support to produce **5.3.6,** because **5.3.4** and other impurities cannot react with **5.3.5**. Of a number of bases [NaOH, KOH, K_2CO_3, $Ba(OH)_2$ and K_3PO_4] and solvents [THF, dimethoxyethane (DME), dimethylacetamide (DMA), dimethylformamide (DMF), dioxane, and toluene], a combination of aqueous KOH in DME gives the best results in these reactions. We have found that although both $Pd(PPh_3)_4$ and $PdCl_2(PPh_3)_2$ work equally well, $PdCl_2(PPh_3)_2$ is easier to work with when setting up a number of reactions in a library synthesis. Our general procedure is as follows: A small test tube is charged with **5.3.2** (10 equiv.), organohalide (15 equiv.), $PdCl_2(PPh_3)_2$ (0.3 equiv.), $3M$ KOH (20 equiv.), and enough DME to bring the concentration of **5.3.2** to $0.5M$. The test tube is covered with a septum and flushed with N_2. The reaction mixture is heated overnight in a sand bath under N_2. Another test tube is charged with 100 equivalents KOH and 1 equivalent of **5.3.5** and flushed with N_2. The DME/KOH solution is syringed into the tube containing the polymer and heated overnight. The polymer is filtered out of the solution and washed successively with H_2O, MeOH, ethyl acetate, and CH_2Cl_2. The products are cleaved from the polymer with 30% TFA in CH_2Cl_2.

The opposite order of addition of halides produced resin-bound boronate **5.3.7** very efficiently (Scheme 8.16). However, subsequent condensation with solution aryl halides occurred in unacceptable yields.

We have synthesized a number of tetrasubstituted ethylenes, including several triphenylethylenes as described in Table 8.8. Using the symmetrical aryl–aryl and alkyl–alkyl boronates **5.3.8** (90,91) and **5.3.9** (Fig. 8.14), we obtained products in high yield and purity after TFA cleavage. We note that this methodology also provides sterically hindered tetraphenylethylenes in high yield (see Table 8.8).

When using unsymmetrical bis(boryl)alkenes, regioisomers are produced. When **5.3.10** is reacted with **5.3.5**, a 2.3-to-1 ratio of **5.3.11b** to **5.3.11a** is obtained in >95% yield (Fig. 8.15). **5.3.11b** is the result of hydrolytic deboration of **5.3.7**

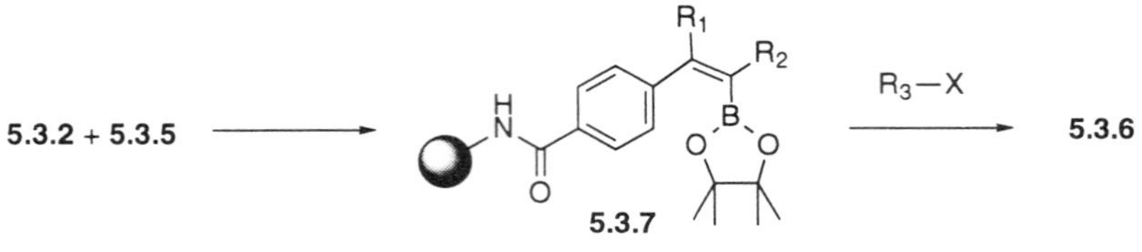

$5.3.2 + 5.3.5 \longrightarrow$ **5.3.7** $\xrightarrow{R_3-X}$ **5.3.6**

Scheme 8.16

during the Suzuki reaction. Resin capture minimizes the amount of deborated material that collects on the polymer since it avoids resin-bound vinyl boronates such as **5.3.7**.

We have also found that the reaction of **5.3.10** with 4-iodo-[2-(N,N-dimethylamino)ethoxy]benzene gives the tamoxifen benzamide **5.3.12b** in a 2.5-to-1 ratio with its regioisomer **5.3.12a** in a >95% yield (Fig. 8.16).

After resin capture, further synthetic transformations may be carried out. For instance, the use of 2-(4-bromophenoxy)-ethanol in the condensation with **5.3.8** and **5.3.5** affords tetraphenylethylene **5.3.13** with an additional reactive functional group. Condensation of **5.3.13** with 3,5-dimethyl phenol using Mitsunobu condi-

TABLE 8.8   Tetrasubstituted Ethylenes Synthesized by Resin Capture

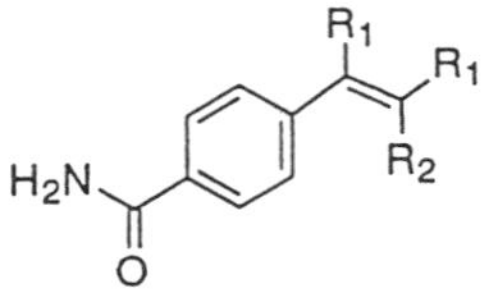

R_1	R_2	% Yield
Phenyl	Methyl	>95
Phenyl	2-Methyl-1-propenyl	78[a]
Phenyl	2-Propenyl	>95[c]
Phenyl	Benzyl	>95
Phenyl	4-Tolyl	83[a]
Ethyl	Methyl	>95
Ethyl	2-Methyl-1-propenyl	75[b]
Ethyl	2-Propenyl	>95[a]
Ethyl	Benzyl	83[b]
Ethyl	4-Tolyl	85[a]

[a]Contains small percentage of 4-iodobenzamide.
[b]Contains small percentage of deborated material.
[c]Partial isomerization to conjugated diene.

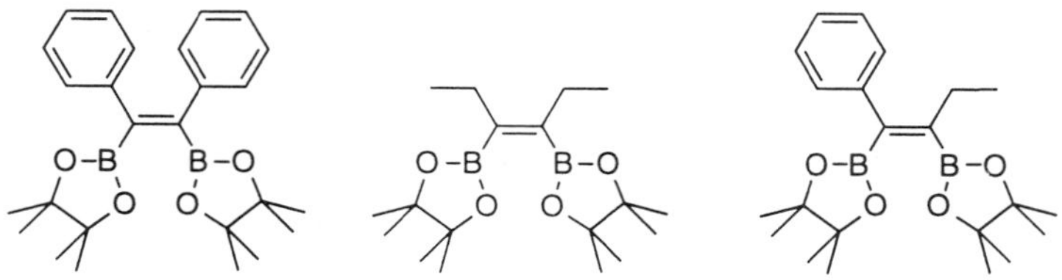

Figure 8.14

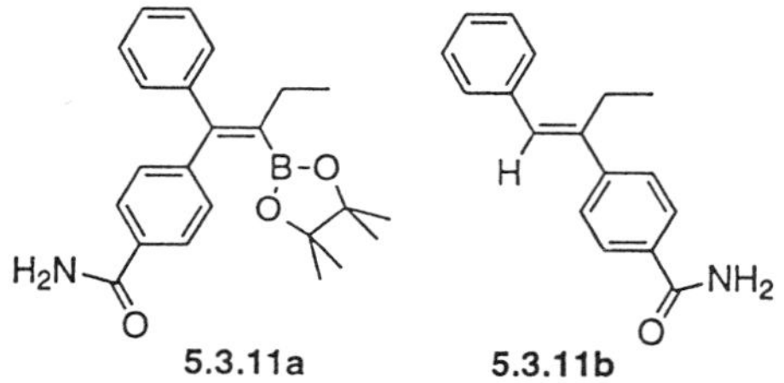

Figure 8.15

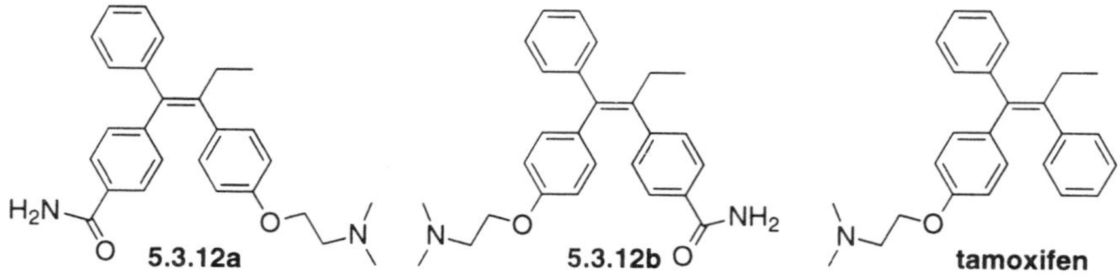

Figure 8.16

tions (94) leads to the formation of **5.3.14** after resin cleavage (Scheme 8.17). Reagent **5.3.1** has also been reported to facilitate the conversion of aryl halides to aryl boronic esters (95). Thus, Pt-catalyzed reaction of **5.3.5** with reagent **5.3.1** afforded aryl boronic ester **5.3.15**, which could be coupled to *N*-benzyl-4-iodobenz-amide in >95% yield (Scheme 8.18). Thus, in contrast to resin bound vinyl boronates, the resin bound aryl boronates readily react with aryl halides in solution.

Resin capture represents a new strategy for solid-phase synthesis in which the first step is not the attachment of the first input to the solid support but is rather a solution reaction whose products are amenable to subsequent attachment to the resin. Resin capture allows flexibility with the solution reactions because the reac-

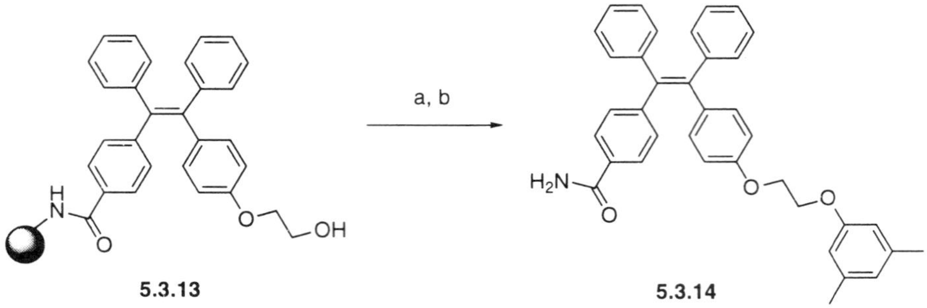

5.3.13 **5.3.14**

Scheme 8.17 (a) 3,5-Dimethylphenol, diisopropylazodicarboxylate, triphenylphosphine, *N*-ethyl morpholine, 16 h; (b) 30% TFA in CH_2Cl_2; >95% yield based on loading of polymer.

tions do not need to be adapted or maximized for solid support and because low-yielding reactions or reactions with several side products may be run in solution to prevent side products from collecting on the polymer. As these examples demonstrate, solution products can be efficiently and selectively incorporated on solid support for further transformation. We believe that resin capture is an efficient strategy for library generation that combines the ease of solution synthesis with the ease of isolation and purification of solid supported products.

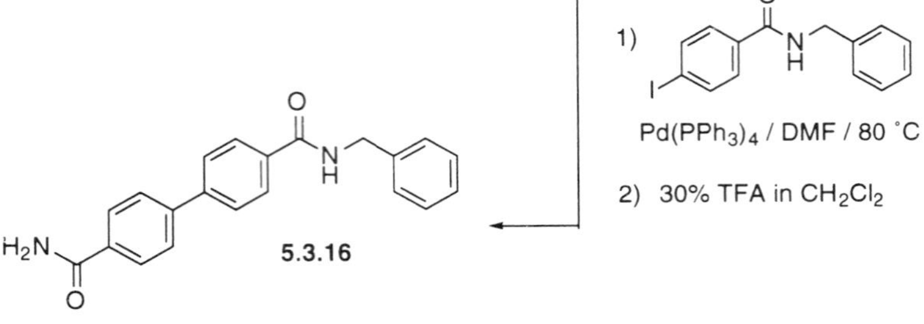

Scheme 8.18

REFERENCES

1. Pinella, C., Appel, J., Blondelle, S., Dooley, C., Dorner, B., Eichler, J., Ostresh, J., and Houghten, R. A., *Biopolymers* **37**, 221–240 (1995).
2. Gallop, M. A., Barrett, R. W., Dower, W. J., Fodor, S. P. A., and Gordon, E. M., *J. Med. Chem.* **37**, 1233–1251 (1994).
3. Pavia, M. R., Sawyer, T. K., and Moos, W. H., *Bioorg. Med. Chem. Lett.* **3**, 387–396 (1993).
4. Jung, G., and Beck-Sickinger, A. G., *Angew. Chem., Int. Ed. Engl.* **31**, 367–383 (1992).
5. Gold, L., Polisky, B., Uhlenbeck, O., and Yarus, M., *Annu. Rev. Biochem.* **64**, 763–797 (1995).
6. Ecker, D. J., Vickers, T. A., Hanecak, R., Driver, V., and Anderson, K., *Nucleic Acids Res.* **21**, 1853–1856 (1993).
7. Furka, Á., Sebestyén, F., Asgedom, M., and Dibó, G., *Int. J. Peptide Protein Res.* **37**, 487–493 (1991).
8. Strecker, A., *Justus Liebigs Ann. Chem.* **75**, 27 (1850).
9. Strecker, A., *Justus Liebigs Ann. Chem.* **91**, 349 (1854).
10. Hantzsch, A., *Ber. Dtsch. Chem. Ges.* **23**, 1474 (1890).
11. Biginelli, P., *Ber. Dtsch. Chem. Ges.* **24**, 2962 (1891).
12. Biginelli, P., *Ber. Dtsch. Chem. Ges.* **26**, 447 (1893).
13. Mannich, C., and Krosche, W., *Arch. Pharm. (Weinheim, Ger.)* **250**, 647 (1912).
14. Passerini, M., *Gazz. Chim. Ital.* **51**, 126, 181 (1921).
15. Bucherer, H. T., and Fischbeck, H. T., *J. Prakt. Chem.* **140**, 69 (1934).
16. Bucherer, H. T., Steiner, W., *J. Prakt. Chem.* **140**, 24 (1934).
17. Bergs, H., Ger. Patent 566 094, 1929.
18. Khand, I. U., Knox, G. R., Pauson, P. L., Watts, W. E., and Foreman, M. I., *J. Chem. Soc., Perkin Trans. 1* **9**, 977–981 (1973).
19. Wipf, P., and Cunningham, A., *Tetrahedron Lett.* **36**, 7819–7822 (1995).
20. Armstrong, R. W., Combs, A. P., Tempest, P. A., Brown, S. D., and Keating, T. A., *Acc. Chem. Res.* **29**, 123–131 (1996).
21. Combs, A. P., Ph.D. Thesis, University of California, Los Angeles, 1993.
22. Ugi, I., Lohberger, S., and Karl, R., in *Comprehensive Organic Synthesis,* Vol. 2, B. M. Trost and I. Fleming (Eds.), Pergamon, New York, 1991, pp. 1083–1109.
23. Moran, E. J., Tellew, J. E., Zhao, Z., and Armstrong, R. W., *J. Org. Chem.* **58**, 7848 (1993).
24. Armstrong, R. W., Tellew, J. E., and Moran, E. J., *J. Org. Chem.* **57**, 2208 (1992).
25. Armstrong, R. W., Salvati, M. E., and Nguyen, M., *J. Am. Chem. Soc.* **114**, 3145 (1992).
26. Pillai, V. N. R., *Synthesis* 1–26 (1980).
27. Williams, P. L., Gairi, M., Albericio, F., and Giralt, E., *Tetrahedron* **47**, 9867–9880 (1991).
28. Rich, D. H., and Gurwara, S. K., *Tetrahedron Lett.* **26**, 301–304 (1975).

29. Atherton, E., and Sheppard, R. C. *Solid Phase Synthesis; A Practical Approach*, IRL, Oxford 1989, pp. 63–74.

30. Tempest, P. A., Brown, S. D., and Armstrong, R. W., *Angew. Chem., Int. Ed. Engl.* **35,** 640 (1996).

31. Posner, G., *Chem. Rev.* **86,** 831–844 (1986).

32. (a) Ugi, I., *Isonitrile Chemistry,* Academic, London, 1971. (b) Ugi, I., Dömling, A., and Hörl, W., *Endeavour* **18,** 115–123 (1994).

33. Rink, H., *Tetrahedron Lett.* **28,** 3787–3789 (1987).

34. Keating, T. A., and Armstrong, R. W., *J. Am. Chem. Soc.* **117,** 7842–7843 (1995).

35. Keating, T. A., and Armstrong, R. W., *J. Am. Chem. Soc.* **118,** 2574–2583 (1996).

36. Ugi, I., *Angew. Chem., Int. Ed. Engl.* **21,** 810–819 (1982).

37. Geller, J., and Ugi, I., *Chem. Scr.* **22,** 85–89 (1983).

38. Rosendahl, F. K., and Ugi, I., *Ann. Chem.* **666,** 65–67 (1963).

39. Fukuyama, T., presented at the 35th Annual Buffalo Medicinal Chemistry Symposium, Buffalo, NY, May 1994.

40. Barton, D. H. R., Bowles, T., Huisnec, S., Forbes, J. E., Llobera, A., Porter, A. E. A., and Zard, S. Z., *Tetrahedron Lett.* **29,** 3343–3346 (1988).

41. Baldwin, J. E., and Yamaguchi, Y., *Tetrahedron Lett.* **30,** 3335–3338 (1989).

42. Brossi, A., Dolan, L. A., and Teitel, S., in *Organic Syntheses,* Vol. VI, Wiley, New York, 1988, pp. 1–4.

43. Greene, T. W., and Wuts, P. G. M., *Protective Groups in Organic Synthesis,* 2nd ed.; Wiley-Interscience, New York, 1991, pp. 349–350.

44. Coppola, B. P., Noe, M. C., Schwartz, D. J., Il Abdon, R. L., and Trost, B. M., *Tetrahedron* **50,** 93–116 (1994).

45. Dalla Croce, P., and Rosa, C. L., *Heterocycles* **27,** 2825–2832 (1988).

46. Padwa, A., Burgess, E. M., Gingrich, H. L., and Roush, D. M., *J. Org. Chem.* **47,** 786–791 (1982).

47. Potts, K. T., in *1,3-Dipolar Cycloaddition Chemistry,* Vol. 2, A. Padwa (Ed.), Wiley-Interscience, New York, 1984, pp. 1–82.

48. Lown, J. W., in *1,3-Dipolar Cycloaddition Chemistry,* Vol. 1, A. Padwa (Ed.), Wiley-Interscience, New York, 1984, pp. 653–732.

49. Gokel, G., Lüdke, G., and Ugi, I., in *Isonitrile Chemistry,* I. Ugi (Ed.), Academic, New York, 1971, pp. 145–199.

50. Huisgen, R., Gotthardt, H., Bayer, H. O., and Schafer, F. C., *Angew. Chem., Int. Ed. Engl.* **3,** 136–137 (1964).

51. Brunn, E., Funke, E., Gotthardt, H., Huisgen, R., *Chem. Ber.* **104,** 1562 (1971).

52. Santiago, B., Dalton, C. R., Huber, E. W., and Kane, J. M., *J. Org. Chem* **60,** 4947–4950 (1995).

53. Horton, D., and Varela, O., *Carbohydr. Res.* **134,** 205–214 (1984).

54. Armstrong, R. W., and Teegarden, B. R., *J. Org. Chem.* **56,** 915 (1992).

55. Teegarden, B. R., Ph.D. Thesis, University of California, Los Angeles, 1991.

56. Sternbach, L. H., *J. Med. Chem.* **22,** 1 (1979).

57. Bunin, B. A., and Ellman, J. A., *J. Am. Chem. Soc.* **114,** 10997–10998 (1992).

58. Bunin, B. A., Plunkett, M. J., and Ellman, J. A., *Proc. Natl. Acad. Sci. U.S.A.* **91,** 4708–4712 (1994).

59. DeWitt, S. H., Kiely, J. S., Stankovic, C. J., Schroeder, M. C., Reynolds Cody, D. M., and Pavia, M. R., *Proc. Natl. Acad. Sci. U.S.A.* **90,** 6909–6913 (1993).

60. Plunkett, M. J., and Ellman, J. A., *J. Am. Chem. Soc.* **117,** 3306–3307 (1995).

61. Cho, N. S., Song, K. Y., and Párkányi, C., *J. Heterocycl. Chem.* **26,** 1807–1810 (1989).

62. Jones, G. B., Davey, C. L., Jenkins, T. C., Kamal, A., Kneale, G. G., Neidle, S., Webster, G. D., and Thurston, D. E., *Anti-Cancer Drug Des.* **5,** 249 (1990).

63. McDowell, R. S., Blackburn, B. K., Gadek, T. R., McGee, L. R., Rawson, T., Reynolds, M. E., Robarge, K. D., Somers, T. C., Thorsett, E. D., Tischler, M., Webb II., R. R., and Venuti, M. C., *J. Am. Chem. Soc.* **116,** 5077 (1994).

64. Moroder, L., Lutz, J., Grams, F., Rudolph-Böhner, S., Ösapay, G., Goodman, M., and Kolbeck, W., *Biopolymers* **38,** 295–300 (1996).

65. Boojamra, C. G., Burrow, K. M., and Ellman, J. A., *J. Org. Chem.* **60,** 5742–5743 (1995).

66. Goff, D. A., and Zuckermann, R. N., *J. Org. Chem.* **60,** 5744–5745 (1995).

67. Karp, G. M., *J. Org. Chem.* **60,** 5814–5819 (1995).

68. Armstrong, R. W., Tempest, P. A., and Cargill, J. F., *Chimia* **50,** 258–260 (1996).

69. Lam, K., Salmon, S., Hersh, E., Hruby, V., Kazmeierski, W., and Knapp, R., *Nature* **360,** 768 (1992).

70. Sebestyén, F., Dibó, G., Kovacs, A., and Furka, Á., *Bio. Med. Chem. Lett.* **3,** 413 (1993).

71. Dooley, C., Chung, N., Wilkes, B., Schiller, P., Bidlack, J., Pasternak, G., and Houghten, R., *Science* **266,** 2019 (1994).

72. Brenner, S., and Lenner, R., *Proc. Natl. Acad. Sci. U.S.A.* **89,** 5381 (1992).

73. Kerr, J., Banville, S., and Zuckermann, R., *J. Am. Chem. Soc.* **115,** 2529 (1993).

74. Ohlmeyer, M., Swanson, R., Dillard, L., Reader, J., Asouline, G., Kobayashi, R., Wigler, M., and Still, W., *Proc. Natl. Acad. Sci. U.S.A.* **90,** 10922 (1993).

75. (a) Urbas, D. J., and Ellwood, D., U.S. Pat. 5,252,962 (1993). (Held by Bio Medic Data Systems, Maywood, NJ.) (b) D'Hont, L., Tip, A., and Meier, H., U.S. Pat. 5,351,052 (1994). (Held by Texas Instruments, Inc., Dallas, TX.) (c) We employed the Implantable Micro Identification (IMI) System from Bio Medic Data Systems, Maywood, NJ. The transponders were scanned with a DAS-4004 pocket scanner.

76. Nicolaou, K. C., Xiao, X. Y., Parandoosh, Z., Senyei, A., and Nova, M. P., *Angew. Chem. Intl. Ed. Eng.* **34,** 2289 (1995).

77. Moran, E. J., Sarshar, S., Cargill, J. F., Shahbaz, M. M., Lio, A., Mjalli, A. M. M., and Armstrong, R. W., *J. Am. Chem. Soc.* **117,** 10787 (1995).

78. Wang, S.-S., *J. Am. Chem. Soc.* **95,** 1328 (1973).

79. Lu, G., Mojsov, S., Tam, J., and Merrifield, R., *J. Org. Chem.* **46,** 3433 (1981).

80. Cheng, S., Comer, D. D., Williams, J. P., Meyers, P. L., and Boger, D. L., *J. Am. Chem. Soc.* **118,** 2567 (1996).

81. Zuckermann, R. N., Martin, E. J., Spellmeyer, D. C., Stauber, G. B., Shoemaker, K. R., Kerr, J. M., Figliozzi, G. M., Goff, D. A., Siani, M. A., Simon, R. J., Banville,

S. C., Brown, E. G., Wang, L., Richter, L. S., and Moos, W. H., *J. Med. Chem.* **37,** 2678 (1994).

82. Murphy, M. M., Schullek, J. R., Gordon, E. M., and Gallop, M. A., *J. Am. Chem. Soc.* **117,** 7029–7030 (1995).

83. Brown, S. D., and Armstrong, R. W., *J. Am. Chem. Soc.* **118,** 6331–6332 (1996).

84. van den Koedijk, C. D., Blankenstein, M. A., and Thijssen, J. H., *Biochem. Pharmacol.* **47,** 1927 (1994).

85. Harper, M. J. K., and Walpole, A. L., *Nature (London)* **212,** 87 (1966).

86. Callaghan, R., and Higgins, C. F., *Br. J. Cancer* **71,** 294 (1995).

87. Kirk, J., Syed, S. K., Harris, A. L., Jarman, M., Roufogalis, B. D., Stratford, I. J., and Carmichael, J., *Biochem. Pharmacol.* **48,** 277 (1994).

88. Nephew, K. P., Polek, T. C., and Khan, S. A., *Endocrinology* **137,** 219 (1996).

89. Ishiyama, T., Matsuda, N., Miyaura, N., and Suzuki, A., *J. Am. Chem. Soc.* **115,** 11018 (1993).

90. Ishiyama, T., Matsuda, N., Murata, M., Ozawa, F., Suzuki, A., and Miyaura, N., *Organometallics* **15,** 713 (1996).

91. Backes, B. J., and Ellman, J. A., *J. Am. Chem. Soc.* **116,** 11171–11172 (1994).

92. Frenette, R., and Friesen, R. W., *Tetrahedron Lett.* **35,** 9177 (1994).

93. Johnson, S. G., presented at the 211th National Meeting of the American Chemical Society, New Orleans, LA, March 1996.

94. Richter, L. S., and Gadek, T. R., *Tetrahedron Lett.* **35,** 4705 (1994).

95. Ishiyama, T., Murata, M., and Miyaura, N., *J. Org. Chem.* **60,** 7508 (1995).

9

INDEXED COMBINATORIAL LIBRARIES: NONOLIGOMERIC CHEMICAL DIVERSITY FOR THE DISCOVERY OF NOVEL ENZYME INHIBITORS

MICHAEL C. PIRRUNG, JOSEPH H.-L. CHAU, AND JRLUNG CHEN

Department of Chemistry, P. M. Gross Chemical Laboratory, Duke University, Durham, North Carolina 27708-0346

9.1 INTRODUCTION

As the assembly of this volume attests, interest in the preparation of large libraries of organic molecules for the purpose of screening them for biological activity has grown greatly in recent years. The principles by which stupendous mixtures of compounds can be used to discover new pharmacologically active agents are well established, since natural products screening (1) has made major contributions to the current pharmacopoeia. One of the disadvantages of natural products as drug leads is that determination of their structures is required, though the powerful chemical and physical methods available today make that a relatively certain proposition. Often, the molecules discovered are present in vanishingly small amounts and are quite complex, providing a challenge in obtaining, either by isolation or synthesis, the quantities of product necessary to reach the market through the long and tortuous development process. A recent example of a powerful new drug where this has been an issue is taxol (2). Finally, accessing totally novel chemical entities through natural products screening can be difficult because of the parsimony and commonalty of biosynthetic pathways; molecules discovered in this way often fall into one of the major known structural classes (terpenoids, steroids, alkaloids, polyketides, etc.). However, a radically different structure is occasionally discovered, as has occurred with the enediyne natural products (3).

Rational design is another means to discover novel drugs that has received a great deal of attention (4). Although the intellectual appeal of this approach is undeniable, one problem in its application is that many factors controlling the interactions of macromolecules with "micromolecules" are still incompletely understood (5). Furthermore, many of the interactions dictating the function of drugs [pharmacokinetics (6) e.g.] are not between molecules but between a molecule and a complex system that cannot be analyzed by solely chemical principles, making design one of the most challenging problems facing organic and medicinal chemists.

Combinatorial chemistry is really a hybrid of two classical approaches to drug discovery, screening and rational chemical synthesis. It may be useful to define the term combinatorial chemistry, since its usage until now has been rather loose. In a combinatorial chemistry experiment, an ensemble of molecules is prepared by a method that permits the chemical steps to be performed in parallel, such that the number of compounds prepared far exceeds the number of steps. Further, the compounds are prepared in a format that facilitates their assay, also in parallel, against a biological recognition molecule of interest. The aim of combinatorial chemistry is to provide economies of scale in the screening of synthesized compounds for activity. Its goal at the molecular level is to discover a compound that fits tightly within some receptor (using the term broadly to include enzymes, cell-surface receptors, nucleic acids, carbohydrates, etc.) site of an a priori unknown structure. Access to a comprehensive collection of molecular shapes and distributions of charge in space should make it possible to fit *any* receptor site. This assertion need not be made recklessly since an example of the development of powerful binding interactions in a way complementary to this proposal already exists in the mammalian immune system. It is capable of producing macromolecules that can bind to virtually any antigen by using the 20 amino acids in a primary antibody repertoire of $\sim 10^8$ different types of molecules [notably, assembled in a combinatorial (vide infra) synthesis from approximately 100 V and 5 J light-chain and 200 V, 30 D, and 6 J heavy-chain germ-line gene sequences] (7). Therefore, it is reasonable that a library of millions of molecules should be capable of fitting *any* binding site. Of course, methods of preparing and screening up to 10^8 molecules are not readily available; efforts toward this goal drive much of today's research in combinatorial chemistry.

Determining the structures of the active compounds, like in natural products screening, is a key issue in library screening. However, when molecular libraries are chemically prepared, they can be engineered to make structural determination straightforward by incorporation of some sort of code or tag ("encoding") that can be easily read. Means of identification of elements in libraries have included: physical isolation on macroscopic pins (8); microscopic localization on a surface, (9); sequencing of the peptides themselves (10); sequencing of polymers coding for peptide sequences, including DNA (11) or peptides (12); and sequencing by organic identifying groups (13). Another option to identify active compounds is "deconvolution," wherein pools are first screened to find actives and then individual components within active pools are synthesized for testing (14). A hybrid of encoding and deconvolution involves preparing pools of compounds on a solid phase but cleaving a portion of them from the support for assay (15). When active pools are discovered, the original support is divided such that individual elements can be tested. It is worth emphasis that different methods to determine the structures of actives are appropriate to different types of libraries, and that these considerations are further influenced by the types of assays to be used (vide infra).

The rationality in the creation of a library comes in the choice of the building blocks and the chemistry used for its construction. The ingredients can be chosen so as to provide molecules that can be easily synthesized or have known pharmacophoric groups. The tremendous efforts that have gone into perfecting solid-phase peptide synthesis and the known biological activities of peptides made their initial use in library syntheses natural. Furthermore, the novel concept of resin splitting, or "split synthesis," as originally applied to peptides, permits a mixed library of molecules to be prepared on solid phase even though each individual support particle bears but one sequence (10,16). Of course, most current drugs are not oligomeric molecules. There is therefore interest in preparing more recognizable pharmacologically active structures in library format, in most cases on solid phase (17).

The assays to be used to screen a library are an important consideration from the earliest moments in its design. Obviously, if a molecule is attached to a bulky solid support, it will be impossible to screen it against a biological recognition molecule that is also immobilized. However, in one case, an antibody has been used in an affinity purification scheme where the most powerfully bound elements of a library, with tags attached, were retained on an immunoaffinity column (12). They were then eluted and decoded. Generally, a choice must be made between immobilizing the molecular diversity, which facilitates the synthesis of large libraries and identification of the active molecules, or the biological recognition element, which can permit affinity enrichment of the active molecules within a large library. The partial cleavage method circumvents the problem of linking an identifier to a molecule while still permitting solution-phase assays, but requires more manipulations. The Scylla and Charybdis of combinatorial chemistry is the choice between library size and assay ease. While it is in principle possible to make very large libraries of compounds, it can be impractical to screen larger libraries using some methods while still enabling the identification of actives.

Two different types of syntheses can be and have been performed. Their distinction is based on the number of building block sets, which further influences the library size (vide infra) and the protocol for synthesis. Syntheses can be combinatorial or permutational: (18) The former produces compounds of defined connectivity [Eq. (9.1)], (19)* and the latter can produce compounds of variable length, ordered in all possible sequences.

---

*Mathematical set notations are used in these equations and figures. Names of sets are italicized; members of a set are bracketed, and in some cases referred to through subscripted Roman letters of the set name. The number of elements in a set is $|X|$.

$$A \times B \times C \Longrightarrow A_i\text{---}B_j\text{---}C_k \tag{9.1}$$

They need not be limited to the preparation of linear molecules; indeed, cyclization [Eq. (9.2)] may be possible and even desirable.

$$A \times B \times C \Longrightarrow \begin{array}{c} A_i\text{---}B_j \\ \diagdown \diagup \\ C_k \end{array} \tag{9.2}$$

It is not necessary that the **A–B** linkage in a combinatorial synthesis be chemically related in any way to the **B–C** (or **C–A**) linkage, but permutational syntheses require the same linking chemistry throughout the oligomer; this makes possible the preparation of molecules of any length. Peptides come immediately to mind as an example of the latter [Eq. (9.3)].

$$P = \{F, Q, R\} \Longrightarrow \begin{array}{l} \text{FF, FQ, FR, QF, QQ,} \\ \text{QR, RF, RQ, RR} \end{array} \tag{9.3}$$

A useful analogy for a combinatorial synthesis is the assembly of bicycles from sets including front wheels, rear wheels (with gear sets), and frames [Eq. (9.4)].

$$\tag{9.4}$$

One and only one member of each set is needed to complete a bicycle, but a number of possibilities within each set might produce a bike that works. One advantage of combinatorial syntheses is that compounds from chemically distinct building block sets are united to form substances that could never be obtained by a permutational synthesis, no matter how diverse the set. Returning to the bicycle analogy, it would never be possible to complete a working bicycle from a set containing only wheels, no matter how large. A more chemically relevant example illustrates the creation of a library using combinatorial synthesis [Eq. (9.5)].

$$\tag{9.5}$$

Three sets of compounds, phenethylamines (**A**), aldehydes (**B**), and acyl halides (**C**), could be condensed, first in a Pictet–Spengler reaction and then in an acylation to form *N*-acyl tetrahydroisoquinolines. With 10 each of the phenethylamines and aldehydes and three acyl halides, this would constitute a three-dimensional combinatorial synthesis to produce a library of 300 compounds (Fig. 9.1).

It is important to recognize the difference between library size and chemical diversity, which are not necessarily the same. While the former can be readily calculated, the latter is harder to quantify (20). If prepared by a combinatorial synthesis, the library size is $N_1 \times N_2 \times \cdots \times N_x$, where N_x is the number of elements

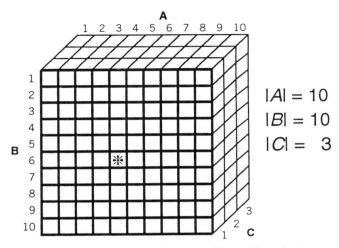

Figure 9.1   Three-dimensional combinatorial synthesis.

in building block set *x;* if prepared by a permutational synthesis, the library size is N^l, where *N* is the number of building blocks in the (single) set and *l* is the length of the molecules prepared. Even though a (permutational) synthesis of octapeptides using Phe, Trp, Met, Val, Leu, and Ile as building blocks would produce a library of over 46,000 members, it is difficult to argue that it possesses much chemical diversity because of the repeating peptide backbone and the hydrophobic character of each of the building blocks. On the contrary, a combinatorial (synthesis) of 400 esters formed from 40 diverse alcohols and 10 diverse acids might be able to sample a much wider variation of shape and charge in space.

It is also important to recognize the limitations of any novel method and apply it to problems for which it is well suited. It is unlikely that combinatorial chemistry in its current state could have been used to discover a taxol, for instance. However, it is certainly reasonable that optimized peptide therapeutics, such as octreotide, (21) might have been. As the chemistry for preparing other structural classes is adapted for library synthesis, discoveries of lead compounds for more diverse targets will be made.

Development of a new library/identification methodology and its application to two structural classes known to possess biological activity was the focus of this research. A method we refer to as *indexing,* which is similar to deconvolution but avoids iterative synthesis, was used in the preparation and screening of pools containing candidate carbamates (22) and tetrahydroacridines (23) against acetylcholinesterase (24). Members of each of these classes, physostigmine (a natural product) and tacrine (a synthetic compound), are known inhibitors of acetylcholinesterase and have been used in the treatment of myasthenia gravis and glaucoma and proposed as possible therapeutics for Alzheimer's disease (25). Another cholinesterase inhibitor class, the huperzines, has been discovered by natural products screening and is of particular interest for the Alzheimer's application (26).

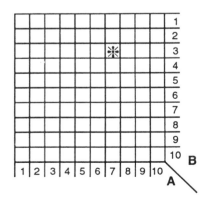

physostigmine   tacrine   huperzine

9.2 THEORY

The testing of a library prepared by combinatorial synthesis can be conceptually represented as an N-dimensional matrix, wherein each axis has as many elements as are present in each set (n). The simplest case is a library of molecules composed from two sets of substructures A and B, each of which has 10 structural variants (the number of elements in each building block set, a, $b = 10$). They can be envisioned to compose a 10×10 grid (Fig. 9.2). The assay value for each combination is contained in a cell indexed by (A_x, B_y). To assay all of the cells as pure compounds would require 100 experiments. One cell possesses the maximum response function ($R_{x,y}$) in the grid; the task is to find it without actually looking at them all. By screening the rows and the columns, which are indices to the cells at their intersections, as well-defined sublibrary mixtures, only 20 reactions and assays are required to find the maximum response. Each compound is tested twice, once each as a component of an A mixture and a B mixture. The index to the maximum cell in this example is its *row* reaction, composed of one reagent B_3 and an equimolar mixture of A reagents A_1–A_{10}, and its *column* reaction, composed of the reagent A_7 and an

Figure 9.2   Conceptual matrix for an indexed combinatorial synthesis.

equimolar mixture of B reagents B_1–B_{10}. Because all combinations are tested, an assumption that parameters A and B do not interact is not required. This example shows a five-fold improvement in the synthesis and data collection efficiency for the library compared to one-at-a-time processing. Clearly, this process can be conducted with more sets and with more elements in each set, leading to higher-dimensional arrays and to higher efficiency in data collection.

Screening of any pool of compounds, whether it is derived from nature or combinatorial synthesis, is limited by the precision and sensitivity of the assay, the potency of the "hits," and the number of elements in each pool. Consider one scenario, a single potent compound that is diluted by mediocre combinations, for row B_3. If its combination with A_7 has a value ($R_{7,3}$) (27)* of 10^9 in the assay in question, and all of its other A combinations are 10^6, the response function for the row should be their average, or 10^8. The increase of the row average due to the inclusion of the "hit" must be greater than the error in the assay to reliably identify an active row (28).[†] Based on this idea, we derived Eq. (9.6) using straightforward experimental statistics, and in the limit of large n, this expression reduces to Eq. (9.7).

$$R_{hit} - R_{ave} > t\sigma \sqrt{\frac{(2n-1)(n-1)}{n}} \qquad (9.6)$$

$$R_{hit} - R_{ave} > 2\sqrt{2}\sigma\sqrt{n} \qquad (9.7)$$

It shows characteristics of the screening of pools consistent with intuition. Greater potency (R_{hit} large) will obviously make hits more likely to be detected. A significant population of mediocre compounds (R_{ave} large) will have the opposite effect, raising the background and making it more difficult to identify actives (29).* Precise assays (σ small) will make actives easier to find. Lone active compounds are more likely to be missed with larger building block sets ($n \to \infty$) because they are "diluted" by inactive components, (30)[†] but the contribution from this term rises

---

*The response function (= assay value) for each cell is indexed by its A column and B row ($R_{A,B}$). The assay value for a row is given by $R_{A,y}$ where y is the row number, and for a column is given by $R_{x,B}$ where x is the column number.

[†]This is simply the comparison of the experimental means (Student's t-test) with and without the potent compound. The same criterion applies to columns. Of course, the only experimental values accessible at the stage of library screening were the row and column averages with the potent compound, as well as their standard deviations. Once actives were identified and individual pure compounds synthesized for testing, hits were validated statistically using Eq. 9.6.

*However, since each compound is tested twice, once as a component of an A mixture and once as a component of a B mixture, the likelihood that it will be missed is reduced compared to single testing. The probability, p_i, of an active compound in dimension i being in a pool with compounds of comparable activity is likely to be <1.0. Therefore, the probability of it being in a comparable-activity pool in both dimensions i and j is $p_i \times p_j$, which is even smaller.

[†]The right-hand side of Eq. (9.6) is only a mildly increasing function of n because it explicitly scales with the root of n and t gently decreases with increasing n. At the 95% confidence level, t is ~2 for > 10 degrees of freedom, corresponding to $n > 6$.

only with the square root of the set size. Larger building block sets are therefore desirable, since they increase the probability that at least one active is present in the library but do not decrease by a corresponding amount the sensitivity for finding the hit. It is impossible to quantify the relationship between set size and the likelihood of finding a hit a priori; it will be unique to each possible library chemistry and assay.

9.3   RESULTS

A library of carbamates [which should inhibit acetylcholinesterase by carbamoylation of the active site serine (24)] was prepared using indexed combinatorial synthesis. A basis set of the nine alcohols in Figure 9.3 was used in reactions with the basis set of 6 isocyanates in Figure 9.4. These building block set sizes were chosen so that the library would be large enough to demonstrate the principle but small enough to verify the composition of the library by analytical methods. The alcohol building blocks were particularly chosen with the target in mind, knowing that relatively good leaving groups facilitate reaction with the serine hydroxyl. It is worth emphasizing that the chemistry of the reaction(s) used in the preparation of a library must be investigated on single, pure compounds before any pool synthesis can be contemplated. The reaction must be optimized with the building blocks expected to fall at both ends of the range of reactivity within each set, and the assay must be validated with a diversity of structural types. Problems with certain compounds will be discerned during this process, and they must be eliminated from the building block set. For example, in the alcohol set in this combinatorial synthesis, naphthol was initially included because naphthyl methyl carbamate is known as an acetylcholinesterase inhibitor and insecticide (Sevin). However, it hydrolyzes too

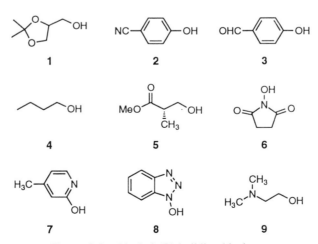

Figure 9.3   Alcohol (O) building blocks.

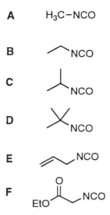

Figure 9.4 Isocyanate (N) building blocks.

rapidly in the assay buffer used to provide valid inhibition data. We also had wished to use choline since methylcarbamylcholine would be a good mimic of acetylcholine. However, the complete insolubility of choline in any of the solvents useful for the carbamylation made this impossible. We initially planned to use the dozen or so isocyanates available from Aldrich, but several of these led to completely inactive carbamates. Carbamates derived from (trichloromethyl)isocyanate could not be used because they are unstable, losing chloride and eventually undergoing hydrolysis.

Each of the 15 row and column reactions utilized a *unitary reagent* and a *mixed reagent* [Eqs. (9.8) and (9.9)].

$$\text{R-NCO} \; + \; \Sigma \; \text{R'OH} \quad \longrightarrow \quad \Sigma \; \underset{\underset{\text{H}}{|}}{\text{R}_{\text{N}}} \overset{\overset{\text{O}}{\|}}{\text{C}}_{\text{OR'}} \quad \text{N-dimension} \qquad\qquad (9.8)$$

$$\Sigma \text{R-NCO} \; + \quad \text{R'OH} \quad \longrightarrow \quad \Sigma \; \underset{\underset{\text{H}}{|}}{\text{R}_{\text{N}}} \overset{\overset{\text{O}}{\|}}{\text{C}}_{\text{OR'}} \quad \text{O-dimension} \qquad\qquad (9.9)$$

Each of the basis set molecules was the unitary reagent in only one reaction of the 15; it was present in a mixed reagent equimolar with the members of its basis set in all reactions where the other basis set members were unitary reagents. To eliminate kinetic effects, reactions were forced to completion for each component in the reaction by conducting them with a stoichiometric quantity of the unitary reagent relative to the total of the mixed reagents. The resulting 15 mixtures were used to determine aggregate IC_{50} values against acetylcholinesterase. Select compounds in the active rows and columns (vide infra) were individually synthesized and characterized and their presence in row and column reactions was verified by high-pressure liquid chromatography (HPLC).

The data are presented graphically in Figure 9.5. In the N dimension, the inhibi-

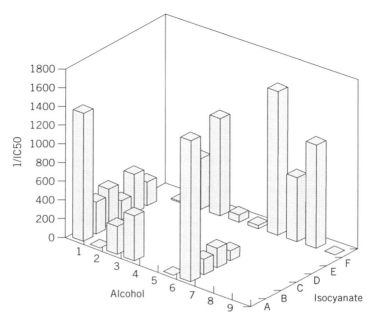

Figure 9.5   Inhibition of acetylcholinesterase by carbamates displayed as $1/IC_{50}$.

tory potency decreases in the order Me > *i*-Pr > Et > *tert*-Bu. The same order was found when the carbamates from column 6 were individually prepared, purified, and analyzed. In the O dimension, the potency decreases in the order succinimide > benzotriazole > benzaldehyde. Synthesis and assay of both active and inactive components from row A showed potencies that closely reflected those obtained in the mixed assays (31).* It also permitted the presence in the sublibrary of low activity components to be established by HPLC as a control that the row reaction indeed possesses all imputed members. The most potent inhibitor in this library is *O*-succinimidyl-*N*-methylcarbamate (**6A**), a heretofore unknown compound.

6A

These initial results were encouraging, but a more potent class of inhibitors was sought. Tetrahydroacridines are known to bind tightly to acetylcholinesterase,

*The parallels between the assay results with pure compounds and sublibraries suggest that the contributions of the O residue and the N residue are independent.

which is believed to be the molecular basis of action of tacrine, marketed as a cognition-enhancing drug (27) for Alzheimer's disease, Cognex. A known route to aminoquinolines shown in Eq. (9.10) had earlier been applied to the preparation of tetrahydroacridines from cyclohexanone (28).

$$\qquad (9.10)$$

A basis set of the 12 cyclic ketones in Figure 9.6 was used in these reactions with the basis set of 5 cyanoanilines in Figure 9.7. Symmetrical ketones were chosen to eliminate ambiguity concerning the site of cyclization from the imine intermediate ($R_1 = R_2$). The cyanoanilines are all commercially available. The presence of the imputed number of members in each row and column reaction was verified by HPLC. The 17 mixtures resulting from the pool syntheses were used to determine aggregate IC_{50} values against acetylcholinesterase. The data are summarized in Figure 9.8. Select compounds in the active rows and columns were individually synthesized and assayed. The most active compound in this library was **13I**, which

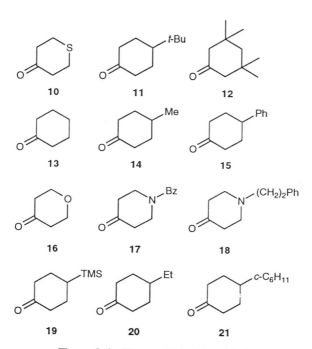

Figure 9.6 Ketone (K) building blocks.

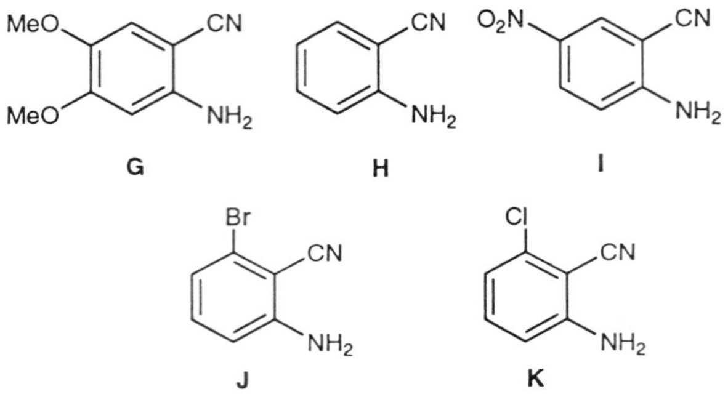

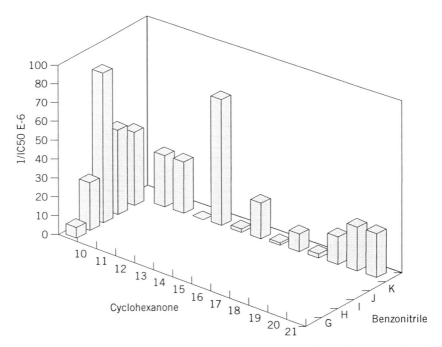

Figure 9.7   Cyanoaniline (C) building blocks.

when tested as the pure compound shows 10-fold greater potency than the parent compound, tacrine.

Because the structure of the complex between acetylcholinesterase and tacrine has recently been reported (29), it can be used to interpret some of the data from the second library experiment. In Figure 9.9 shows the active site region of this struc-

Figure 9.8   Inhibition of acetylcholinesterase by tetrahydroacridines displayed as % inhibition relative to the most potent compound.

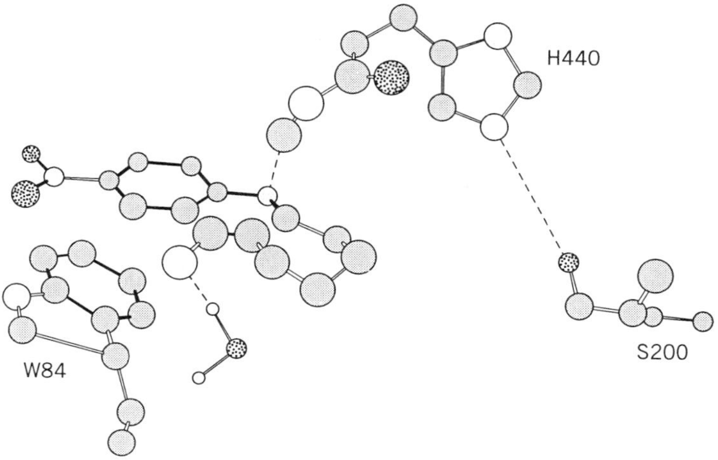

Figure 9.9   Proposed three-dimensional structure of acetylcholinesterase-**13I** complex.

ture, modified by the inclusion of the nitro group at the appropriate position on the tetrahydroacridine ring. A rather obvious juxtaposition of Trp-84 and the benzene ring of the quinoline substructure of the tetrahydroacridine suggests that π-stacking and/or charge-transfer interactions may play an important role in the interaction of tetrahydroacridines with the enzyme. Such interactions would likely be enhanced in the complex with the nitroaryl compound **13I**.

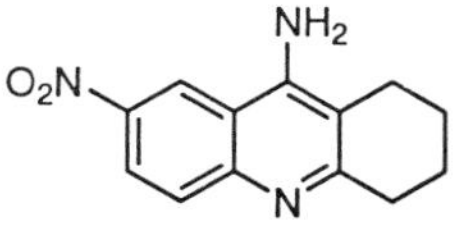

$$K_i = 0.7 \text{ nM}$$
13I

9.4   DISCUSSION

A key issue in the use of combinatorial methods based on pooled synthesis is the pool size in which a hit can be reliably found. The statistical formalism of Eq. (9.6) has been applied to the data obtained in both of these library experiments. The result suggests that subpools of carbamates formed from as many as 70 building blocks or a total library size of over 800 would still have permitted the active compound to be reliably identified using this assay. In the case of the tetrahydroacridines, because the activity was relatively unresponsive to the structural changes in the cyclohexane ring, the pool size could only have been as large as 25 while still maintaining the

95% confidence level for the superior activity of the pool. As is obvious from Eq. (9.7), hits are most easily identified when the components of the pools have widely divergent activities and the average activity is low. In this instance, the average activity was relatively high. A spread of activities is most likely with chemical diversity in the building blocks as wide as possible.

An almost trivial point that is nevertheless a key influence on the size of a library that can be effectively screened is the solubility of the pool in the assay mixture. Consider a symmetrical library that is composed of D dimensions with N components in each. Each pool therefore contains N^{D-1} members. If the maximum concentration of a pool that can be obtained is C_{max}, then the concentration of a lone active in an assay of that pool will be C_{max}/N^{D-1}. The concentration at which an active can be detected should be around its dissociation constant for the target. Therefore, for a C_{max} of 100 mM, a compound with millimolar potency could be found in a pool as large as 100 (i.e., a three-dimensional library of 10^3 compounds). The limit on potency scales directly with C_{max}, so that if the solubility of the pool is 10-fold lower, the potency of an active necessary for its discovery is 10-fold greater (i.e., the compound must be active at a 10-fold lower concentration). If a compound has micromolar potency and the C_{max} is 100 mM, the library could be as large as 10^7, and the active could still be found provided other assay criteria [Eq. (9.7)] were adequate. Since compounds that provoke the most interest for pharmaceutical development have micromolar or even nanomolar potency, solubility should not limit the utility of pool screening. Unlike the situation in natural products screening, combinatorial chemistry offers the opportunity to control the number and concentration of drug candidates so that only the most potent hits will be found.

9.5   CONCLUSION

Indexed combinatorial libraries permit the preparation and identification of active nonoligomeric compounds and the use of any type of assay. A similar concept, "orthogonal combinatorial libraries," wherein subpools containing only a single common member are created and screened, has recently been utilized to discover a novel tripeptide ligand for the vasopressin V2 receptor (30). It is worth emphasis that the goals of library methods such as these are not so much synthetic as analytic. Their purpose is to gain information on as wide a universe of structures as possible in the shortest time and with the smallest cost. Once interesting molecules are identified from among the many in the library, conventional macroscopic synthesis techniques can be used to obtain them in quantities necessary for further study. It is important to recognize that the testing of mixtures makes possible interactions between compounds that could lead either to an increase (synergism) or decrease (antagonism) of the measured potency compared to the pure compounds. The latter is a "false negative" possible in any pooled screening effort. Provided that the library is diverse enough to find a sufficient number of interesting leads, such antagonism can be tolerated.

ACKNOWLEDGMENT

This work was financially supported by the NIH (GM43816) and ONR (N00014-94-1-0364). The assistance of B. Blackburn in administrative support of this work is greatly appreciated.

REFERENCES

1. Silver, L., and Bostian, K., *Eur. J. Clin. Microbiol. Infect. Dis.* **9,** 455–461 (1990).

2. (a) Wender, P. A., *Chemtracts: Org. Chem.* **7,** 160–171 (1994); (b) Stierle, A., Strobel, G., and Stierle, D., *Science* **260,** 214–217 (1993).

3. (a) Skrydstrup, T., Ulibarri, G., Audrain, H., and Grierson, D. S., *Recent Prog. Chem. Synth. Antibiot. Relat. Microb. Prod.* 213–291 (1993); Ed.: Lukacs, G. Springer, Berlin. (b) Nicolaou, K. C., and Dai, W. M., *Angew. Chem., Int. Ed. Engl.* **30,** 1387–1416 (1991); (c) Lee, M. D., Ellestad, G. A.; Borders, D. B., *Acc. Chem. Res.* **24,** 235–243 (1991).

4. (a) Olson, A. J., and Morris, G. M., *Perspect. Drug Discovery Des.* **1,** 329–344 (1993); (b) Kieber-Emmons, T., *Biomed. Appl. Biotechnol.* **1,** 3–34 (1993); (c) Martin, Y. C., *Methods Enzymol.* **203,** 587–613 (1991).

5. Chervenak, M. C., and Toone, E. J., *J. Am. Chem. Soc.* **116,** 10533–10539 (1994).

6. Gumbleton, M., and Sneader, W., *Clin. Pharmacokinet.* **26,** 161–168 (1994).

7. (a) Hillson, J. L., and Perlmutter, R. M., *Int. Rev. Immunol.* **5,** 215–229 (1990); (b) Kuby, J., *Immunology,* W. H. Freeman, New York, 1991.

8. Geysen, H. M., Meloen, R. H., and Barteling, S. J., *Proc. Natl. Acad. Sci., U.S.A.* **81,** 3998–4002 (1984).

9. (a) Fodor, S. P. A., Read, J. L., Pirrung, M. C., Stryer, L., Liu, A. T., and Solas, D., *Science* **251,** 767–773 (1991); (b) Jacobs, J. W., and Fodor, S. P. A., *Trends Biotechnol.* **12,** 19–26 (1994); (c) Holmes, C. P., Adams, C. L., Fodor, S. P. A., and Yu-Yang, P., *Perspect. Med. Chem.* 489–500 (1993); Ed.: Testa, B. Verlag Helvetica Chim. Acta, Basel. (d) Holmes, C. P., and Fodor, S. P. A., *Harnessing Biotechnol. 21st Century, Proc. Int. Biotechnol. Symp. Expo., 9th,* M. R. Ladisch, and A. Bose, ACS, Washington, DC, 1992, pp. 241–243.

10. Lam, K. S., Salmon, S. E., Hersh, E. M., Hruby, V. J., Kazmierski, W. M., and Knapp, R. J., *Nature (London)* **354,** 82–84 (1991).

11. (a) Cwirla, S. E., Peters, E. A., Barrett, R. W., and Dower, W. J., *Proc. Natl. Acad. Sci., U.S.A.* **87,** 6378–6382 (1990); (b) Scott, J. K., and Smith, G., *Science* **249,** 386–390 (1990); Devlin, J. J., Panganiban, L. C., and Devlin, P. E., *Science* **249,** 404–406 (1990); (c) Brenner, S., and Lerner, R. A., *Proc. Natl. Acad. Sci., U.S.A.* **89,** 5381–5383 (1992); (d) Needels, M. C., Jones, D. G., Tate, E. H., Heinkel, G. L., Kochersperger, L. M., Dower, W. J., Barrett, R. W., and Gallop, M. A., *Proc. Natl. Acad. Sci., U.S.A.* **90,** 10700–10704 (1993); (e) Nielsen, J., Brenner, S., and Janda, K. D., *J. Am. Chem. Soc.* **115,** 9812–9813 (1993).

12. Kerr, J. M., Banville, S. C., and Zuckermann, R. N., *J. Am. Chem. Soc.* **115,** 2529–2531 (1993).

13. (a) Ohlmeyer, M. H. J., Swanson, R. N., Dillard, L. W., Reader, J. C., Asouline, G.,

Kobayashi, R., Wigler, M., and Still, W. C., *Proc. Natl. Acad. Sci., U.S.A.* **90,** 10922–10926 (1993); (b) Borchardt, A., and Still, W. C., *J. Am. Chem. Soc.* **116,** 373–374 (1994).

14. Houghten, R. A., Pinilla, C., Blondelle, S. E., Appel, J. R., Dooley, C. T., and Cuervo, J. H., *Nature (London)* **354,** 84–86 (1991).

15. Jayawickreme, C. K., Graminski, G. F., Quillan, J. M., and Lerner, M. R., *Proc. Natl. Acad. Sci., U.S.A.* **91,** 1614–1618 (1994).

16. Furka, A., Sebestyen, F., Asgedom, M., and Dibo, G., *Int. J. Pept. Protein. Res.* **37,** 487–493 (1991).

17. (a) Bunin, B. A., and Ellman, J. *J. Am. Chem. Soc.* **114,** 10997–10998 (1992); (b) DeWitt, S. H., Kiely, J. S., Stankovic, C. J., Schroeder, M. C., Cody, D. M. R., and Pavia, M. R., *Proc. Natl. Acad. Sci., U.S.A.* **90,** 6909–6913 (1993).

18. Pirrung, M. C., *Chemtracts: Org. Chem.* **6,** 88–91 (1993).

19. Bryant, V., *Aspects of Combinatorics,* Cambridge University Press, Cambridge, 1993.

20. Martin, E. J., Blaney, J. M., Siani, M. A., Spellmeyer, D. C., Wong, A. K., and Moos, W. H., *J. Med. Chem.* **38,** 1431–1436 (1995).

21. Pless, J., *Digestion* **54**(Suppl. 1), 7–8 (1993).

22. Pirrung, M. C., and Chen, J., *J. Am. Chem. Soc.* **117,** 1240–1245 (1995).

23. Pirrung, M. C., Chau, J. H.-L., and Chen, J., *Chem. Biol.* **2,** 621–626 (1995).

24. Quinn, D. M., *Chem. Rev.* **87,** 955–979 (1987).

25. (a) Taylor, P., in *The Pharmacological Basis of Therapeutics,* A. G. Gilman, T. W. Rall, A. Nies, P. Taylor (Eds.), Pergamon, New York, 1990, pp. 131–149; (b) Hallak, M., and Giacobini, E., *Neuropharmacology* **28,** 199–206 (1989); (c) Sano, M., Bell, K., Marder, K., and Stricks, L., *Clinical Pharm.* **16,** 61 (1993).

26. Hanin, I., Tang, X. C., and Kozikowski, A. P., in *Cholinergic Basis for Alzheimers Therapy,* R. Berker and E. Giacobini (Eds.), Birkhauser, Boston, 1991, pp. 305–313.

27. Holford, N. H. G., and Peace, K. E., *Proc. Natl. Acad. Sci., U.S.A.* **89,** 11466–11470 (1992).

28. (a) Meyers, A. I., Sircar, J. C., and Singh, S., *J. Heterocyclic Chem.* **4,** 461–462 (1967); (b) Singh, S., and Meyers, A. I., *J. Heterocyclic Chem.* **5,** 737–739 (1968).

29. Harel, M., Schalk, I., Ehret-Sabatier, L., Bouet, F., Goeldner, M., Hirth, C., Axelsen, P. H., Silman, I., and Sussman, J. L., *Proc. Natl. Acad. Sci., U.S.A.* **90,** 9031–9035 (1993).

30. Deprez, B., Williard, X., Bourel, L., Coste, H., Hyafil, F., and Tartar, A., *J. Am. Chem. Soc.* **117,** 5405–5406 (1995).

10

STRATEGIES FOR COMBINATORIAL LIBRARIES OF OLIGOSACCHARIDES

CAROL M. TAYLOR

Department of Chemistry, University of Auckland, Private Bag 92019, Auckland, New Zealand

10.1 INTRODUCTION

There are three major classes of biopolymers—oligonucleotides, oligopeptides, and oligosaccharides. The most advanced and well-documented combinatorial libraries are those of peptides (1) and nucleotides (2). Throughout this chapter, oligosaccharides will be compared with these other two classes of biopolymers to emphasize that much effort is required to bring oligosaccharides "up-to-speed" in terms of synthesis and potential to study their roles in biology.

It has long been appreciated that oligonucleotides (the building blocks of heredity) and oligopeptides (enzymes, hormones, and other receptors) play important roles in a wide range of biochemical processes. As a consequence, considerable effort has been, and continues to be, expended developing methods for the synthesis of these oligomers. Oligopeptides and oligonucleotides are now available by *almost* routine methods—either chemically (via automated solid-phase synthesis) or via recombinant technology using the polymerase chain reaction (PCR) (3). These techniques have had a tremendous impact on science, and their development has led to several Nobel prizes (4). Once oligopeptides and oligonucleotides became readily available, the pace at which we could study their involvement in biochemical processes escalated. It has been the success of these synthetic and genetic strategies, coupled with the ability to sequence oligopeptides and oligonucleotides, that has been responsible for the rapid development of combinatorial libraries of these compounds.

The scientific community has been slower to discover the roles of oligosaccharides in biochemical processes. For many years, carbohydrates were seen to serve two major functions: as structural materials (e.g., cellulose) and as energy storage compounds (e.g., glucose and starch). However, it has become clear that oligosaccharides play more "intelligent" roles in the processes of life. In essence, oligosaccharides are important recognition elements, most noteably on the surface of cells. They are important in intercellular communication, and thereby the control of cell growth and development (5).

Progress toward understanding the molecular basis of the functions of oligosaccharides has been slower than researchers would like and the field has been described as "the last frontier in macromolecular chemistry and function" (6). This slow progress is attributable to the fact that oligosaccharides are not readily available in homogeneous form from natural sources, and synthesis is nontrivial.

Within the past 6–7 years, the scientific community has been overwhelmed by discoveries indicating the tremendous importance of oligosaccharides. A pivotal development was the discovery, in 1990, that sialyl Lewis^x (Fig. 10.1) is the natural ligand for E-selectin (7). The discovery of this role that sialyl Lewis^x plays in cell adhesion has given researchers the potential to mediate the inflammatory response. This could lead to new therapies for inflammatory disorders, including rheumatoid arthritis, septic shock, and reperfusion tissue injury. This excitement has led to the revitalization of carbohydrate research and a sense of urgency and competition to develop new therapies based on what is described as "glycotechnology."

Another important family of oligosaccharides is the gangliosides. Tay-Sachs disease is a ganglioside breakdown disorder that typically kills afflicted children before they are 3 years old. The concentration of the oligosaccharide, known as GM_2, in the brain of an infant with Tay-Sach's disease, is many times higher than normal. This arises because the child has a β-N-acetylhexosaminidase deficiency that limits normal metabolism of GM_2 to GM_3. There are a host of other fatal, related diseases that reflect abnormal ganglioside metabolism. Understanding the function of these oligosaccharides in the brain, and the potential to manipulate their behavior, has obvious medical applications.

Oligosaccharide "markers" also appear to play a key role in oncogenic transformation—the metastasis by which normal cells become cancerous ones. The identification of tumor antigens, absent from normal cells, permits the exploration of new avenues for the detection and therapy of cancer. An example of this is the breast cancer antigen MBr1 (8), whose presence is limited in normal adult human tissue.

Oligosaccharides are typically composed of less than 20 monosaccharide units. They usually occur in nature as conjugates of lipids and proteins (9). The carbohydrate portion of these molecules possesses a "rather rigid topography which derives from the interplay of a number of factors, including configuration, points of attachment, oxidation states and substitution patterns within the oligosaccharide" (10). It is this topography that is responsible for the recognition of and interaction with other molecules.

As alluded to earlier, the major barrier to studying the interaction of oligosaccharides with their receptors is the availability of the oligosaccharides in homogeneous form and in milligram quantities. At present, the synthesis of oligosaccharides of any complexity is attempted only by experts in the field. This is an

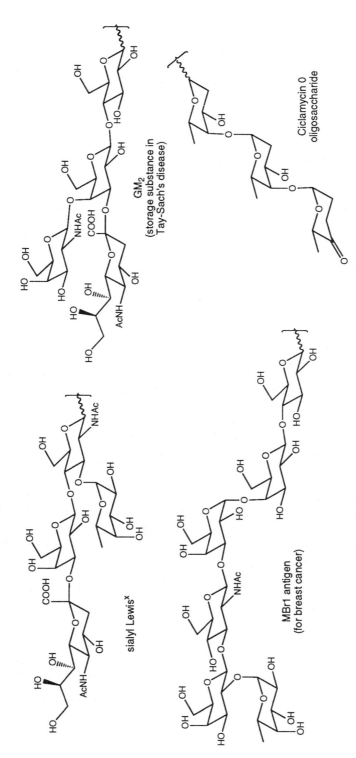

Figure 10.1 Selected oligosaccharides of biological significance.

sialyl Lewis^x

GM$_2$
(storage substance in Tay-Sach's disease)

MBr1 antigen
(for breast cancer)

Ciclamycin 0
oligosaccharide

209

unfortunate situation because many scientists, without extensive experience in carbohydrate synthesis, would like to perform experiments using synthetic oligosaccharides. There is a dire need for more ready access to oligosaccharides, ideally in the form of combinatorial libraries, to investigate the many vital roles of these molecules in nature.

10.2   APPLICATIONS OF OLIGOSACCHARIDE LIBRARIES

While libraries of carbohydrates cannot yet be produced by simultaneous synthesis,* they have been accessed in other ways. The following two examples illustrate the tremendous potential of libraries of compounds in the identification of biologically active molecules, and in gaining insight into the relationship between structure and function.

The selectins (11) are a family of cell adhesion molecules with a calcium-dependent carbohydrate recognition domain. The natural ligands identified so far (e.g., sialyl Lewis^x), have a low affinity for their selectins (K_d in the millimolar range). In a search for selectin ligands with higher binding affinities, Patel et al. (12) expressed new sialylated, fucose-containing structures on the surface of cells that do not normally bind E-selectin. Using nature to produce such a library of compounds, these workers identified three high-affinity ligands ($K_d < \mu M$), of which the tetraantennary glycan in Figure 10.2(b) is representative. These high-affinity ligands were subsequently identified, in *extremely* low concentrations, on the surface of cells that *do* bind selectins.

Lemieux (10), over the course of many years, has made a sustained effort to probe the combining sites of antibodies and lectins and to gain an understanding of the interactions that are important in carbohydrate–protein binding. A comprehensive study of the binding of the Lewis^b tetrasaccharide by GS4 (lectin 4 of *Griffonia simplificolia*) involved the synthesis of many analogs of the tetrasaccharide. This endeavor included ALL the monodeoxy derivatives, to determine the importance of hydrogen bonding within the oligosaccharide and in the interaction with the protein. Figure 10.3 shows the variations that were made to the Lewis^b tetrasaccharide. Access to this highly sophisticated analysis of structure–activity relationships (SARs) built upon a synthetic strategy that gave them access not only to the native structure but to a wide range of chemically modified compounds. It must be emphasized that this seminal piece of work was made possible only by *expertise in carbohydrate synthesis*.

---

*During the preparation of this manuscript, considerable progress has been made in this area. See, for example: (a) Kanie, O., Barresi, F., Ding, Y. L., Labbe, J., Otter, A., Forsberg, L. S., Ernst, B., and Hindsgaul, O. *Angew. Chem. Intl. Ed. Engl.* **34**, 2720–2722 (1996); (b) Liang, R., Yan, L., Loebach, J., Uozumi, Y., Ge, M., Horan, N., Gildersleeve, J., Thompson, C., Smith, A., Biswas, K., Sekanina, K., Still, W. C., and Kahne, D. E. *Science* **274** 1520–1522 (1996).

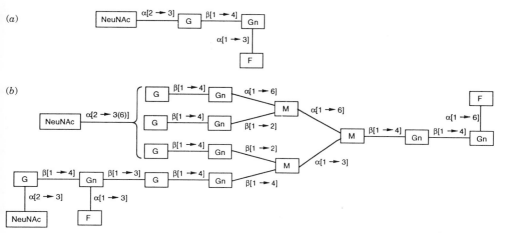

Figure 10.2 (a) Sialyl Lewis^x; (b) a high-affinity ligand for E-selectin, identified by Patel et al. (12). Abbreviations: NeuNAc = N-acetylneuraminic acid, G = galactose, Gn = N-acetylglucosamine, F = fucose, M = mannose.

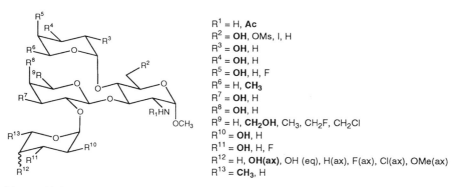

R^1 = H, **Ac**
R^2 = **OH**, OMs, I, H
R^3 = **OH**, H
R^4 = **OH**, H
R^5 = **OH**, H, F
R^6 = H, **CH$_3$**
R^7 = **OH**, H
R^8 = **OH**, H
R^9 = H, **CH$_2$OH**, CH$_3$, CH$_2$F, CH$_2$Cl
R^{10} = **OH**, H
R^{11} = **OH**, H, F
R^{12} = H, **OH(ax)**, OH (eq), H(ax), F(ax), Cl(ax), OMe(ax)
R^{13} = **CH$_3$**, H

Figure 10.3 Tetrasaccharides synthesized by Lemieux (10). Bold type indicates the native structure of the Lewis^b determinant; other substituents reflect modifications made to study SARs.

10.3   CHALLENGE PRESENTED BY OLIGOSACCHARIDE SYNTHESIS (13)

The synthesis of polypeptides (up to about 100 residues) (14) and oligonucleotides (15) has become almost routine, using automated solid-phase techniques. Both are iterative processes whereby each monomer is added, in a linear fashion, to a growing oligomer in two chemical steps. The first step involves unmasking of a nucleophile on the growing oligomer, the second is the coupling of this functionality with an activated form of the next monomer.

Perhaps, like oligonucleotides and oligopeptides, oligosaccharides might be constructed by a stepwise assembly of monomers. Unfortunately the situation is far more complex for oligosaccharides, as shown in Figure 10.4. There are a number of factors that make the synthesis of oligosaccharides a particularly difficult task—both in solution and, more so, in the solid phase. The formation of glycosidic bonds is typically more troublesome than the formation of peptide bonds (oligopeptides) and phosphodiester linkages (oligonucleotides). The glycosylation process is sensitive to water, there are many side reactions, and there is the issue of stereochemistry. These major issues related to synthesis will be discussed briefly, as they are primary considerations in any attempt to produce libraries of sugar molecules.

10.3.1. Glycosylation Reaction

With a view to making libraries of compounds, a glycosylation method is required that would permit the essentially quantitative formation of either α- or β-glycosidic linkages to any position on any sugar residue.

There are two broad classes of methods available for the formation of glycosidic linkages: those employing glycosyltransferase enzymes and those based on chemical methods. Enzymes have proven extremely useful in the arena of carbohydrate synthesis (16). Their use obviates the need for protecting groups (see Section 10.3.2). Moreover, the reactions are substrate specific and stereospecific. A crowning achievement was the recent synthesis of sialyl Lewis[x] on a silica support (17).

A serious limitation of enzymatic carbohydrate synthesis is the availability of enzymes. There are an increasing number now available; however, enzymatic synthesis will *always* be limited by nature's repertoire of enzymes. Glycosyltransferases are specific for natural sugars and are rarely useful for the incorporation of modified sugars or the formation of linkages not found in nature. Enzymatic methods will therefore have some boundaries in the arena of combinatorial libraries. Chemical methods, in principle at least, have no such limitations and it should be possible to make any chosen target—natural or unnatural.

An extremely high-yielding glycosylation reaction is essential for library development. As Figure 10.5 shows, an incomplete glycosylation leaves a percentage of unreacted nucleophile on the growing oligomer. Thus, in the next coupling cycle there are *two* possible products. In any synthesis, each time a glycosylation does not go to completion it leads to an increasingly *complex mixture* of products. This is highly undesirable because in screening a library of oligosaccharides we want to attribute activity to a *single chemical entity*.

Hundreds of chemical methods have been used to form glycosidic bonds (18). However, for the purposes of building libraries, a method with wide applicability is required, a method that will give high yields regardless of the nature of the substrates. This general method must also be able to generate, by variation in some reaction parameter(s), either an α- or a β-glycosidic linkage. The reality is that no such ideal method exists.

For several years now, the Kahne group has been exploring the scope and limitations of the sulfoxide glycosylation method (19). This method involves activation of

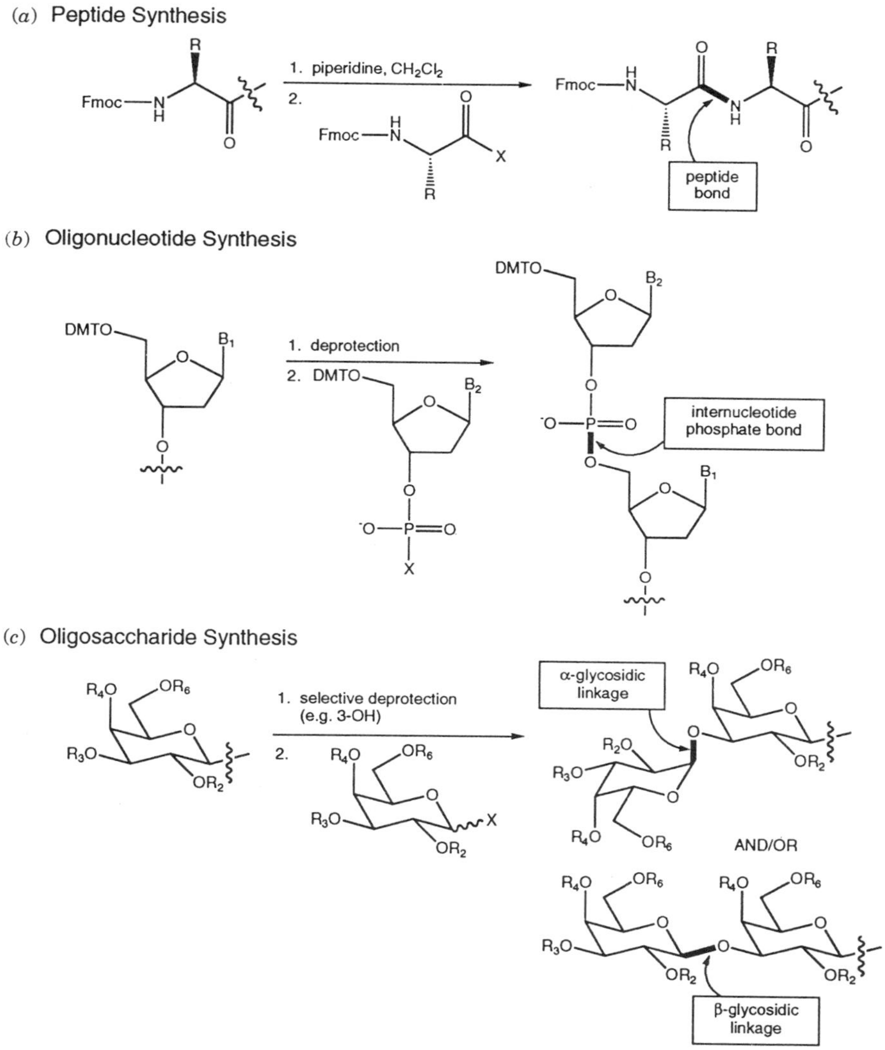

(*a*) Peptide Synthesis

(*b*) Oligonucleotide Synthesis

(*c*) Oligosaccharide Synthesis

Figure 10.4 Chemical synthesis of nature's biopolymers. Abbreviations: X = activating group, Fmoc = fluorenylmethoxycarbonyl, B = base, DMT = dimethoxytrityl, P³ = protecting group at C_3, etc.

an anomeric sulfoxide by triflic anhydride. An activated species is then trapped by a nucleophile (glycosyl acceptor) to form a glycosidic bond. Figure 10.6 shows that good yields can usually be obtained with the sulfoxide glycosylation method, even with a sterically hindered alcohol like the steroid depicted, and that the stereochemistry of the glycosidic linkage can be varied by changing the protecting groups on the glycosyl donor. At low temperature, there is highly stereoselective formation

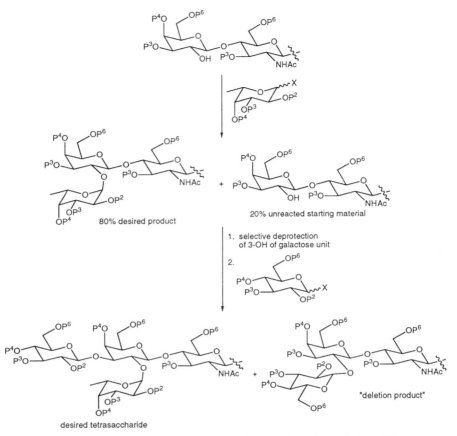

Figure 10.5   Deletion products: the end result of incomplete glycosylations. P^2 = protecting group at C_2, P^3 = protecting group at C_3, etc.

of α-glycosidic linkages. A β-glycosidic bond can be formed by incorporating a protecting group at C-2 that has the capacity to undergo neighboring group participation; the pivaloyl group has proven particularly useful (20). This method thus shows potential generality, but much work has yet to be done.

10.3.2   Protection Strategies

Many amino acids have side chain functionality that must be protected during the synthesis of a peptide. However, most contain only a single amino group (the only coded amino acids that possess a second amine in their side chains are Lys and Arg). In peptide synthesis, the protection of functional groups is achieved by two classes of protecting groups: permanent/side chain protection and temporary protection. The latter serves to protect the α-amino group during each coupling (Fig. 10.4); it is

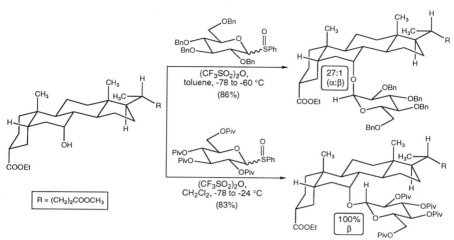

Figure 10.6 Glycosylation of a sterically hindered alcohol using the sulfoxide method (19a).

then removed and the next residue added. This is described as an orthogonal protecting group strategy.

By comparison, each monosaccharide of an oligosaccharide bears several hydroxyl groups that are nearly equivalent chemically. These alcohols need to be differentially protected. It is not trivial, for example, to protect the C_2-OH, C_4-OH, and C_6-OH of a glucose residue, leaving the C_3-OH free or protected in a different way. Moreover, oligosaccharides are rarely linear; the majority of structures involve branching. This further complicates the requirements of a protecting group strategy.

To illustrate these complexities, the synthesis of a hypothetical, branched trisaccharide is outlined in Figure 10.7. Initially, a set of reaction conditions is required that will selectively deprotect the C_3-OH (condition A). A stereospecific glycosylation with an N-acetylglucosamine residue would then give the disaccharide. To attach the fucose unit at C_2 of the galactose, another set of reaction conditions (condition B) is necessary to unmask the C_2-OH. Finally, if only a trisaccharide is desired, a third set of reaction conditions (condition C) is needed that will remove all other protecting group functionality but leave the glycosidic linkages intact and with their stereochemical integrity.

If peptide synthesis utilizes an orthogonal protecting group strategy, then it would not be an exaggeration to claim the need for a *three-dimensional protecting group strategy* for oligosaccharide synthesis. For the initial galactose building block in the above example, we would seek a solution wherein P[2], P[3], P[4], and P[6] might each be selectively removed under reaction conditions to which the growing oligosaccharide and the other three protecting groups are stable.

At present there is no perfect solution to the protecting group problems that plague the carbohydrate chemist. There is certainly no strategy that can be gener-

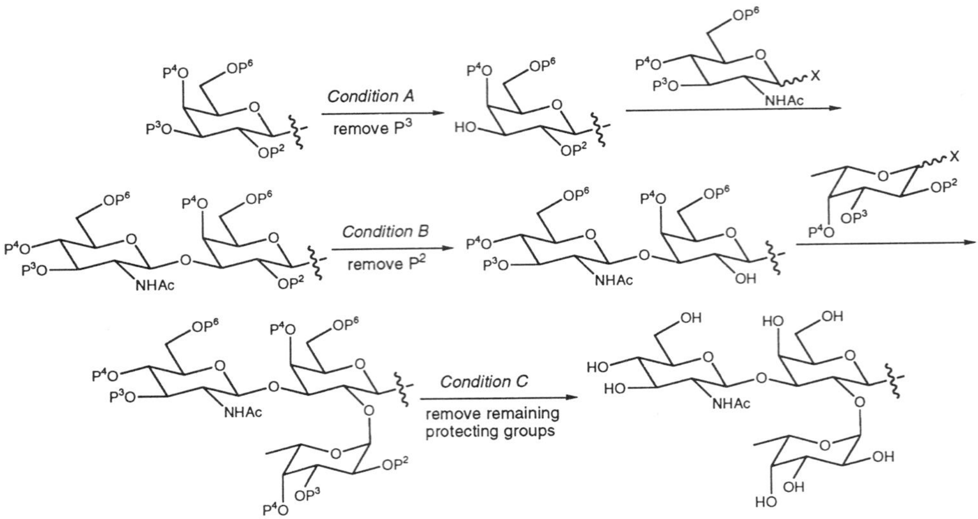

Figure 10.7 Three-dimensional protecting group strategy for the synthesis of branched oligosaccharides. P^2 = protecting group at C_2, P^3 = protecting group at C_3, etc.

alized, each oligosaccharide that is synthesized requires the development of a unique protection strategy that is arrived at largely by experimentation.

It is clear that more predictable and versatile approaches to the protection of the hydroxyl groups on sugar monomers are needed before combinatorial libraries of oligosaccharides can become a reality. This will likely involve the development of some new protecting groups that can be removed under mild and specific reaction conditions.

10.4   SOLUTION- VERSUS SOLID-PHASE APPROACHES TO SYNTHESIS

It is possible that small libraries of oligosaccharides might be prepared in solution. In fact, glycosylation reactions often produce a plethora of products that might well be considered a "library!"

An example of the possibility of solution-based libraries of oligosaccharides was based on the remarkable one-step synthesis of the ciclamycin trisaccharide (Fig. 10.1) by Raghavan and Kahne (21). These workers began to investigate the controlled polymerization of 2,6-dideoxysugars (Fig. 10.8). When a 2:1 ratio of A:B was employed the disaccharide ($n = 0$) was obtained in 45% yield, along with a 20% yield of the trisaccharide ($n = 1$). On increasing the A:B ratio to 5:1, a statistical mixture of the di-, tri-, tetra-, penta-, and hexasaccharides was obtained, and these five compounds were separable by chromatography (22).

While it is certainly possible to generate such libraries of oligosaccharides in solution, the issue of screening and isolation makes solution-based libraries less attractive than syntheses carried out on a polymeric support. It is a fact that most combinatorial chemistry to date has utilized solid-phase synthesis. The advantages of such an approach are many, including:

1. Yields of coupling reactions can be maximized by the use of excess solution-based reagents, relative to the precious, growing oligomer attached to the solid support. Moreover, repetitive couplings can be used to force difficult reactions to completion.
2. Beads of a resin can be sorted so that the reaction history of each group of beads is known.
3. Tags can be independently attached to beads of resin, which carry, in coded form, the identity of the chemical species present (see Section 10.5.2).

Considerable effort has been directed toward the development of methods for solid-phase oligosaccharide synthesis, and several approaches have emerged. During the 1970s, the groups of Schuerch, Fréchet, Anderson, Gagnaire, Zehavi, and Guthrie were the pioneers of solid-phase oligosaccharide synthesis. Their contributions were reviewed in 1980 by Fréchet (23) who concluded, at that time, that "[the solid phase] approach is not competitive with the more classical solution chemistry methods, due mainly to the lack of suitable glycosidation reactions." Things have changed since 1980, and there has been a renaissance in solid-phase oligosaccharide synthesis in recent years, as a direct response to the growing recognition of the tremendous biological importance of oligosaccharides. For example, Westerduin and co-workers used a solid-phase approach to produce oligomers of β(1-5)-lined-D-galactofuranose to investigate the relationship between polymer length and immunogenecity (24).

A full discussion of the research being performed in the field of solid-phase oligosaccharide synthesis is beyond the scope of this chapter. The essence of three chemical approaches is captured in Figure 10.9.

Danishefsky and co-workers have explored an approach based on glycal chemis-

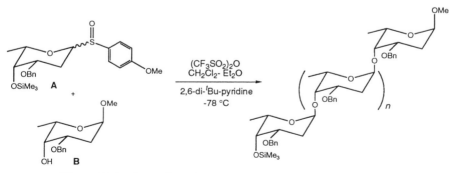

Figure 10.8 Controlled oligomerization of 2,6-dideoxy sugars (22).

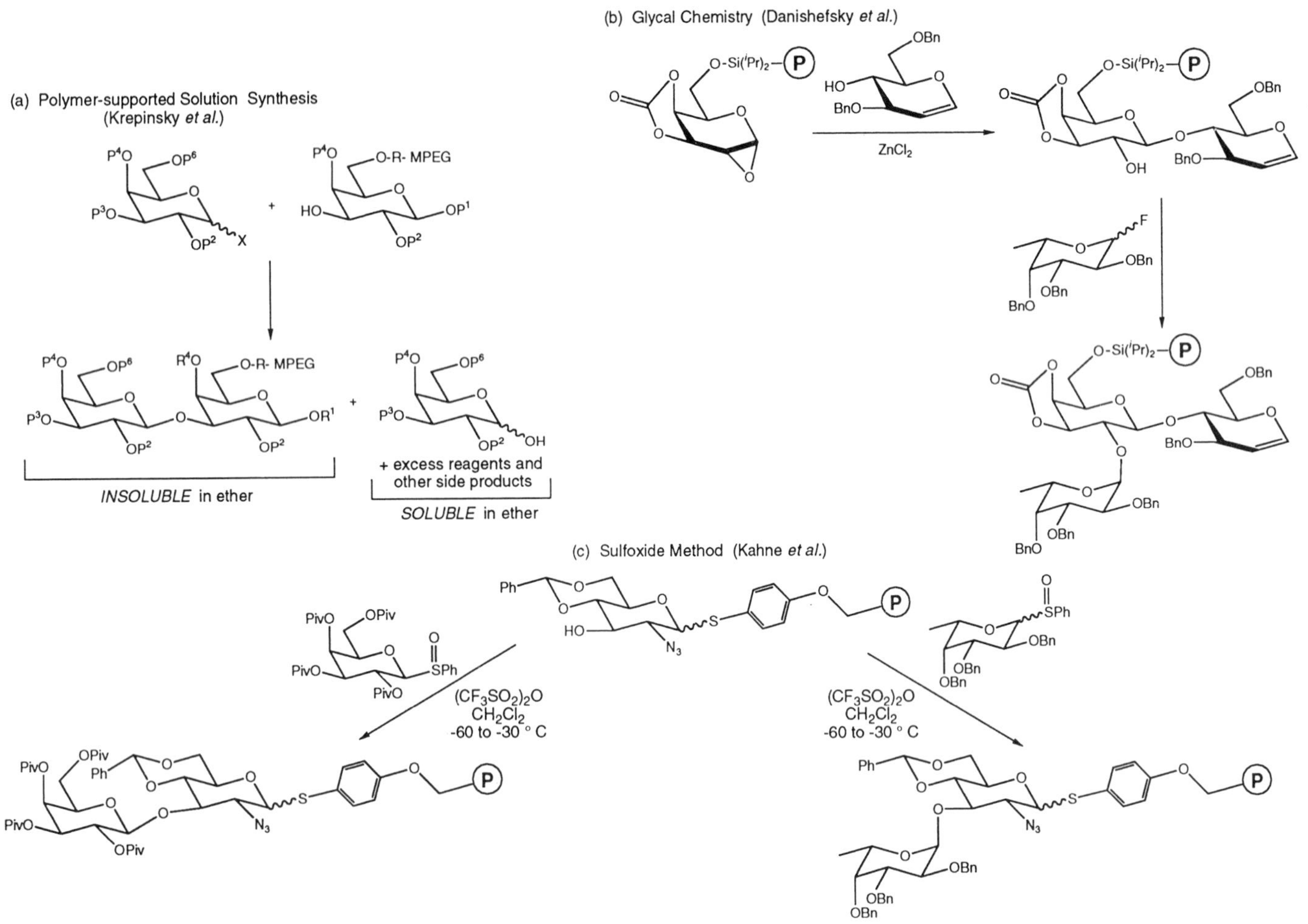

(a) Polymer-supported Solution Synthesis
(Krepinsky et al.)
INSOLUBLE in ether
+ excess reagents and other side products
SOLUBLE in ether
(b) Glycal Chemistry (Danishefsky et al.)
ZnCl2
(c) Sulfoxide Method (Kahne et al.)
(CF3SO2)2O
CH2Cl2
-60 to -30 ° C

Figure 10.9 Chemical strategies for the solid-phase synthesis of oligosaccharides (19c,25,26).

try (25). A polymer-bound glycal is activated for glycosyl donation by formation of the 1,2-epoxide. Reaction with a solution-based nucleophile generates a free hydroxyl at C_2 that has proven useful in the construction of the Lewis[b] skelton. A selling-point for this methodology has been the system's "self-policing" nature: Any unreacted glycosyl donor is hydrolyzed during the rinsing procedure of each glycosylation cycle and can therefore not lead to deletions.

Among the problems to be overcome in the transposition of a glycosylation method from solution to the solid phase is that the reaction rates are slower. Douglas and co-workers' approach to overcoming this problem has been to employ a polymeric support that is soluble under glycosylation reaction conditions but can subsequently be purified by crystallization (26).

Yan and co-workers have used the sulfoxide glycosylation method to form both α- and β-glycosidic linkages to the 3-position of an N-acetylglucosamine precursor (19c). Repetitive couplings were employed to good effect.

Schuster and co-workers (17) have reported a "chemoenzymatic" solid-phase synthesis of sialyl Lewis[x] linked to a dipeptide. According to their strategy, peptide bonds are formed using chemical methods and the oligosaccharide portion of the glycopeptide is assembled with glycosyltransferase enzymes. These researchers have alluded to studying the interactions of immobilized oligosaccharide libraries with carbohydrate binding proteins.

Although solid-phase synthesis of oligosaccharides is an active area of research, it must be conceded that no current method has reached a level of sophistication where the development of an automated synthesizer is a possibility. Without doubt, however, this is the aim of those working in the field.

10.5   IDENTIFICATION OF THE ACTIVE INGREDIENT

The ultimate goal of producing combinatorial libraries is to discover compounds that have some desired behavior and, associated with this behavior, the potential to serve as a drug. A major challenge in developing a library of compounds is screening the library for activity and identifying the chemical species responsible. This has been likened to finding the proverbial needle in the haystack (27).

10.5.1   Assays for Biological Activity

There are no limitations to the kinds of activity for which oligosaccharide libraries will be screened. However, given the importance of oligosaccharides in recognition processes, it is likely that the screening of many oligosaccharide libraries will involve binding assays. Methods need to be sufficiently sensitive to detect the compounds at the low levels at which they are produced.

One recently developed technique involves the tagging of oligosaccharides with biotinylated diaminopyridine (28) (Fig. 10.10). The resulting adducts are fluorescent and can be quantitated in picomolar concentrations at pHs less than 5. The adducts are also well resolved by standard reversed phase high performance liquid

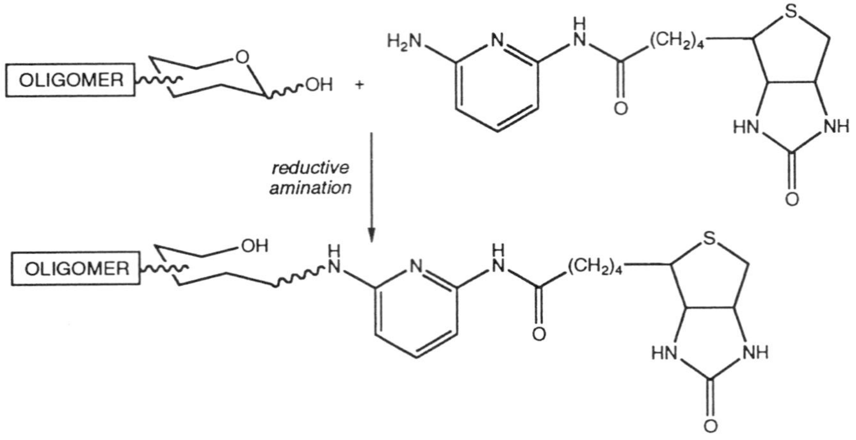

Figure 10.10   Tagging of oligosaccharides with biotinylated aminopyridine (28).

chromatography (RP-HPLC) methods. This procedure could provide a sensitive means of detection or analysis.

As discussed, it seems likely that combinatorial libraries will involve oligosaccharides attached to a solid support. Based on experiences with peptide and nucleotide libraries, it may be possible to screen compounds while still attached to the resin. Particularly for binding assays, inert spacers of a suitable length will be required to ensure that the polymer does not interfere with binding.

It must be borne in mind, however, that oligosaccharides tend to exist in nature as glycoconjugates (i.e., glycoproteins and glycolipids). In some cases, this may require that oligosaccharides in a library be presented in a form ready for conjugation to a carrier protein or lipid, and that this conjugation be carried out prior to performing an assay. One example of derivatization and conjugation is that used by Danishefsky and co-workers, both in their solution synthesis of Lewis[y] and in the solid-phase synthesis of Lewis[b] (Fig. 10.11) (25b,29). The reducing end of the oligosaccharide is protected as an allyl ether that serves as a masked aldehyde.

10.5.2   Identifying the Chemical Species Responsible for Biological Activity

When a positive assay result is obtained, it becomes vital that we are able to link the observed behavior with a discrete chemical species. There are three general approaches that might be used to determine the chemical makeup of an oligosaccharide from a library:

1. *Isolation and classical structure determination* using techniques such as nuclear magnetic resonance (NMR) and mass spectrometry
2. *Spatial resolution of* library components (i.e., a single chemical species exists in a given reaction well or on a bead of resin)

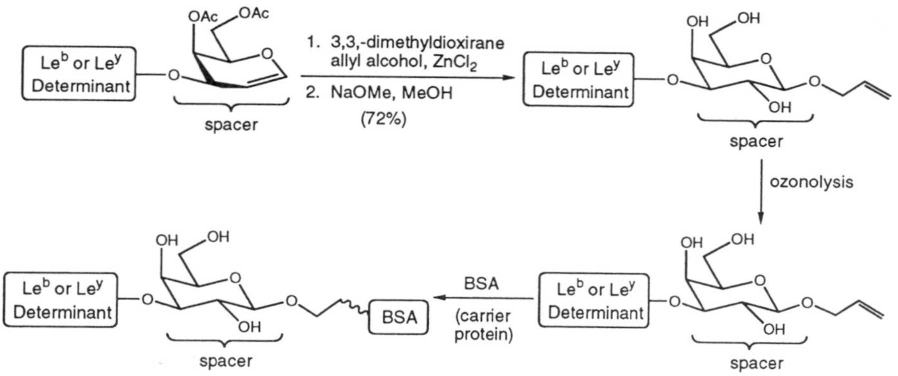

Figure 10.11 Synthesis of an oligosaccharide in bioconjugatable form according to Dani-shefsky and co-workers (25b,29).

3. *Encoding*, whereby a more readily sequenced molecular tag is used to encode for the structure of the library component

Typically, only very small amounts of each compound in the library are produced. Techniques that require sizable quantities, such as NMR, are inappropriate. Mass spectrometry (30) may provide some useful information. A technique that might well prove useful is oligosaccharide microscale analysis by circular dichroic (CD) spectroscopy. This is being developed by Ikemoto and co-workers (31) and is based on the derivatization of monosaccharides with two chromophores suitable for exciton coupling. Comparison of this library of CD data, with the curves obtained from suitably derivatized fragments of an unknown, then permit determination of the monosaccharides, linkage positions, and absolute configurations.

A "polysaccharide sequencer" was marketed by Oxford Glycosystems in 1993 (32). This sequencer is based on the so-called reagent array analysis method. The polysaccharide is radiolabeled and then subjected to batteries of glycosylhydrolase enzymes to produce radioactive fragments that can then be separated by HPLC and detected by measuring their radioactivity. A computer program then suggests possible sequences for the original polysaccharide and assigns a statistical likelihood to each. This could well be useful, however, as with synthesis that employs enzymes, the technique is restricted to the available repertoire of enzymes.

The basis of encoding a combinatorial library is the attachment of molecular tags to beads of resin, which provide a record of the reaction history of that bead. Ohlmeyer and co-workers (33) have introduced a binary code for libraries of peptides. When a pool of seven amino acids are employed to build a library, three tags are required to code for each amino acid. An analogous code for an oligosaccharide library would necessarily be more complex. More information is required for each chemical step: the identity of the monosaccharide being added, the stereochemistry of the glycosidic linkage being formed, and the site of attachment of the monosaccharide to the growing oligomer. This required increase in complexity of a code is conceptually related to the protecting group problems in synthesis (see Section 10.3.2).

Given the complexity of oligosaccharide structure determination, and the challenge that a "code" for oligosaccharides presents, it is probable spatial resolution will be most applicable to libraries of oligosaccharides.

10.6 PROSPECTUS

It is clear that there is tremendous potential for combinatorial libraries of oligosaccharides, but that current technology falls a long way short of making them a reality.

It is imperative that further effort be directed toward the development of efficient strategies for the synthesis of oligosaccharides, particularly in the solid phase. Inherent in this goal are the following: (a) improving the efficiency of glycosylation reactions, (b) asserting control over the stereochemistry of glycosidic linkages, and (c) development of generalizable protecting group strategies.

It will take years to realize these ambitions. However, it seems almost certain that the controlled synthesis of combinatorial libraries of oligosaccharides will play a key role in developing our understanding of what Lemieux has described as "the rich mosaic of carbohydrate structures which . . . play key roles in both the maintenance of health and the establishment of disease" (10).

ACKNOWLEDGMENT

I would like to thank Professor Daniel Kahne of Princeton University for stimulating discussions on many and varied aspects of chemistry and in particular the potential for combinatorial libraries of oligosaccharides, during my time in his laboratory.

REFERENCES

1. Jung, G., and Beck-Sickinger, A. G., *Angew. Chem. Int. Ed. Engl.* **31,** 367–383 (1992).
2. (a) Ecker, D. J., Vickers, T. A., Hanecak, R., Driver, V., and Anderson, K., *Nucleic Acids Res.* **21,** 1853–1856 (1993); (b) Latham, J. A., Johnson, R., Toole, J. J., *Nucleic Acids Res.* **22,** 2817–22 (1994); (c) Wyatt, J. R., Vickers, T. A., Roberson, J. L., Buckheit, Jr., R. W., Klimkait, T., DeBaets, E., Davis, P. W., Rayner, B., Imback, J. L., and Ecker, D. J., *Proc. Natl. Acad. Sci. U.S.A.* **91,** 1356–1360 (1994).
3. Mullis, K. B., *The Polymerase Chain Reaction,* Birkhauser, Boston, 1994.
4. Khorana, H. G., 1968 Nobel Prize in Medicine, for nucleotide synthesis; Merrifield, R. B., 1984 Nobel Prize in Chemistry, for solid-phase peptide synthesis; Mullis, K. B., and Smith, M., 1993 Nobel Prize in Chemistry for the development of the polymerase chain reaction (PCR).
5. Hakomori, S., *Ann. Rev. Biochem.* **50,** 733–764 (1981).

6. Ruoslahti, E., in *Carbohydrate Recognition in Cellular Function,* Wiley, Chichester, Ciba Foundation Symposium 145, 1989.

7. Phillips, M. L., Nudelman, E., Gaeta, F. C. A., Perez, M., Singhal, A. K., Hakamori, S., and Paulson, J. C., *Science* **250,** 1130–1132 (1990); (b) Walz, G., Aruffo, A., Kolanus, W., Bevilacqua, M., and Seed, B., *Science* **250,** 1132–1135 (1990); (c) Lowe, J. B., Stoolman, L. M., Nair, R. P., Larsen, R. D., Berhend, T. L., and Marks, R. M., *Cell* **63,** 475 (1990).

8. Bremer, E. G., Levery, S. B., Sonnino, S., Ghidoni, R., Canevari, S., Kannagi, R., and Hakomori, S., *J. Biol. Chem.* **259,** 14773–14777 (1984).

9. Paulsen, H., *Angew. Chem. Int. Ed. Engl.* **29,** 823–839 (1990).

10. Lemieux, R. U., *Chem. Soc. Rev.* **18,** 347–374 (1989).

11. Lasky, L. A., *Science* **258,** 964–969 (1992).

12. Patel, T. P., Goelz, S. E., Lobb, R. R., and Parekh, R. B., *Biochemistry* **33,** 14815–14824 (1994).

13. (a) Garegg, P. J., *Acc. Chem. Res.* **25,** 575–580 (1992); (b) Halcomb, R. L., and Wong, C.-H., *Curr. Opin. Struct. Biol.* **3,** 694–700 (1993).

14. (a) Merrifield, R. B., *J. Am. Chem. Soc.* **85,** 2149 (1963); (b) Merrifield, R. B., *Science* **232,** 341 (1986).

15. (a) Letsinger, R. L., and Mahadevan, V., *J. Am. Chem. Soc.* **87,** 3526–3527 (1965); (b) Carruthers, M. H., *Science* **230,** 281–285 (1985).

16. Toone, E. J., Simon, E. S., Bednarski, M. D., and Whitesides, G. M., *Tetrahedron* **45,** 5365–5422 (1989).

17. Schuster, M., Wang, P., Wong, C.-H., and Paulson, J., *J. Am. Chem. Soc.* **116,** 1135–1136 (1994).

18. (a) Toshima, K., and Tatsuta, K., *Chem. Rev.* **93,** 1503–1531 (1993); (b) Schmidt, R. R., *Angew. Chem. Int. Ed. Engl.* **25,** 212–235 (1986); (c) Paulsen, H., *Angew. Chem. Int. Ed. Engl.* **21,** 155–173 (1982).

19. (a) Kahne, D., Walker, S., Cheng, Y., and Van Engen, D., *J. Am. Chem. Soc.* **111,** 6881–6882 (1989); (b) Kim, S.-H., Augeri, D., Yang, D., and Kahne, D. *J. Am. Chem. Soc.* **116,** 1766–1775 (1994); (c) Yan, L., Taylor, C. M., Goodnow, Jr., R., and Kahne, D., *J. Am. Chem. Soc.* **116,** 6953–6954 (1994).

20. Kunz, H., and Harreus, A., *Liebigs Ann. Chem.* 41–48 (1982).

21. Raghavan, S., and Kahne, D., *J. Am. Chem. Soc.* **115,** 1580–1581 (1993).

22. Raghavan, S., Ph.D. Thesis, Princeton University, 1993.

23. Fréchet, J. M. J., in *Polymer-supported Reactions in Organic Synthesis,* P. Hodge and D. C. Sherrington, (Eds.), Wiley, New York 1980.

24. (a) Westerduin, P., Veeneman, G. H., Pennings, Y., van der Marel, G. A., and van Boom, J. H., *Tetrahedron Lett.* **28,** 1557 (1987); (b) Veeneman, G. H., Notermans, S., Liskamp, R. M. J., van der Marel, G. A., and van Boom, J. H., *Tetrahedron Lett.* **28,** 6695 (1987); (c) Veeneman, G. H., Brugghe, H. F., van den Elst, H., and van Boom, J. H., *Carbohydr. Res.* **195,** C1 (1990).

25. (a) Danishefsky, S. J., McClure, K. F., Randolph, J. T., and Ruggieri, R. B., *Science* **260,** 1307 (1993); (b) Randolph, J. T., and Danishefsky, S. J., *Angew. Chem. Intl. Ed. Engl.* **33,** 1470–1473 (1994); (c) Timmers, C. M., van der Marel, G. A., and van Boom, J. H., *Recl. Trav. Chim. Pays-Bas* **112,** 609–610 (1993).

26. (a) Douglas, S. P., Whitfield, D. M., and Krepinsky, J. J., *J. Am. Chem. Soc.* **113,** 5095–5097 (1991); (b) Douglas, S. P., Whitfield, D. M., and Krepinsky, J. J., *J. Am. Chem. Soc.* **117,** 2116–2117 (1995); (c) Krepinsky, J. J., Douglas, S. P., and Whitfield, D. M., *Methods Enzymol.* **242,** 280–293 (1994).

27. Houghten, R. A., *Curr. Biology* **4,** 564–567 (1994).

28. Rothenberg, B. E., Hayes, B. K., Toomre, D., Manzi, A. E., and Varki, A., *Proc. Natl. Acad. Sci. U.S.A.* **90,** 11939–11943 (1993).

29. Behar, V., and Danishefsky, S. J., *Angew. Chem. Int. Ed. Engl.* **33,** 1468–1470 (1994).

30. Brummel, C. L., Lee, I. N. W., Zhou, Y., Benkovic, S. J., and Winograd, N., *Science* **264,** 399–402 (1994).

31. Ikemoto, N., Lo, L.-C., Kim, O. K., Berova, N., and Nakanishi, K., *Carbohydrate Res.* **239,** 11–33 (1993).

32. (a) Stinson, S., *Chem. Eng. News,* Oct. 18, 30, 32 (1993); (b) Edge, C. J., Rademacher, T. W., Wormald, M. R., Parekh, R. B., Butters, T. D., Wing, D. R., and Dwyer, R. A., *Proc. Natl. Acad. Sci. U.S.A.* **89,** 6338 (1992).

33. (a) Ohlmeyer, M. H. J., Swanson, R. N., Dillard, L. W., Reader, J. C., Asouline, G., Kobayashi, R., Wigler, M., and Still, W. C., *Proc. Natl. Acad. Sci. U.S.A.* **90,** 10922–10926 (1993); (b) Nestler, H. P., Bartlett, P. A., and Still, W. C., *J. Org. Chem.* **59,** 4723–4724 (1994); (c) Eckes, P., *Angew. Chem. Int. Ed. Engl.* **33,** 1573–1575 (1994).

11

SOLUBLE COMBINATORIAL LIBRARIES OF PEPTIDES, PEPTIDOMIMETICS, AND ORGANICS: FUNDAMENTAL TOOLS FOR BASIC RESEARCH AND DRUG DISCOVERY

JOHN M. OSTRESH, BARBARA DÖRNER, SYLVIE E. BLONDELLE, AND RICHARD A. HOUGHTEN
Torrey Pines Institute for Molecular Studies, 3550 General Atomics Court, San Diego, California 92121

11.1 INTRODUCTION

The recent emergence of combinatorial libraries, which originated in the field of peptide chemistry, represents a seminal breakthrough in all areas of basic research and drug discovery. Despite the long history of success in synthesizing individual compounds for drug discovery, the tremendous productivity increases associated with combinatorial chemistry have prompted the pharmaceutical industry to embrace the concept for the rapid identification of lead compounds and the study of structure-activity relationships. Historically, the concept of combinatorial chemistry arose from the need for ever-increasing numbers of compounds. The development of solid-phase techniques (1), followed by their application to simultaneous multiple multiple synthesis (2,3), led to the first practical and broadly applicable validation of the combinatorial concept by two groups in 1991 (4,5). Although combinatorial chemistry has been used, in many instances, for the identification of individual active peptides [reviewed in (6)] from mixtures of millions of peptides, the common perception that peptides have undesirable properties such as poor oral bioavailability and short half-life has prompted recent efforts to apply the concept to peptidomimetic and small organic compounds.

Within the pharmaceutical industry, libraries have traditionally been regarded as the thousands of discrete compounds that have been accumulated by years of methodical synthesis and characterization within laboratories. More recently, those involved in the field of combinatorial chemistry have extended the meaning of libraries to describe collections of individual or mixtures of compounds ranging in number from tens to millions that are prepared in a highly systematic manner. Although combinatorial libraries of peptides have been prepared using both molecular biology and chemistry approaches (7), the application of the concept to small organic compounds, using currently available techniques, can only be realized using chemical approaches. Chemically prepared combinatorial libraries can be broadly divided into three main categories: pooled soluble combinatorial libraries (4,8), support-bound libraries (5), and tagged libraries (9–12). The strength of the pooled soluble combinatorial library approach over other methods is that the chemical structure of active compounds is easily determined based upon deconvolution of the structural similarities of the compounds within each of the active pools (4,8). Therefore, this approach appears to be easily applicable to the screening of organic and peptidomimetic libraries. In contrast, the use of support-bound libraries has two disadvantages: the influence of the solid support on activity inherent to the method and the difficulty of structural determination. The tagged library approach, which eliminates the problem of structure determination, also has the disadvantage of the influence of the tag on activity.

The first reported progress made in the transition from peptide libraries to peptidomimetic and organic libraries occurred with the stepwise generation of "peptoid" libraries, based on N-alkylated polyglycine subunits (13,14). In addition to the increased stability of these compounds to proteolytic enzymes, peptoids closely mimic the structural features of peptides, increasing the likelihood of finding active compounds in assays in which the native ligand is a protein or peptide. In this laboratory, chemical transformations have been used to prepare similar peptidomimetic libraries by the exhaustive alkylation of existing peptide libraries. This concept has been termed "libraries from libraries" (15). A wide array of chemical diversities can be easily generated using this method. Thus, organic polyamine libraries have also been prepared by the exhaustive reduction of existing peptide and peptidomimetic libraries (16). Several groups have reported the stepwise synthesis of nonpolymeric organic libraries of limited diversity, such as benzodiazepines (17) [reviewed in (18)].

11.2 LIBRARY PREPARATION

11.2.1 Resin Mixing Approach

Figure 11.1 shows one of two approaches used in the chemical synthesis of combinatorial libraries. Known as the "divide, couple and recombine" (DCR) (4) or "split resin" (5) method, this approach has been the most popular choice for the development of combinatorial libraries because of its ease of application to many different

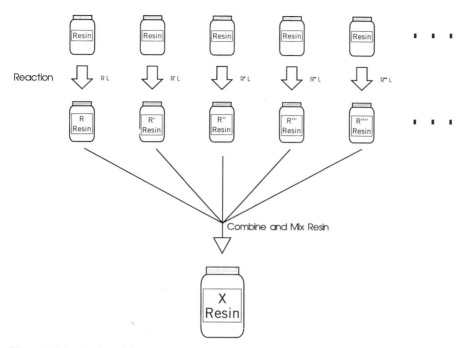

Figure 11.1 Resin mixing approach for the generation of approximately equimolar resin mixtures. Individual reagents (RL, where R is the incoming substituent and L is a leaving group) are reacted with aliquots of resin. The aliquots are then mixed to generate X resin (where X represents resin incorporating approximately equimolar amounts of each substituent).

solid-phase reactions. This approach consists of dividing the solid-phase resin into discrete portions, which are then coupled to individual protected amino acids or other substituents, followed by thorough mixing of the resin portions. This process is repeated until the mixtures of choice are obtained. Because of the physical process used to prepare such mixtures, a single compound is attached to each individual bead. When screening support-bound libraries, these resins are deprotected, assayed, and analyzed. In the case of pooled soluble libraries, the resin portions from the last one or two steps are not recombined in order to provide individual defined groups of compounds having structural similarities, which are the basis for the deconvolution of the compounds responsible for activity. Because of the physical process of dividing, mixing, and recombining the resins, the individual compounds making up each group are present in approximately equimolar amounts. Equimolar representation is necessary to determine the relative activity of each compound in the library and is ensured only as long as the number of compounds per final aliquot of resin synthesized is much less (10–100 times) than the number of resin beads used (7). The straightforward weighing of resin aliquots, which

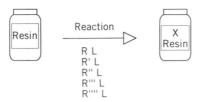

Figure 11.2 Chemical mixture approach for the generation of approximately equimolar resin mixtures. Resin mixtures are obtained by reacting mixtures of individual reagents, which can be incorporated using an excess or as limiting reagents. The ratio of each individual reagent is based on their reaction kinetics. RL and X are defined as described in Figure 11.1.

results in the approximate equimolar representation of each compound within the library, makes this approach easily applicable to the solid-phase synthesis of combinatorial libraries composed of small organic molecules.

11.2.2 Chemical Mixture Approach

The second approach to the synthesis of combinatorial libraries is outlined in Figure 11.2. In this approach, mixtures of protected amino acids or other building blocks are added simultaneously. The approximate equimolarity of individual compounds can be achieved either by using a large excess of reagent in which the concentration of each individual incoming building block is based on its relative coupling rate (8,19) or by incorporating equimolar amounts of the incoming building blocks as limiting reagents (2). One advantage of these chemical methods over the DCR approach is that any individual building block(s) (i.e., location or number of defined substituents) making up the library can be used as the basis for the deconvolution of active compounds. In addition, these methods are much less labor intensive than the resin mixing approach. The simplest application of the chemical mixture approach to the generation of small molecule organic libraries would incorporate individual building blocks as limiting reagents. However, the expected wide variation in kinetics and mechanisms can lead to preferential incorporation of incoming substituents onto the different resin-bound templates, since the concentration of each component changes as the reaction proceeds. On the other hand, the use of a large excess of incoming reagents allows one to assume pseudo first order reaction kinetics in many cases. Nevertheless, a thorough knowledge of the kinetics and mechanism of the reaction is required.

11.3 DECONVOLUTION METHODS

11.3.1 Support-bound Combinatorial Libraries

The first report of the screening of combinatorial libraries involved support-bound mixtures of tens to hundreds of thousands of octapeptides on polystyrene pins arranged in a microtiter plate format (2). These original libraries were used in conjunction with an iterative deconvolution process to identify individual sequences, termed "mimotopes," having high affinity for a monoclonal antibody. Although conceptually sound, the limited success of this approach appeared to be due to, at least initially, the nature of the support, the incompleteness of the synthetic steps in the process, the linkage to the solid support, and the interference of the solid support. Recently, these limitations have been minimized, especially with the use of cleavable linkers (20,21).

The use of support-bound libraries in combinatorial chemistry was furthered by the realization, which was obvious in hindsight, that the split resin approach leads to one compound per resin bead (5). When millions of peptides, each attached to an individual resin bead, were assayed for antibody or receptor binding, colorimetric visualization of the beads with the attached antibodies or receptors allowed the specific beads to be microsequenced. Several groups have since reported the use of tags that code for the structure of interest, adding the potential for structural determination of nonproteogenic compounds and/or eliminating the need for microsequencing. Using this method, the structures of attached polynucleotides (9), peptides (10,11), or other chemicals (22) that code for the compounds of interest are easily determined.

11.3.2 Nonsupport-bound Combinatorial Libraries

A direct method for the synthesis of large diversities of compounds that are not attached to any solid support was developed in our laboratory. These soluble libraries can be used in virtually any in vitro, or even in vivo, assay (4,8). The generation of these libraries uses the simultaneous multiple-peptide synthesis method, also known as the "tea-bag" approach (3). Using this approach, solid-phase resin beads are contained within individual mesh packets. Resin mixtures are then obtained using either the resin mixing (4,5) or chemical mixture methods (8,19). Following deprotection and cleavage, individual pooled mixtures having at least one substituent in common are then assayed.

Two methods for the determination of the active sequences or structures from the millions present within a combinatorial library are used in our laboratory. Using either method, the library is synthesized in subsets (or pools) such that the structural similarities of the compounds within each subset lead to the identification of active compounds. In the first method, the chemical structure of an active compound is obtained by an iterative process of selection and synthesis (the deconvolution process). In this method, subsets of the mixtures of compounds are sequentially synthesized and assayed such that the number of compounds within each pool is made smaller and smaller until a single active compound of interest is obtained (4). Figure 11.3 illustrates a generic representation of the repetitive steps necessary for the iterative determination of the chemical structure of an active compound from a combinatorial library split into four mixtures of 64 compounds. Figure 11.4 illustrates the same iterative process, using hexapeptides for comparison and ease of comprehension, to identify a single active compound starting from 400 mixtures in

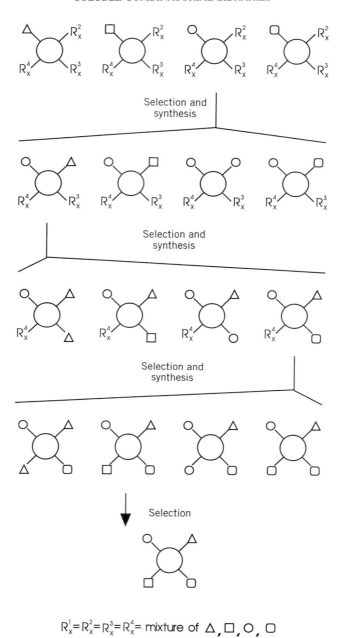

Figure 11.3 Iterative process for the identification of defined compounds from a pooled combinatorial library where R_x^1 through R_x^4 represents mixtures of individual substituents.

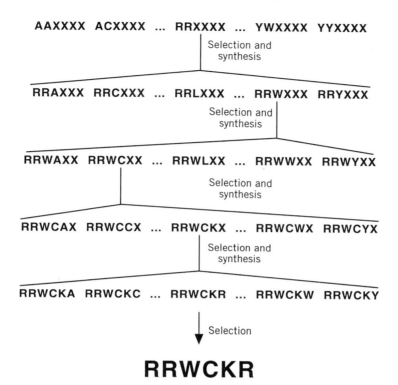

Figure 11.4   Example of the iterative process as described in Figure 11.3 for the case of hexapeptides. X refers to an approximately equimolar mixture of the 20 proteogenic amino acids.

which two amino acids are defined (23). In most cases, the iterative process would be carried out simultaneously from several of the active starting mixtures to identify different active compounds. The cutoff in the selection process is subjective depending on the assay and the overall activity of the mixtures within that assay. This method for deconvoluting structural information is readily applied to organic and peptidomimetic libraries.

In the second method for deconvolution of structural information, the library is pooled such that structural information can be obtained in a single assay (8). Using this method, termed the positional scanning approach, compounds within the combinatorial library are pooled such that at each position in a compound, each subset contains only a single defined substituent or building block. Figure 11.5 illustrates the generic representation of the positional scanning deconvolution process used for the 256 compounds described in Figure 11.3. Again, for comparison and ease of comprehension, Figure 11.6 shows the 120 mixtures and the deconvolution process used for a hexapeptide library. When used in concert, the structural similarities of

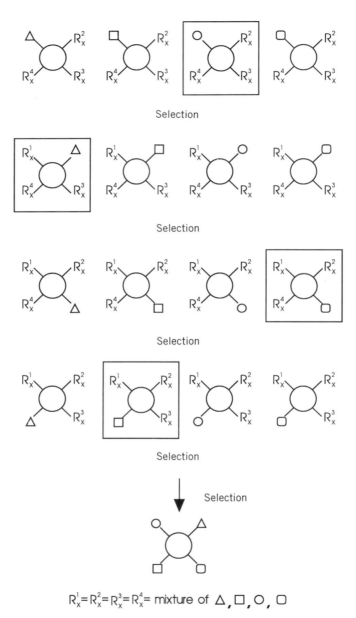

Figure 11.5   Positional scanning process for the identification of defined compounds from a pooled combinatorial library where R_x^1 through R_x^4 represents mixtures of individual substituents.

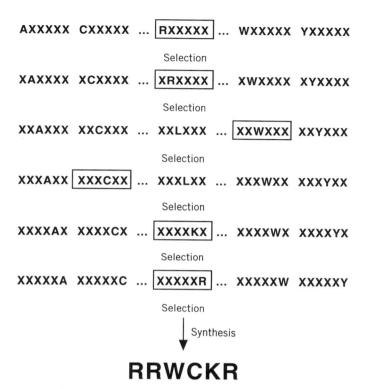

Figure 11.6 Example of the positional scanning process as described in Figure 11.5 for the case of hexapeptides. X represents an approximately equimolar mixture of the 20 proteogenic amino acids.

the most active pools yield information that allows the determination of the active compounds. The resulting individual compounds are synthesized separately to confirm the results of the screening assay. If the chemical mixture approach is used for synthesis, this method can be readily applied to any compound template in which substituents are added.

11.4 COMBINATORIAL LIBRARIES

11.4.1 Peptidic Soluble Combinatorial Libraries

Figure 11.7 describes a number of the peptide combinatorial libraries that have been synthesized and screened in this laboratory using competitive enzyme linked immunosorbent assay (ELISA), receptor-binding assays, antimicrobial microdilution assays, and enzyme inhibition assays [reviewed in (6)]. In most cases, the different library formats yield complementary information depending on the relative redun-

1. Positional Scanning Libraries

    A. Single position hexamers (acetylated and non-acetylated using 20 L-amino acids)

    OXXXXX   XOXXXX   XXOXXX   XXXOXX   XXXXOX   XXXXXO

    B. Dual position hexamers (acetylated and non-acetylated using 20 L-amino acids)

    OOXXXX   XXOOXX   XXOOXX

    C. Single position tetramers (non-acetylated using 52 amino acids)

    OXXX   XOXX   XXOX   XXXO

    D. Single position decamers (acetylated and non-acetylated using 20 L-amino acids)

    OXXXXXXXXX   XOXXXXXXXX   XXOXXXXXXX   XXXOXXXXXX   XXXXOXXXXX

    XXXXXOXXXX   XXXXXXOXXX   XXXXXXXOXX   XXXXXXXXOX   XXXXXXXXXO

2. Iterative Libraries

    A. Dual position hexamers (acetylated and non-acetylated using 20 D-amino acids)

    OOXXXX

    B. Tetramers (acetylated and non-acetylated using 78 amino acids)

    OXXX

Figure 11.7   Different formats for some of the peptide combinatorial libraries used in our laboratory. Note that the iterative process can also be used with each of the positional scanning libraries for deconvolution of active compounds.

dancy of the position being studied, the ligand concentrations necessary for a particular assay, and so forth.

Although L-amino acid peptides are not traditionally considered effective therapeutic agents because of their lack of oral bioavailability and rapid enzymatic degradation, a number of peptide antibiotics have been shown to be of great value as intravenous or topical therapeutics (24,25). In addition, insects and mammals appear to use peptides as a primary host defense system (26) to counter bacterial infections. Compared to classical antibiotics, the different modes of action of peptide antibiotics, which generally affect the permeability of bacterial membranes (27), offer potential against resistant strains of bacteria. In addition, the characterization of new antimicrobial peptides and the design of analogs with improved activities yield a better understanding of the structure–activity relationships involved [reviewed in (27)]. Furthermore, peptide libraries made up of L-amino acids have been proven useful in many antigen/antibody studies (8,28–30), which could lead to the development of new immunodiagnostics.

The cyclization of L-amino acid peptides has been shown to increase their resistance to enzymatic degradation (31,32) because of their reduced conformational flexibility. In addition, cyclic peptides have been used for the construction of conformationally defined templates (33). Therefore, this laboratory has prepared a positional scanning cyclic template combinatorial library in which the active compounds were found to be stable to proteolytic enzymes (34).

To circumvent the potential therapeutic limitations relevant to the active compounds found in the L-amino acid libraries, libraries consisting of D- and/or unnatural amino acid peptides have been used to identify active compounds having much greater enzymatic stability (35).

11.4.2 Peptidomimetic Soluble Combinatorial Libraries

The preparation of libraries of oligomeric N-alkylated glycines (13,14), termed peptoids, was the first report of the generation of peptidomimetic libraries. Favorable changes in the physical and chemical properties of the peptidomimetic compounds relative to peptides, such as enhanced resistance to proteolytic enzymes, increased acid stability, favorable aqueous-organic partitioning characteristics, and so forth, are possible with such libraries.

A simpler approach, which greatly expands the diversity of combinatorial libraries, termed the "libraries from libraries" concept, has been developed in our laboratory (15). With this concept, an existing peptide library was exhaustively permethylated while still attached to the solid support used in its synthesis. Since this approach is based on the transformation of a well-defined peptide combinatorial library, and since the chemical transformation is performed using solid-phase methods, equimolarity of the compounds within the peptidomimetic library is easily ensured. A range of chemical transformations can be envisioned to generate a number of peptidomimetic libraries. Thus, a number of peptide libraries, such as those described in Figure 11.7, have been peralkylated using a variety of alkylating agents, including methyl iodide, allyl bromide, and benzyl bromide (36). An example of the chemical structure of one of these peralkylated libraries composed of permethylated hexapeptides is shown in Figure 11.8. The effect of these modifications is that the resulting compounds have very different physical, chemical, and biological properties than their parent compounds. The screening of each peralkylated library in various bioassays led to the identification of highly active compounds derived from completely different parent peptides.

An illustration of the utility of such libraries is presented in Figure 11.9, in which

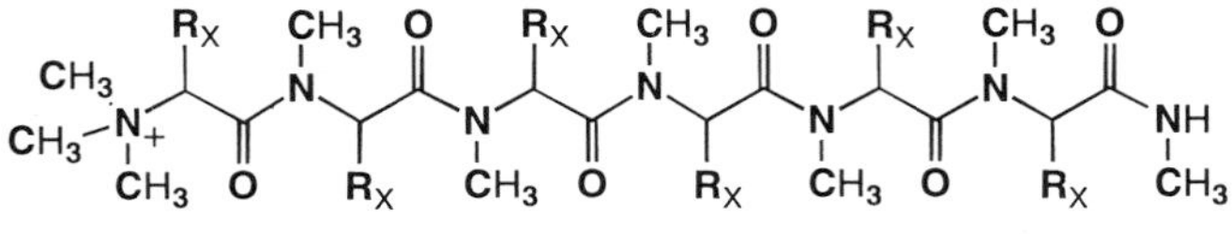

Figure 11.8 N-permethylated hexapeptide combinatorial library. R_x represents the side chains of a mixture of the 20 proteogenic amino acids. The side chains of C, D, E, H, K, N, Q, R, W, and Y have also been modified.

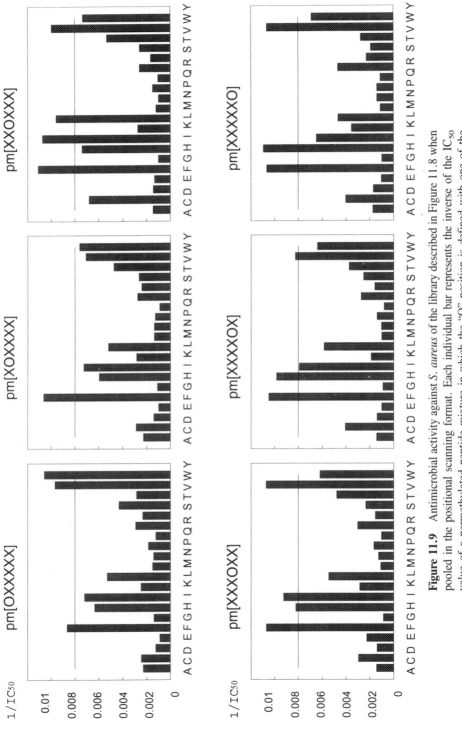

Figure 11.9 Antimicrobial activity against *S. aureus* of the library described in Figure 11.8 when pooled in the positional scanning format. Each individual bar represents the inverse of the IC_{50} value of a permethylated peptide mixture in which the "O" position is defined with one of the 20 proteogenic amino acids.

a permethylated positional scanning hexamer library was screened in a standard microdilution assay to identify individual permethylated compounds having potent antimicrobial activity against *Staphylococcus aureus*. Using the structural information from the most active of the 120 permethylated mixtures in this library, 72 individual peptides were synthesized, permethylated, and cleaved. The permethylated form of LFIFFF-NH$_2$ was found to be the most active compound (IC$_{50}$ = 6 μg/mL and MIC = 11 to 15 μg/mL, where the IC$_{50}$ and MIC values represent the concentrations necessary to inhibit 50 and 100% cell growth, respectively). These compounds showed similar activities against a methicillin-resistant strain of *S. aureus*.

11.4.3 Organic Chemical Libraries

Organic chemical libraries fall into two categories: polymer based and nonpolymer based. In the first category, the synthesis of a small library of oligocarbamates (256 discrete compounds) and its screening against a monoclonal antibody have been reported (37). In our laboratory, polymer-based organic chemical libraries of large diversity have been synthesized using the libraries from libraries approach. The initial application of this concept to form organic libraries was through the generation of a library of substituted polyamines (34 million) (16). To generate the library, a well-characterized hexapeptide library was exhaustively reduced to generate millions of substituted polyamines. This library was found to have substantial activity in both receptor-binding and antimicrobial microdilution assays. Related polyamine libraries have also been synthesized from the exhaustive reduction of peralkylated libraries. Current projects in our laboratory involve the extension of the libraries from libraries concept to form libraries of hydroxylamines, nitrosamines, hydrazines, and so forth.

Advances in the application of chemical reactions to the solid phase initially led to the multiple synthesis (<200 compounds) of discrete nonoligomeric compounds. The synthesis of benzodiazepines (192 compounds) on plastic pins using the microtiter plate format has been reported (17,38), as well as the related syntheses of benzodiazepines and hydantoins (40 compounds) using fritted glass chambers (39). It should be noted that, in each case, these compounds were prepared as discrete products, eliminating the productivity advantage of combinatorial libraries during the assay portion of the process. The feasibility of using pooled combinatorial chemical libraries was first validated by the synthesis of mixtures of β-mercaptoketones (9 compounds) (40) and the synthesis and screening of potential antioxidants (27 compounds) (41). However, validation of the ability of individual assays to distinguish between compounds having the potential for multiple opposing properties remains to be proven when using combinatorial mixtures containing a large diversity of nonpolymeric compounds. The screening of a library consisting of 7600 acylated and alkylated amino acids, which yielded compounds with an affinity for streptavidin, has been reported (42). Similar strategies using diverse chemical reactions such as alkylations, acylations, reductions, and oxidations have been used in our laboratory to sequentially generate large combinatorial libraries (>10,000 compounds) consisting of small organic molecules. More recently, a large number of reports in both solid phase organic and combinatorial synthesis have been published [see review (43)].

11.5 CONCLUSION

Many methods developed for use in the field of peptide chemistry are currently being applied to the solid-phase synthesis, simultaneous multiple synthesis, and combinatorial synthesis of peptidomimetic and organic compounds. The tremendous increase in productivity associated with the various methods for combinatorial synthesis and screening is the motivating factor behind their expanding use. These combinatorial methods will play a progressively more important role in the search for novel pharmacophores and for the development of new methods useful in all areas of basic research and drug discovery.

ACKNOWLEDGMENT

We would like to thank Eileen Weiler for her editorial assistance. The work performed in this laboratory was funded by Houghten Pharmaceuticals, Inc., San Diego, California.

REFERENCES

1. Merrifield, R. B., *J. Am. Chem. Soc.* **85**, 2149–2154 (1963).
2. Geysen, H. M., Rodda, S. J., and Mason, T. J., *Mol. Immunol.* **23**, 709–715 (1986).
3. Houghten, R. A., *Proc. Natl. Acad. Sci. U.S.A.* **82**, 5131–5135 (1985).
4. Houghten, R. A., Pinilla, C., Blondelle, S. E., Appel, J. R., Dooley, C. T., and Cuervo, J. H., *Nature* **354**, 84–86 (1991).
5. Lam, K. S., Salmon, S. E., Hersh, E. M., Hruby, V. J., Kazmierski, W. M., and Knapp, R. J., *Nature* **354**, 82–84 (1991).
6. Pinilla, C., Appel, J., Blondelle, S. E., Dooley, C. T., Dörner, B., Eichler, J., Ostresh, J. M., and Houghten, R. A., *Biopolymers (Peptide Sci.)* **37**, 221–240 (1995).
7. Gallop, M. A., Barrett, R. W., Dower, W. J., Fodor, S. P. A., and Gordon, E. M., *J. Med. Chem.* **37**, 1233–1251 (1994).
8. Pinilla, C., Appel, J. R., Blanc, P., and Houghten, R. A., *Biotechniques* **13**, 901–905 (1992).
9. Needels, M. C., Jones, D. G., Tate, E. H., Heinkel, G. L., Kochersperger, L. M., Dower, W. J., Barrett, R. W., and Gallop, M. A., *Proc. Natl. Acad. Sci. U.S.A.* **90**, 10700–10704 (1993).
10. Kerr, J. M., Banville, S. C., and Zuckermann, R. N., *J. Am. Chem. Soc.* **115**, 2529–2531 (1993).
11. Nikolaiev, V., Stierandová, A., Krchňák, V., Seligmann, B., Lam, K. S., Salmon, S. E., and Lebl, M., *Peptide Res.* **6**, 161–170 (1993).

12. Chen, C. M., and Benoiton, N. L., *Can. J. Chem.* **54**, 3310–3311 (1976).

13. Simon, R. J., Kania, R. S., Zuckermann, R. N., Huebner, V. D., Jewell, D. A., Banville, S., Ng, S., Wang, L., Rosenberg, S., Marlowe, C. K., Spellmeyer, D. C., Tan, R., Frankel, A. D., Santi, D. V., Cohen, F. E., and Bartlett, P. A., *Proc. Natl. Acad. Sci. U.S.A.* **89**, 9367–9371 (1992).

14. Zuckermann, R. N., Martin, E. J., Spellmayer, D. C., Stauber, G. B., Shoemaker, K. R., Kerr, J. M., Figliozzi, G. M., Goff, D. A., Siani, M. A., Simon, R. J., Banville, S. C., Brown, E. G., Wang, L., Richter, L. S., and Moos, W. H., *J. Med. Chem.* **37**, 2678–2685 (1994).

15. Ostresh, J. M., Husar, G. M., Blondelle, S. E., Dörner, B., Weber, P. A., and Houghten, R. A., *Proc. Natl. Acad. Sci. U.S.A.* **91**, 11138–11142 (1994).

16. Cuervo, J. H., Weitl, F., Ostresh, J. M., Hamashin, V. T., Hannah, A. L., and Houghten, R. A., in *Peptides 1994: Proceedings of the 23rd European Peptide Symposium*, H. L. S. Maia (Ed.), Escom, Leiden, 465–466 (1995).

17. Bunin, B. A., and Ellman, J. A., *J. Am. Chem. Soc.* **114**, 10997–10998 (1992).

18. Gordon, E. M., Barrett, R. W., Dower, W. J., Fodor, S. P. A., and Gallop, M. A., *J. Med. Chem.* **37**, 1385–1401 (1994).

19. Ostresh, J. M., Winkle, J. H., Hamashin, V. T., and Houghten, R. A., *Biopolymers* **34**, 1681–1689 (1994).

20. Bray, A. M., Maeji, N. J., Valerio, R. M., Campbell, R. A., and Geysen, H. M., *J. Org. Chem.* **56**, 6659–6666 (1991).

21. Valerio, R. M., Bray, A. M., Campbell, R. A., Dipasquale, A., Margellis, C., Rodda, S. J., Geysen, H. M., and Maeji, N. J., *Int. J. Peptide Protein Res.* **42**, 1–9 (1993).

22. Ohlmeyer, M. H. J., Swanson, R. N., Dillard, L. W., Reader, J. C., Asouline, G., Kobayashi, R., Wigler, M., and Still, W. C., *Proc. Natl. Acad. Sci. U.S.A.* **90**, 10922–10926 (1993).

23. Blondelle, S. E., Pérez-Payá, E., Dooley, C. T., Pinilla, C., and Houghten, R. A., *Trends Anal Chem.* **14**, 83–92 (1995).

24. Verhoef, J. C., Bodde, H. E., DeBoer, A. G., Bouwstra, J. A., Junginger, H. E., Merkus, F. W. H. M., and Breimer, D. D., *Eur. J. Drug Metab. Pharmacok.* **15**, 83–93 (1990).

25. Jawetz, E., *Pediat. Clin. N. Am.* **8**, 1057–1071 (1961).

26. Zasloff, M., *Curr. Opin. Immunol.* **4**, 3–7 (1992).

27. Saberwal, G., and Nagaraj, R., *Biochim. Biophys. Acta Rev. Biomembr.* **1197**, 109–131 (1994).

28. Pinilla, C., Appel, J. R., and Houghten, R. A., *Biochem. J.* **301**, 847–853 (1994).

29. Pinilla, C., Appel, J. R., and Houghten, R. A., *Gene* **128**, 71–76 (1993).

30. Appel, J. R., Pinilla, C., and Houghten, R. A., *Immunomethods* **1**, 17–23 (1992).

31. DiMaio, J., and Schiller, P. W., *Proc. Natl. Acad. Sci. U.S.A.* **77**, 7162–7166 (1980).

32. Sham, H. L., Bolis, G., Stein, H. H., Fesik, S. W., Marcotte, P. A., Plattner, J. J., Rempel, C. A., and Greer, J., *J. Med. Chem.* **31**, 284–295 (1988).

33. Tuchscherer, G., Dörner, B., Sila, U., Kamber, B., and Mutter, M., *Tetrahedron* **49**, 3559–3575 (1993).

34. Eichler, J., Lucka, A. W., and Houghten, R. A., *Peptide Res.* **7**, 300–307 (1994).

35. Dooley, C. T., Chung, N. N., Wilkes, B. C., Schiller, P. W., Bidlack, J. M., Pasternak, G. W., and Houghten, R. A., *Science* **266**, 2019–2022 (1994).

36. Dörner, B., Ostresh, J. M., Husar, G. M., and Houghten, R. A., in *Peptides 1994: Proceedings of the 23rd European Peptide Symposium,* H. L. S. Maia (Ed.), Escom, Leiden, 463–464 (1995).

37. Cho, Y. C., Moran, E. J., Cherry, S. R., Stephans, J. C., Fodor, S. P. A., Adams, C. L., Sundaram, A., Jacobs, J. W., and Schultz, P. G., *Science* **261,** 1303–1305 (1993).

38. Bunin, B. A., Plunkett, M. J., and Ellman, J. A., *Proc. Natl. Acad. Sci. U.S.A.* **91,** 4708–4712 (1994).

39. DeWitt, S. H., Kiely, J. S., Stankovic, C. J., Schroeder, M. C., Cody, D. M. R., and Pavia, M. R., *Proc. Natl. Acad. Sci. U.S.A.* **90,** 6909–6913 (1993).

40. Chen, C., Ahlberg-Randall, L. A., Miller, R. B., Jones, A. D., and Kurth, M. J., *J. Am. Chem. Soc.* **116,** 2661–2662 (1994).

41. Kurth, M. J., Randall, L. A. A., Chen, C., Melander, C., Miller, R. B., McAlister, K., Reitz, G., Kang, R., Nakatsu, T., and Green, C., *J. Org. Chem.* **59,** 5862–5864 (1994).

42. Staňková, M., Issakova, O., Sepetov, N. F., Krchňák, V., Lam, K. S., and Lebl, M., *Drug Dev. Res.* **33,** 146–156 (1994).

43. Thompson, L. A., and Ellman, J. A., *Chem. Rev.* **96,** 555–600 (1996).

12

COMBINATORIAL LIBRARIES OF PEPTIDES, PROTEINS, AND ANTIBODIES USING BIOLOGICAL SYSTEMS

GROVER P. MILLER, WENYAN ZHONG, JEFF SMILEY, AND STEPHEN J. BENKOVIC

Pennsylvania State University, Chemistry Department, University Park, PA 16802 (G.P.M., W.Z., S.J.B.)

Youngstown State University, Chemistry Department, Youngstown, OH 44555 (J.S.)

12.1 INTRODUCTION

Proteins and peptides are the results of nature's ongoing experiment in combinatorial libraries. The polymeric character of peptides and their generally larger, more structurally elaborate relatives, the proteins, provides an ideal experimental system for creating a collection of genetically encoded macromolecules, from which those with desired properties can be selected. With a naturally occurring set of 20 amino acids, any of which can be incorporated into any position in a linear polypeptide, a cell's protein synthesizing machinery can create a huge array of different molecules. A combinatorial library of decapeptides, for example, would consist of 20^{10}, or 10,240,000,000,000 members; the number of permutations possible in large proteins is even more astronomical.

Protein chemists have recently devised methods for tapping the wealth of molecular structural properties that can be found in biological systems. Our discussion will focus on the methods used in creating libraries of peptides and proteins (and the highly specialized proteins, recombinant antibodies) using biochemical techniques. In addition, we will survey some of the unique molecular species that have been selected from such libraries due to their desired binding, conformational, or catalytic properties.

In all of the experimental methods discussed herein, the concept essential to define a biological system is that the structurally or catalytically significant peptide or protein is encoded by a nucleic acid—usually DNA but in rare instances RNA serves as the starting point. An investigator thus creates the collection of randomized proteins by manipulating the DNA, using recombinant DNA techniques, and using cells (usually bacteria) to produce the protein from the genetic information. By randomizing a trinucleotide codon in a DNA sequence, a collection of sequences is obtained that can theoretically encode a collection of peptides or proteins in which any of the 20 naturally occurring amino acids is incorporated into the given position corresponding to the altered codon. Randomization at n codon positions results in a combinatorial library of 20^n members.

A powerful advantage exclusive to biological systems is that a single DNA molecule, encoding a desired peptide or protein, can be amplified into an amount of material necessary for DNA sequence determination, and thus the peptide or protein sequence determination. (Currently there are no methods available for similar amplification of a peptide molecule alone, although methods for sequence determination of minuscule amounts of polypeptide are advancing with impressive results.) For this biological advantage to be realized, there must exist a connection between the polypeptide of interest and the DNA encoding it. This connection can be a physical link in which the polypeptide and the DNA are attached to each other or a biological link in which a cell carrying the DNA produces the polypeptide using its protein synthesis machinery. In each case the protein–DNA complex or the cell producing the peptide or protein can be selected from the mixed population of which it is a member by virtue of a structural or catalytic property of that polypeptide. We begin our discussion of biological combinatorial libraries with an outline of the recombinant DNA methods used for constructing these various populations of encoded proteins.

12.2   CONSTRUCTING A BIOLOGICAL COMBINATORIAL LIBRARY

The essential starting point for a library is the creation of a repertoire of genes encoding peptides. The task involves combinatorial synthesis of a mixture of oligonucleotides, which can then be incorporated into the gene of interest. For a short peptide, this synthesis may produce the genetic code for the entire span of amino acids. For larger proteins, the amino acid substitutions are usually confined to a specified region, and the degenerate oligonucleotides are either directly ligated into the gene as in cassette mutagenesis (1) or the oligonucleotides are used as primers in the polymerase chain reaction (2) and the amplified product serves as the cassette. More random methods of creating mutant genes include chemical mutagenesis (3) and error-prone polymerase chain reaction (PCR) (4).

The ability to tightly control oligonucleotide synthesis permits the creation of a library with desired characteristics; for example, substitutions at a given amino acid in a peptide may be totally random or limited to certain types of amino acids. The essence of the genetic code is such that similar codons often encode similar amino acids; thus, techniques such as parsimonious mutagenesis (5) are used to limit randomization to desired types of amino acids. Oligonucleotide synthesis using trinucleotide phosphoramidites (6) and mixtures of these customized reagents offers the possibility to control the degree of variation at a modified site even more precisely.

An example of limiting the randomization of a peptide sequence is found in the use of cysteines in peptides, which are capable of forming disulfide linkages. Researchers have shown that a constrained peptide can be created by incorporating two cysteines nested in a randomized sequence (7–9). These peptides often exhibit stronger affinity for a receptor than the unconstrained counterpart. In addition, several groups have noted a biological bias against an odd number of cysteines.

When constructing a combinatorial gene library, an important criterion is the diversity of the library. The library must be of sufficient size to afford the possibility of possessing members with desired traits. However, there is little advantage in increasing the library size above that which can be screened practically. Other factors to be considered are whether the polypeptide of interest can be produced as a cytosolic or transmembrane protein in the bacterial host, and whether the amino- or carboxyl-terminus of the protein is important for binding or catalytic activity. To address these issues, it is important to consider which of the various biological systems is best suited for the construction of a desired combinatorial library.

12.3 CHOOSING THE APPROPRIATE BIOLOGICAL SYSTEM

A combinatorial approach offers the attractive idea of testing a large number of potential drug candidates. In a sense this technique imitates the evolutionary process in nature by randomizing and selecting an amino acid sequence for a desired trait, for example, binding. A crucial element is the ability to recover the genetic sequence for the best binders, using the link between gene and product as mentioned above, where, for example, the gene of interest is fused to a viral or bacterial gene. A variety of biological systems are available for library construction; however, choosing the appropriate system depends on the desirability of the features characteristic of that particular type of library.

12.3.1 Phage Display Libraries

Perhaps the most commonly used method for creating biological combinatorial libraries is phage display of peptides and proteins. Bacteriophage—viruses that infect bacteria—are composed of a relatively small DNA genome, plus a protein coat that is encoded by the genome. One of the coat proteins of the phage M13, termed gp3, forms the end of the filamentous phage and has been used successfully for constructing fusion proteins composed of recombinant peptides or proteins situated on the exposed N-terminus of gp3. Ligation of an oligonucleotide to the 5′ end of the gene (*gIII*) yields a recombinant phage with a displayed peptide encoded by the inserted DNA. This particle of biological material is thus composed of a polypeptide linked to the DNA encoding it by nature of the phage architecture, as shown in Figure 12.1.

In 1988, Parmley and Smith published the first example of proteins expressed as a fusion to gp3 (10). They successfully rescued phage-displayed fragments of β-galactosidase from a mostly inert phage library using affinity purification with an anti-β-galactosidase antibody. In this experiment, the collection of phage was applied to an immobilized anti-β-galactosidase antibody. The phage of interest remained bound to the anchored antibody, and the inert phage were washed away. Bound phage were removed from the immobilized support by stringent washing, and the recovered phage were found to contain a population with a proportion of β-galactosidase fragments that was higher than the original phage before selection.

The authors in this original study went further to suggest that the system could be used to define ligands to antibodies. For all intents and purposes, the small size of peptides permits the creation of large libraries of recombinant gp3 and gp8, typically containing 10^6-10^8 members. Understandably, increasing the length of the peptide to the level of proteins raises the probability of disrupting the function of the viral coat proteins. One solution is to produce phage on which only a small fraction of the total gp8 coat protein is recombinant phage protein (11). In many cases, the length of the recombinant protein is not prohibitive to phage production, since entire proteins and even recombinant antibody fragments can be attached to phage surfaces (*vide infra*).

In cases where the recombinant protein is not easily secreted from the bacterial host as an M13 phage fusion product, an alternative phage display system involves fusion of the polypeptide of interest to lambda (λ) phage. Most recombinant λ phage systems did not utilize the phage display concept, producing instead soluble recombinant proteins in phage-infected cells, but the laboratories of Maruyama et al. (12) and Sternberg and Hoess (13) recently reported the development of λ phage display systems utilizing, respectively, fusion to carboxyl- and amino-termini of λ phage coat proteins. Since the traditional application of the λ phage system simply results in a different screening strategy, this type of system is discussed in more detail in the screening section.

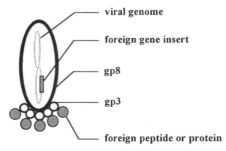

Figure 12.1 This example illustrates one of the attractive features of biological systems, namely, the link between gene and product. The viral genome contains the foreign gene insert (▓), whose expression results in the fusion of the foreign peptide or protein (●) to the viral coat protein (○), gp3.

12.3.2 Peptides on Plasmids

A method for generating peptide libraries that is similar to phage display is termed "peptides-on-plasmids" (14). In this method, the particle of protein–DNA complex is even smaller than a bacteriophage and consists merely of the peptide of interest fused to the C-terminus of the *lac* repressor, which is bound in turn to the plasmid encoding this fusion protein. This method eliminates any possible interference in phage production caused by the presence of the fusion protein and allows a method for selection of peptides in which the presence of a free C-terminus is important. Following selection of a desired peptide–plasmid complex, the DNA is purified and reintroduced into bacteria by electroporation for recovery, amplification, and further rounds of selection or sequencing.

12.3.3 Peptides on Polysomes

One of the major limitations in library construction using phage- or plasmid-based systems is the number of bacterial transformants that can be obtained following ligation of the synthetic DNA to the phage or plasmid DNA. This limitation was circumvented in a technically demanding method described by Mattheakis and colleagues (15). Using an in vitro transcription/translation system, the technique yields polysomes, where newly synthesized polypeptides are still attached to the mRNA from which they were translated. The authors report a library of 10^{12} random decapeptides, which could represent as much as 10% of the entire theoretically possible library. By contrast, electroporation with recombinant DNA can practically yield up to 10^9 individual library members per transformation.

12.3.4 Peptides on Bacteria

Analogous to phage-displayed libraries, this delivery system entails the surface display of peptides as a fused element of the bacterium. Several bacterial systems are available. Some researchers studied peptides and proteins in gram-negative bacteria as a fusion to the flagellar filament of *Escherichia coli* (16) and outer membrane proteins, such as LamB (17), PhoE (18), and OmpA (19) of *E. coli* and *Salmonella typhimurium*. Using gram-positive bacteria, other groups have targeted the outer membrane proteins, such as staphylococcal protein (SpA) of *Staphylococcus xylosusi* (20). Although not used as often as phage display, the recombinant bacteria offer an alternative construct for combinatorial peptide libraries.

12.4 SCREENING THE COMBINATORIAL LIBRARY

With large libraries comes the seemingly daunting task of recovering peptides or proteins with desirable characteristics. Many clever screening techniques have been devised to circumvent this problem. Interestingly, all share at least one characteristic, namely, the immobilization of the receptor or ligand at some point during the assay. Immobilization facilitates the separation of binders from nonbinders. Since each round of selection carries over a fraction of nonspecific binding sequences, multiple rounds of selection are often employed to enrich a favored population. Another tactic involves a two-stage selection scheme. An initial screen yields a general motif, which then serves as a starting point for the creation of a second library (21,22).

12.4.1 Soluble Ligands

The most common screening technique is the immobilization of the target receptor and assaying soluble ligands (23–28), as illustrated in Figure 12.2. With the availability of biotinylating reagents, many groups covalently attach biotin molecules to the receptor. Adding the modified receptor to the phage-displayed library yields receptor-ligand complexes. By utilizing the strong interaction between biotin and streptavidin, these complexes can be recovered using a solid surface, such as plates or beads, displaying streptavidin. Acid then provides a means of eluting the phage-displayed ligand and its genetic sequence. These eluted phage can be sequenced or used in another round of screening.

A more direct approach involves attaching the receptor directly to a solid surface, then assaying the recombinant phage for binding (29). Nonspecific binders are removed by washing with a nonspecific protein, such as bovine serum albumin (BSA). As above, bound phage can be eluted with acid. The selected phage can then be used for another round of screening, termed "panning." This technique enriches the population of interest.

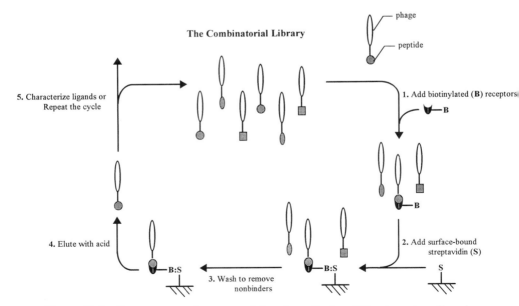

Figure 12.2 Common screening approach for phage-displayed libraries, where ligands remain soluble until screening.

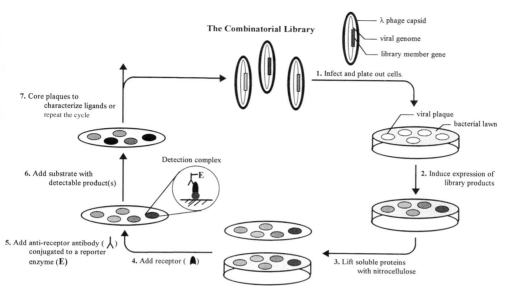

Figure 12.3 Common screening approach using a λ phage library, where ligands are immobilized prior to screening.

12.4.2 Immobilized Ligands

Another common screening technique is immunoblotting, where ligands are bound to a support for screening (30,31). In a typical system the gene of interest is subcloned into the λ phage genome downstream of a *lac* promoter. Packaged recombinant phage are added to *E. coli* cells, and the mixture is plated on agar (Fig. 12.3). Propagating phage lyse cells to create plaques on a bacterial lawn. The expression of the library genes is accomplished upon addition of isopropyl-β-D-thiogalactopyranoside, IPTG, an inducer for the *lac* promoter. After induction, a sheet of nitrocellulose is placed on the plate to absorb all soluble proteins. To assay binding of library members to a receptor, the coated nitrocellulose is treated with the receptor, followed by the addition of an antireceptor antibody conjugated to a reporter enzyme. If the receptor recognizes a member of the library, a complex will form between the ligand, the receptor, and the antibody. To detect this complex, a substrate is added whose product(s) can be easily determined, such as a colored precipitant. To recover the corresponding clones, the plaques are cored, and phage are propagated. These recombinant phage can be characterized or used in another cycle of screening.

12.5 COMBINATORIAL PEPTIDE LIBRARIES

An amino acid can exist in a variety of conformations. With a pool of 20 different amino acids, the sequential addition of each amino acid increases the possible structural and chemical diversity of the polypeptide. Thus, a library of randomized peptides is a formidable source of ligands. Studies have shown that members of combinatorial peptide libraries can compete with natural ligands, both peptides and nonpeptides, for a binding site (*vide infra*). These peptides possess structural contacts critical for target recognition and can affect the physiological action of the natural ligands, such as antigens, hormones, and enzyme substrates. These applications make combinatorial libraries a useful tool in the early stages of drug discovery.

12.5.1 To Define or Mimic Epitopes

One branch of the vertebrate immune system is the humoral response, whose recognition elements are antibodies. These soluble proteins are highly specific detectors of pathogenic microorganisms and transformed cells. The function of antibodies relies on their high specificity and affinity for a foreign particle, the antigen. The antigenic determinant, or epitope, is often a region on a protein, polysaccharide, or nucleic acid. The study of antibody–antigen interactions deepens our understanding of the pathology of diseases and provides new diagnostic and therapeutic approaches.

An effective tool in this pursuit has been combinatorial peptide libraries. Here, the varied types of ligands an antibody may recognize affords an excellent test of the versatility of these libraries to represent or mimic epitopes. Moreover, the high affinity of antibodies for epitopes provides a high selective screen for ligands. To demonstrate the specificity of the ligand for the antibody, researchers employ a variety of assays comparing the binding properties of the peptide and the native antigen. Three common tests for specificity include Western blotting with the particular antibody, competition for the antibody binding site, and the ligand's ability to induce similar immune responses. These techniques have demonstrated the ability of peptides to duplicate the important contacts that mediate binding to an antibody.

An immediate application of combinatorial peptide libraries is the determination of a continuous epitope, often termed epitope scanning. There are a multitude of examples where researchers have elucidated linear epitopes using this approach. A good example is a study performed by Scott and Smith (32). For example, characteristically the gene of the antigenic protein is divided into short overlapping oligonucleotides, encoding typically six to eight amino acids. These oligonucleotides are then subcloned into the expression system. The resulting peptide library carrying potential antigenic determinants can be screened for binders to a particular antibody.

On the other hand, antibodies may recognize a motif that exists only in the native conformation of the protein. In this case, the antigenic determinant is a discontinuous epitope. Unlike above, a linear scan of the target protein would not necessarily yield the string of amino acids that mediate binding. This type of target is not beyond the capabilities of a peptide library (28,33). For example, the monoclonal antibody H107 binds the native conformation of recombinant human H-subunit ferritin. A study employing a phage-displayed nonapeptide library indicated a sequence of amino acids was able to duplicate critical contacts between the antibody and native antigen (28). The peptides contained amino acids that are close in the folded protein but distant in sequence. Removal of these amino acids in the protein did not affect its folding or reactivity to another antibody, yet these changes greatly reduced or abolished binding by the H107 antibody.

The epitope of a protein can include modified amino acids. For example, the MPM2 monoclonal antibody has specificity for a phosphorylated epitope present on more than 40 eukaryotic M-phase proteins (31). In an effort to determine this epitope, Westerdorf and colleagues (31) created a peptide library encoding portions of two M-phase proteins, MPP1 and MPP2, in bacteriophage λ. Peptides recovered from plaque lifts of individual lysed colonies were treated with M-phase kinases to phosphorylate putative ligands, then screened for binding to MPM2 monoclonals. Recovered peptides contained a common motif found in the two M-phase proteins, displaying a preference for phosphorylation by M-phase kinases rather than inter-phase and cytosolic kinases. The construction of a modified peptide library expands the potential application of peptide libraries to identifying or mimicking ligands.

An antigen may be nonproteinaceous. Antibodies have been shown to recognize complex carbohydrates (34). The conformational versatility of a peptide can duplicate critical contacts when nonpeptides serve as ligands. Early studies of phage-displayed peptide libraries produced sequences that could compete with biotin and α-D-mannopyranoside as ligands for streptavidin and concavalin A, respectively (35–38). In regard to drug discovery, the interaction between proteins and carbohydrates plays an important role in many biological processes (39), such as cell adhesion and recognition events. The development of therapeutics targeting this interplay is hampered by the difficulties in synthesizing carbohydrates. One route to overcoming this obstacle is to mimic the important contacts of the carbohydrate with a simpler molecule. Using a phage-displayed peptide library, Hoess and co-workers recovered an eight-amino-acid sequence that competes with an antigenic carbohydrate for binding the monoclonal antibody B3 (27). This antibody recognizes a surface antigen present on many carcinoma cells (34), a target in drug development.

Although many studies have determined the ligand bound by a monoclonal antibody, peptide libraries can identify epitopes from a complex polyclonal antisera or fluid (29,40). The approach characterizes the immune response at the amino acid level of persons infected by a common etiological agent(s). Using a peptide-phage library, Sioud and colleagues screened synovial fluids (SF) of patients with rheumatoid arthritis (40). Selected peptides binding the SF antibodies were further screened using a different set of SF antibodies. The two-stage technique identified three sequences common to SF antibodies. These findings demonstrate that peptide libraries can define common binding motifs of antibodies in sera. Consensus peptide sequences from these types of studies offer a possible route to identifying epitopes recognized in autoimmune diseases.

The combinatorial approach is useful for isolating the epitope of an antigenic protein. Nonetheless, peptides are rarely good antigens themselves and thus are unlikely candidates for vaccines. To overcome this obstacle, the peptide can be coupled to a carrier protein or administered with an adjuvant. The former option is well suited for a surface-exposed peptide attached to an attenuated or nonpathogenic bacterium or the coat proteins of phage. Researchers have proved that coupled peptides retain antigenicity by Western blot studies (33,41,43). Immunization studies using mice (20,33,44) and rabbits (42) demonstrated the ability of peptides to induce a humoral response comparable to the native antigen, even in the absence of external adjuvant (43). Thus, surface-displayed peptide combinatorial libraries can offer a simple and inexpensive route to the production of effective vaccines.

12.5.2   To Define Common Ligand Elements

The diversity of the combinatorial peptide library becomes advantageous when the receptor possesses only moderate selectivity for a ligand. For example, Hammer and co-workers determined a common motif of peptides that bind to HLA-DR1 receptor molecules derived from human lymphoblastoid cell lines (25). This receptor is a member of the major histocompatibility complex (MHC) class II of molecules that bind peptide fragments of proteins and display them for recognition by CD4$^+$ T cells (45). Although these molecules bind a variety of peptide sequences, they do show some selectivity. Employing a phage display library of random nonapeptides, the authors of this study screened for binding to the MHC DR1. The sequences of 60 peptides that bound DR1 indicated trends in the types of amino acids at certain positions, such as hydrophobic anchoring residues, small flexible amino acids, and a general bias against negatively charged residues. This approach demonstrates the potential to determine common motifs of peptides that bind MHC class II molecules and may have applications in the design of antagonists specific to major histocompatibility complexes.

12.5.3   To Modulate Activity

Receptor–ligand interactions play an important role in a multitude of cellular processes. One goal in drug discovery is to antagonize, agonize, or modulate these activities. Smith and co-workers conducted the first study applying the combinatorial approach to target the interaction between a protein and a polypeptide (26). As a model system, they chose the binding of two fragments of bovine pancreatic ribonuclease. Partially digesting the enzyme with subtilisin yields a large molecule, S-protein, and a smaller molecule, S-peptide. Ribonuclease activity requires the reconstitution of these fragments. The researchers used S-protein as a receptor for screening a phage-borne library of hexapeptides. The selected peptides prevented the ability of S-peptide to restore enzymatic activity. Interestingly, the sequences of these ligands bore no homology to S-peptide. This initial work demonstrated the utility of peptide libraries to provide antagonistic ligands.

A recent study by Sparks and colleagues focused on ligands of the Src SH3 domain. Using two phage-displayed peptide libraries, they recovered ligands that showed binding specificity to Src SH3 domain (46). The study demonstrated that tight binding required not only a proline-rich motif but also a number of flanking residues as well. Treatment of *Xenopus laevis* oocytes with the selected peptides accelerated progesterone-induced maturation, suggesting that the peptides are able to interact with Src SH3 to antagonize its negative regulation of Src in vivo.

The efficacy of an administered drug may depend upon the ability to target a particular cell and be internalized. As a starting point toward this goal, investigators have focused on integrins, a superfamily of cell adhesion molecules, often exploited by pathogenic bacteria (47,48) and viruses (49,50) to mediate cell entry. In two separate studies, a phage-displayed library of randomized sequences of amino acids yielded peptides possessing an arg-gly-asp motif known to be an important element recognized by integrins (51,52). The introduction of a disulfide bond to the peptide provided peptides displayed on phage that could outcompete the linearized sequence in inhibiting cell binding to fibronectin (53). Moreover, Hart and co-workers employed confocal and fluorescence microscopy to demonstrate the internalization of phage displaying the selected peptides by mammalian cells (53). These findings provide insight into facilitating cell entry of biomolecules for gene therapy and drug delivery.

12.5.4 To Determine Substrate Specificity

The discovery of protease substrates is often difficult because of a lack of initial substrate information and the cost of synthesizing substrates. Combinatorial peptide libraries have been utilized to determine substrate specificity of proteases. For example, Smith and co-workers attached an epitope tag to a randomized hexamer library (54). After treatment of the phage library with a protease, phage possessing a substrate lost the epitope tag. Phage displaying nonsubstrates are then removed by affinity purification, using an antibody recognizing the tag. This technique yielded the consensus substrate sequences for two metallo-proteases, stromelysin and matrilysin. These peptides proved to be highly active substrates, as determined by kinetic studies. As in the previously discussed studies, combinatorial peptide libraries are a potent source of ligands even in the absence of any a priori assumptions. Utilizing biological systems as a vehicle for libraries simply makes applications less expensive and more efficient.

12.6 COMBINATORIAL LIBRARIES OF PROTEINS

In the same way that an entire peptide of 5–20 amino acids can be randomized to create a combinatorial library, proteins of 100–200 amino acids or more can be randomized to yield libraries of potentially astronomical sizes. In practice, however, it is more common to introduce mutations at a low frequency, instead of complete randomization, in order to yield libraries of a manageable size. It is also possible to alter specific portions of proteins, using information previously obtained on the protein's structure to determine the sites for randomization. The resulting collections of different proteins are composed of fewer different members, often on the order of 10^3–10^6, but are still sufficiently diverse to yield individual members with useful properties.

Applications of combinatorial libraries of proteins toward drug discovery most often involve selection of a member of a protein combinatorial library that can bind or catalyze a chemical transformation of a small molecule that possesses pharmacological activity. The collections of various mutated β-lactamases created by recombinant DNA methods are illustrative examples of combinatorial libraries of enzymes with direct applications to drug development. These enzymes, which hydrolyze cephalosporins and penicillins, generally possess some degree of specificity for various natural and synthetic antibiotics. The specificity and catalytic efficiency can be altered by mutagenesis. From a library of a large number of altered proteins, a small handful may display a desired specificity or improved catalytic efficiency. Selection of desired enzymes is straightforward: plasmids encoding active enzymes confer a growth advantage to bacteria grown on media containing the antibiotic, and can be recovered, amplified, and sequenced.

Viadiu and colleagues (55) randomized selected amino acids in TEM β-lactamase and obtained a mutated variant that was altered at two of the five amino acids targeted. This variant displayed modestly increased activity toward a number of β-lactams, including a 280-fold increase against the potent cephalosporin, cefotaxime. Stemmer (56) used a more elaborate, iterative mutagenesis scheme, termed DNA shuffling, to obtain variants of β-lactamases that contain different combinations of desirable point mutations. Such combinations of mutations can arise easily in DNA shuffling but would be highly unlikely to arise in a more conventional point mutagenesis strategy. The increased diversity in the combinatorial library created by Stemmer resulted in a selected variant with 32,000-fold increased activity toward cefotaxime.

Foreseeable clinical uses for altered enzymes selected from combinatorial libraries on the basis of their ability to catalyze drug transformations would involve administration of a catalyst for the purpose of clearing excess amounts of a drug once its desired pharmacological effects had been realized. This approach was postulated during the development of catalytic antibodies (57–59), "artificial" enzymes for which there are often no naturally occurring counterparts. Much of the attraction of catalytic antibodies lies in the investigator's ability to choose the reaction of interest; in this context one might anticipate the development of antibodies capable of catalyzing the degradation of any number of pharmacological agents.

A field of study involving combinatorial libraries of noncatalytic proteins is the development of DNA binding proteins with structural features called zinc fingers (60–64). The technique involves display of the library of various proteins on the surfaces of phage, as in the phage display of peptides. In this case, the phage display library is exposed to an immobilized ligand, which in these studies consists of a specific sequence of DNA. Purified proteins from selected members of the phage library are found to bind to the specified sequence with high affinity and selectivity. The patterns of amino acid substitutions in the DNA-binding zinc finger protein Zif268 that result in changes in affinity and selectivity suggest that a code, relating the amino acid substitutions in the protein to the sequence of the DNA ligand, might be developed upon the accumulation of sufficient data.

A potential clinical application for zinc finger proteins would require delivery of a gene encoding the recombinant protein into targeted cells, presumably cells in which the expression of an oncogene or a viral gene is deleterious to the cell. Success of the method would depend upon several factors: identification of a unique and highly conserved sequence within the coding or promoter region of the oncogene or viral gene; development of a zinc finger protein, which binds tightly and specifically to the specified sequences; the ability of the protein to obstruct transcription of the gene by blocking the synthesis of RNA by RNA polymerase; and the ability of the protein to withstand intracellular degradation processes.

12.7 COMBINATORIAL ANTIBODY LIBRARIES

Combinatorial antibody libraries are a very useful tool for production of antibodies with predetermined specificity (30,65). By utilizing the phage display or other related techniques, it is possible to select a desired member from a large pool of molecules without knowing the specific sequence of each individual. In order to select a particular antibody that possesses the desired binding or catalytic properties from the library, a powerful screening system becomes very important. Two aforementioned techniques have been used: phage display (66–68) and immunoblotting (69). Moreover, the use of semisynthetic and naive libraries offers a means of obtaining the desired antibody bypassing the immunization step. The development of antibody combinatorial libraries has been applied to prevention or treatment of a series of human viral diseases (70) such as type I human immunodeficiency virus (HIV-I), respiratory syncytial virus (RSV) infection, and herpes simplex viruses 1 and 2 infections.

The original strategy for creating combinatorial antibody libraries involved the random pairing of antibody genes from an immunized mammal (Fig. 12.4). The first step was to use a designed antigen as an immunogen to obtain mRNA encoding antibodies of interest. Converting the mRNA to cDNA by reverse transcription provided templates for PCR recovery of antibody heavy- and light-chain genes. Typically, these amplified genes consisted of the entire light chain but only a portion of the heavy chain. Their expression yielded one binding site of the normally bidentate antibody, hence these proteins were referred to as antibody fragments (Fabs). For the construction of combinatorial libraries, the two pools of chains were paired with each other to generate the combinatorial antibody library. An example of an alternative construction is a semisynthetic antibody, where the CDR3 region of the antibody's heavy chain is randomized synthetically to expand the sequence space (71,72).

The diversity of the combinatorial library depends on the diversity of the mRNA pool obtained after immunization. Further amplification from cDNA and the subcloning and expression in *E. coli* all effect the diversity of the library. How well the final library reflects the original immunized mouse repertoire still remains to be elucidated. The diversity of the final library is normally tested by restriction digestion or sequencing of randomly picked clones from the library (66). In order to

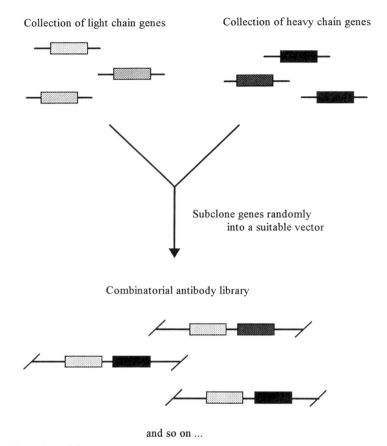

Figure 12.4   Simplified scheme for the construction of a combinatorial antibody library.

cover all the clones of the original library, the final library size is very critical. It is normally 10^7–10^8, restricted by ligation efficiency and transformation efficiency. The K_D of the high-affinity antibody obtained from this library is normally in the micromolar range. Affinity can be improved further by mutation and selection.

With the development of an in vivo recombination approach, the creation of extremely large combinatorial repertoires is now possible (73). This model system involves the Cre- *lox* site-specific recombination system of bacteriophage P1, which combines the heavy-chain and light-chain genes from two different replicons within an infected bacterium. Recombination at *lox*P site is catalyzed by the Cre protein. Light-chain libraries and heavy-chain libraries can be cloned into the "acceptor" fd phage vector (A) and the "donor" plasmid vector (B) separately (Fig. 12.5). In both vectors, the heavy-chain (*HC*) genes are flanked by two *lox*P sites. Mutant *lox*P511 and wt *lox*P were used to avoid the deletion of *HC* gene in the presence of Cre. When Cre recombinase is provided in vivo by infecting *E. coli* with phage P1, A

A. The acceptor fd phage

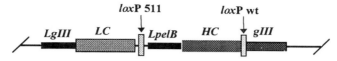

B. The donor plasmid

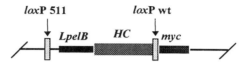

Figure 12.5 Recombination vectors for an in vivo approach to antibody library construction (see text). *LC*, light-chain gene; *HC*, heavy-chain gene; *LgIII*, gIII leader sequence; *LpelB*, pelB leader sequence; *Lox*P wt, wild-type *lox*P site; *lox*P 511, a mutant *lox*P site with a single-point mutation; *gIII*, gene for viral protein gp3; *myc*, gene encoding a peptide from *c-myc* that is recognized by the monoclonal antibody 9E10.

and B can cointegrate by recombination to give an antibody library that encodes light chains from the acceptor library and heavy chains from the donor library. Using this strategy, a library with 6.5×10^{10} members was generated, and from it Fabs were obtained that bound to a range of different antigens and haptens with affinities in the nanomolar range (74).

The diversity of the combinatorial library makes it possible to screen a large number of molecules within a short period of time compared to rational approaches such as site-directed mutagenesis. This property makes it a very attractive approach for drug discovery. Antibodies obtained from combinatorial libraries can be used to study the interaction between biomolecules and also may be used for therapy of all kinds of human diseases (75–81). Fab antibodies specific for RSV selected from a combinatorial Fab library was found to be able to prevent virus infection in the lungs of mice when administered before exposure to the virus and to effect rapid resolution of infection when administered at the height of infection (74). In addition, a recombinant human Fab selected from an IgG1 k phage display library derived from the bone marrow lymphocyte RNA of an HIV-1 positive donor was found to be able to not only neutralize infectivity but also prevent cell-to-cell transmission of herpes simplex virus 1 and 2 in vivo (75). Thus, the combinatorial library provides a very useful tool to select antibodies that could be potential drugs for all kinds of human diseases.

Additional applications of combinatorial antibody libraries can be focused on obtaining a humanized antibody in vitro by resembling in vivo maturation. It also can be applied to obtain the antagonist or agonist of receptors involved in signal transduction and further facilitate the discovery of strategies to control signal transduction pathways.

12.8 CONCLUSIONS

A recent advance in drug discovery has been the development of combinatorial technologies. Unlike the rational approach, where the goal is to target a specific physiological action with a defined strategy, the application of combinatorial libraries requires the creation of a large collection of diverse molecules and the development of an effective screen to isolate molecules possessing a desired activity. The success of combinatorial libraries of biological origin to fulfill these requirements is illustrated in the preceding examples. The strengths of these systems derive from the link between gene and product and the ability to amplify and enrich members of the library to permit easy recovery of selected molecules. This ease of use assures the continued importance of biologically derived combinatorial libraries to provide lead compounds for therapeutic agents.

REFERENCES

1. Hill, D. E., Oliphant, A. R., and Struhl, K., *Methods Enzymol.* **155,** 558–568 (1987).
2. Dillon, P. J., and Rosen, C. A., in *PCR Protocols: Current Methods and Applications,* B. A. White (Ed.), Humana Press, Totowa, NJ, 1995, pp. 263–268.
3. Ausubel, F. M., Brent, R., Kingston, R. E., Moore, D. D., Smith, J. A., Seidman, J. G., and Struhl, K., *Current Protocols in Molecular Biology,* Wiley Interscience, New York, 1987, Chapter 8.
4. Leung, D. W., Chen, E., and Goeddel, D. V., *Tech. J. Methods Cell Mol. Biol.* **1,** 11–15 (1989).
5. Balint, R. F., and Larrick, J. W., *Gene* **137,** 109–118 (1993).
6. Virnekas, B., Ge, L., Pluckthun, A., Schneider, K. C., Wellnhofer, G., and Moroney, S. E., *Nucleic Acids Res.* **22,** 5600–5607 (1994).
7. Lener, D., Benarous, R., and Calogero, R. A., *FEBS Lett.* **361,** 85–88 (1995).
8. McConnell, S. J., Kendall, M. L., Reilly, T. M., and Hoess, R. H., *Gene* **151,** 115–118 (1994).
9. McLafferty, M. A., Kent, R. B., Ladner, R. C., and Markland, W., *Gene* **128,** 29–36 (1993).
10. Parmley, S. F., and Smith, G. P., *Gene* **73,** 305–318 (1988).
11. Greenwood, J., Willis, A. E., and Perham, R. N., *J. Mol. Biol.* **220,** 821–827 (1991).
12. Maruyama, I. N., Maruyama, H. I., and Brenner, S., *Proc. Natl. Acad. Sci. U.S.A.* **91,** 8273–8277 (1994).
13. Sternberg, N., and Hoess, R. H., *Proc. Natl. Acad. Sci. U.S.A.* **92,** 1609–1613 (1995).
14. Cull, M. G., Miller, J. F., and Schatz, P. J., *Proc. Natl. Acad. Sci. U.S.A.* **89,** 1865–1869 (1992).
15. Mattheakis, L. C., Bhatt, R. R., and Dower, W. J., *Proc. Natl. Acad. Sci. U.S.A.* **91,** 9022–9026 (1994).
16. Kuwajima, G., Asaka, J.-L., Fujiwara, T., Nakano, K., and Kondoh, E., *Bio/Tech.* **6,** 1080–1083 (1988).

17. Harbit, A., Boulain, J. C., Ryter, A., and Hofnung, M., *EMBO J.* **5**, 3029–3037 (1986).

18. Agterberg, M., Adriaanse, H., and Tommassen, J., *Gene* **59**, 145–150 (1987).

19. Schorr, J., Knapp, B., Hundt, E., Kupper, H., and Amann, E., in Vaccines 91, R. M. Chanock, H. S. Ginsberg, F. Brown, R. A. Lerner (Eds.), Cold Spring Harbor Laboratory Press, Cold Spring Harbor, NY, 1991, pp. 387–392.

20. Nguyen, T. N., Hansson, M., Stahl, S., Bachi, T., Robert, A., Domzig, W., Binz, H., and Uhlen, M., *Gene* **128**, 89–94 (1993).

21. Miceli, R. M., DeGraaf, M. E., and Fischer, H. D., *J. Immunol. Methods* **167**, 279–287 (1994).

22. Miceli, R. M., DeGraaf, M. E., and Fischer, H. D., *J. Immunol. Methods* **167**, 279–287 (1994).

23. Jellis, C. L., Cradick, T. J., Rennert, P., Salinas, P., Boyd, J., Amirault, T., and Gray, G. S., *Gene* **137**, 63–68 (1993).

24. Saggio, I., and Laufer, R., *Biochem. J.* **293**, 613–616 (1993).

25. Hammer, J., Takacs, B., and Sinigaglia, F., *J. Exp. Med.* **176**, 1007–1013 (1992).

26. Smith, G. P., Schultz, D. A., and Ladbury, J. E., *Gene* **128**, 37–42 (1993).

27. Hoess, R., Brinkamn, U., Handel, T., and Pastan, I., *Gene* **128**, 43–49 (1993).

28. Luzzago, A., Felici, F., Tramontano, A., Pessi, A., and Cortese, R., *Gene* **128**, 51–57 (1993).

29. Motti, C., Nuzzo, M., Meola, A., Galfre, G., Felici, F., Cortese, R., Nicosia, A., and Monaci, P., *Gene* **146**, 191–198 (1994).

30. Persson, M. A. A., *Intern. Rev. Immunol.* **10**, 153–163 (1993).

31. Westerdorf, J. M., Rao, P. N., and Gerace, L., *Proc. Natl. Acad. Sci., U.S.A.* **91**, 714–718 (1994).

32. Scott, J. K., and Smith, G. P., *Science* **249**, 386–390 (1990).

33. Felici, F., Luzzago, A., Folgori, A., and Cortese, R., *Gene* **128**, 21–27 (1993).

34. Pastan, I., Lovelace, E. T., Gallo, M. G., Rutherford, A. V., Magnani, J. L., and Willingham, M. C., *Cancer Res.* **51**, 3781–3787 (1991).

35. Devlin, J. , Panganiban, L. C., and Devlin, P. E., *Science* **249**, 404–406 (1990).

36. Kay, B. K., Adey, N. B., He, Y.-S., Manfredi, J. P., Mataragnon, A. H., and Fowlkes, D. M., *Gene* **128**, 58–65 (1993).

37. Oldenburg, K. R., Loganathan, D., Goldstein, I. J., Schultz, P. G., and Gallop, M. A., *Proc. Natl. Acad. Sci., U.S.A.* **89**, 5393–5397 (1992).

38. Scott, J. K., Loganathan, D., Easley, R. B., Gong, X., and Goldstein, I. J., *Proc. Natl. Acad. Sci., U.S.A.* **89**, 5398–5402 (1992).

39. Springer, T. A., and Lasky, L. A., *Nature* **349**, 196–197 (1991).

40. Dybwad, A., Forre, O., Natvig, J. B., and Sioud, M., *Clin. Immunol. Immunopathol.* **75**, 45–50 (1995).

41. Greenwood, J., Willis, A. E., and Perham, R. N., *J. Mol. Biol.* **220**, 821–827 (1991).

42. Willis, A. E., Perham, R. N., and Wraith, D., *Gene* **128**, 79–83 (1993).

43. Minenkova, O. O., Ilyichev, A. A., Kishchenko, G. P., and Petrenko, V. A., *Gene* **128**, 85–88 (1993).

44. Stoute, J. A., Balou, W. R., Kolodny, N., Deal, C. D., Wirtz, R. A., and Lindler, L. E., *Infection Immunity* **63**, 934–939 (1995).

45. Schwartz, R. H., *Annu. Rev. Immunol.* **3**, 237 (1985).

46. Sparks, A. B., Quilliam, L. A., Thorn, J. M., Der, C. J., and Kay, B. K., *J. Biol. Chem.* **269**, 23853–23856 (1994).

47. Isberg, R. R., *Science* **252**, 934–938 (1991).

48. Relman, D., Tuomanen, E., Falkow, S., Golenbock, D. T., Saukkonen, K., and Wright, S. D., *Cell* **61**, 1375–1382 (1990).

49. Wickham, T. J., Mathias, P., Cheresh, D. A., and Nemerow, G. R., *Cell* **73**, 309–319 (1993).

50. Bergelson, J. M., Shepley, M. P., Chan, B. M., Hemler, M. E., and Finberg, R. W., *Science* **255**, 1718–1720 (1992).

51. Koivunen, E., Gay, A. G., and Ruoslahti, E., *J. Biol. Chem.* **268**, 20205–20210 (1993).

52. Koivunen, E., Bingcheng, W., and Ruoslahti, E., *J. Cell Biol.* **124**, 373–380 (1994).

53. Hart, S. L., Knight, A. M., Harbottle, R. P., Mistry, A., Hunger, H.-D., Cutler, D. F., Williamson, R., and Coutelle, C., *J. Biol. Chem.* **269**, 12468–12474 (1994).

54. Smith, M. M., Shi, L., and Navre, M., *J. Biol. Chem.* **270**, 6440–6449 (1995).

55. Viadiu, H., Osuna, J., Fink, A. L., and Soberon, X., *J. Biol. Chem.* **270**, 781–787 (1995).

56. Stemmer, W. P. C., *Proc. Natl. Acad. Sci., U.S.A.* **91**, 10747–10751 (1994).

57. Lerner, R. A., and Benkovic, S. J., *BioEssays* **9**, 107–112 (1988).

58. Lerner, R. A., and Benkovic, S. J., *Chemtracts–Org. Chem.* **3**, 136 (1990).

59. Schultz, P. G., Lerner, R. A., and Benkovic, S. J., *Chem. Eng. News* **68**(22), 26–40 (1990).

60. Rebar, E. J., and Pabo, C. O., *Science* **263**, 671–673 (1994).

61. Jamieson, A. C., Kim, S.-H., and Wells, J. A., *Biochemistry,* **33**, 6598–5695 (1994).

62. Choo, Y., and Klug, A., *Proc. Natl. Acad. Sci. U.S.A.* **91**, 11163–11167 (1994).

63. Choo, Y., and Klug, A., *Proc. Natl. Acad. Sci. U.S.A.* **91**, 11168–11172 (1994).

64. Wu, H., Yang, W.-P., and Barbas, III, C. F., *Proc. Natl. Acad. Sci. U.S.A.* **92**, 344–348 (1995).

65. Posner, B., Smiley, J., Lee, I., Benkovic, S. J., *TIBS* **19**, 145–150 (1994).

66. Clarkson, T., Hoogenboom, H. R., Griffiths, A. D., and Winter, G., *Nature* **352**, 624–628 (1991).

67. Barbas, C. F. III, Kang, A. S., Lerner, R. A., and Benkovic, S. J., *Proc. Natl. Acad. Sci., U.S.A.* **88**, 7978–7982 (1991).

68. Hoogenboom, H. R., Griffiths, A. D., Johnson, K. S., Chiswell, D. J., Hudson, P., and Winter, G., *Nucleic Acids Res.* **19**, 4133–4137 (1991).

69. Huse, W. D., Sastry, L., Iverson, S. A., Kang, A. S., Alting-Mess, M., Burton, D. R., Benkovic, S. J., and Lerner, R. A., *Science* **246**, 1275–1281 (1989).

70. Chanock, R. M., Crowe, J. E., Jr., Murphy, B. R., and Burton, D. R., *Infect. Agents Disease–Reviews Issues Commentary* **2**, 118–131 (1993).

71. Akamatsu, Y., Cole, M. S., Tso, J. Y., and Tsurushita, N., *J. Immunol.* **151**, 4651–4659 (1993).

72. Barbas, C. F. III, Bain, J. D., Hoekstra, D. M., and Lerner, R. A., *Proc. Natl. Acad. Sci., U.S.A.* **89**, 4457–4461 (1992).

73. Waterhouse, P., Griffiths, A. D., Johnson, K. S., and Winter, G., *Nucleic Acids. Res.* **21**, 2265–2266 (1993).

74. Griffiths, A. D., Williams, S. C., Hartley, O., Tomlinson, I. M., Waterhouse, P., Crosby, W. L., Kontermann, R. E., Jones, P. T., Low, N. M., Allison, T. J., Prospero, T. D., Hoogenboom, H. R., Nissim, A., Cox, J. P. L., Harrison, J. L., Zaccolo, M., Gherardi, E., and Winter, G., *EMBO J.* **13**, 3245–3260 (1994).

75. Burioni, R., Williamson, R. A., Sanna, P. P., Bloom, F. E., and Burton, D. R., *Proc. Natl. Acad. Sci., U.S.A.* **91**, 355–359 (1994).

76. Crowe, J. E., Jr., Murphy, B. R., Chanock, R. M., Williamson, R. A., Babaras, C. F., and Burton, D. R., *Proc. Natl. Acad. Sci., U.S.A.*, **91**, 1386–1390 (1994).

77. Cha, S., Leung, P. S., Gershwin, M. E., Fletcher, M. P., Ansari, A. A., and Coppel, R. L., *Proc. Natl. Acad. Sci., U.S.A.* **90**, 2527–2531 (1993).

78. Orfanoudakis, G., Karim, B., Bourel, D., and Weiss, E., *Mol. Immunol.* **30**, 1519–1528 (1993).

79. Zebedee, S. L., Barbas, C. F. III, Hom, Y. Y., Caothien, R. H., Gaff, R., DeGraw, J., Pyati, J., LaPolla, R., Burton, D. R., and Lerner, R. A., *Proc. Natl. Acad. Sci., U.S.A.* **89**, 3175–3719 (1992).

80. Williamson, R. A., Burioni, R., Sanna, P. P., Partridge, L. J., Barbas, C. F. III, and Burton, D. R., *Proc. Natl. Acad. Sci., U.S.A.* **90**, 4141–4145 (1993).

81. Burton, D. R., Barbas, C. F. III, Persson, M. A., Koening, S., Chanock, R. M., and Lerner, R. A., *Proc. Natl. Acad., Sci. U.S.A.* **88**, 10134–10137 (1991).

INDEX